America's First Vaccination

This book explores the response to a new scientific advance in medicine three hundred years ago to understand how this discourse revealed religious, racial, anti-intellectual, and other ideologies the first time documented vaccinations were introduced in America.

This text serves as a case study that examines the historic discourses surrounding the implementation of a new prevention technique, smallpox inoculation, to prevent the devastating epidemics of smallpox that had visited the new colonies since their start on the American continent. Using this detailed analysis of the arguments surrounding the project in early America, the author examines the various arguments that circulated in the 1720s regarding the project. When compared to today's pandemic, this study argues that Americans over-react and complicate scientific applications not with logical scientific perspectives or even with ethical views, but instead bring exaggerated claims founded on uniquely American historical, religious, racial, territorial, and political ideologies.

America's First Vaccination will be of interest to anyone interested in American history, the history of medicine, cultural studies, and a comparison to current pandemic events.

Barbara Heifferon was one of the initiators of a sub-field in the rhetoric of health of medicine (RHM) in the U.S. This is her sixth book. Her love of medicine began as a cardio-pulmonary technician and continued to a longer career in RHM, technical and scientific writing, pandemics, and writing studies.

Routledge Advances in American History

Education and the Racial Dynamics of Settler Colonialism in Early America
Georgia and South Carolina, ca. 1700–ca. 1820
James O'Neil Spady

The Overseers of Early American Slavery
Supervisors, Enslaved Labourers, and the Plantation Enterprise
Laura R. Sandy

An Unfamiliar America
Essays in American Studies
Edited by Ari Helo and Mikko Saikku

George W Bush Administration Propaganda for an Invasion of Iraq
The Absence of Evidence
Larry Hartenian

Redefining Irishness in a Coastal Maine City, 1770–1870
Bridget's Belfast
Kay Retzlaff

James Monroe, John Marshall, and "The Excellence of Our Institutions", 1817–1825
How Monroe's Presidency Became "An Important Epoch in the History of the Civilized World"
Peter J. Aschenbrenner

Politics, Police and Crime in New York During Prohibition
Gotham and the Age of Recklessness, 1920–1933
Francesco Landolfi

America's First Vaccination
The Controversy of 1721–1722
Barbara Heifferon

For more information about this series, please visit: https://www.routledge.com/Routledge-Advances-in-American-History/book-series/RAAH

America's First Vaccination

The Controversy of 1721–22

Barbara Heifferon

Routledge
Taylor & Francis Group
NEW YORK AND LONDON

First published 2023
by Routledge
605 Third Avenue, New York, NY 10158

and by Routledge
4 Park Square, Milton Park, Abingdon, Oxon, OX14 4RN

Routledge is an imprint of the Taylor & Francis Group, an informa business

ISBN: 978-1-032-32012-0 (hbk)
ISBN: 978-1-032-32013-7 (pbk)
ISBN: 978-1-003-31236-9 (ebk)

DOI: 10.4324/9781003312369

Typeset in Sabon
by MPS Limited, Dehradun

Contents

Figures

Tables

Acknowledgments

Many thanks to Professor Duane Roen who first inspired me to consider Rhetoric and Writing Studies for my doctorate at University of Arizona and to Professor Thomas P. Miller who suggested I might want to combine my career in medical technology with rhetorical studies. Numerous mentors, colleagues, and friends have also inspired me, showed much support for the project, and clarified medical and other issues throughout: Judy Melton, Ph.D.; Lora Anderson, Ph.D.; Terry Jones, M.D.; Harriet Jones, R.N.; Kirk St. Amant, Ph.D.; Brooke Rollins, Ph.D.; Albert Sullivan, M.D.; Peter Gold, Ph.D.; Barbara Bunker, Ph.D.; Liz Zausmer, M.D.; Stanley McKenzie, Ph.D.; Monica and Stephen Spaulding, M.D.s; a wonderfully supportive Dean, and many others. I'm also grateful to the American Antiquarian Society Library and its many Mather holdings, as well as to Harvard's Houghton Library archives. Most of all, I thank and offer my deepest gratitude to my children and grandchildren: Elizabeth, Leah, Cassius, Sophie, and Isla.

Preface

Years ago as a graduate student, I discovered Cotton Mather's medical compendium in the University of Arizona Medical School Library. As a former cardio-pulmonary technician, I had geared my Ph.D. studies toward medical rhetoric. With four history of rhetoric seminars in the rhetoric program, I needed a text to write a paper on a topic in 18th- and 19th-century rhetoric. After learning about the smallpox inoculation project in 1721 and 1722, I could never let my fascination with the topic go. This inquiry needed extensive research, and I adopted for publishing more timely books in most of my academic career. Finally, and especially with the convergence 300 years later of a pandemic in my lifetime, I could finish this book and release it for others to ponder. I approached the 1700s epidemic with as open a mind as I could. One bias I did have was hindsight, in that I knew smallpox had been eradicated as an active disease in the world through judicious use of a vaccination process. On the other hand, my only familiarity with the historical figure of Cotton Mather was a negative one, so there I had a bias in the opposite direction rather than sympathy for the initiator of the smallpox inoculation. As an academic and a feminist, I had read texts about the witchcraft trials and particularly how they might have been used to disenfranchise land-owning widows, etc. but I wanted to let all the texts speak to see what they had to say. The various themes that emerged have been at many times surprising to me, especially as they converged and indeed mapped onto the current Covid-19 pandemic 300 years later.

Barbara Heifferon

Introduction

In the early morning of November 14, 1721, a firebomb with the attached note "Cotton Mather, you dog, dam you! I'll inoculate you with this; with a pox to you" was tossed into a downstairs room of Mather's home reportedly holding one of his nephews, who was recovering from a smallpox inoculation.[1] Fortunately, the "granado" went out when it hit the floor and did minimal damage. As Mather wrote about the incident in his 1724 medical compendium, *The Angel of Bethesda:*

> The Vilest Arts were used, and with such Efficacy, that not only the Physician, but also the Patients under the *Small-Pox Inoculated* were in hazard of their very Lives from an Infuriated People. But I myself had thrown into my House in the Dead of the Night, a fired *Granado*, charged with Combustible Matter, and in such a Manner, that upon its going off, it must probably have killed them there were near it, and would have certainly fired the Chamber and speedily have laid the House in Ashes."[2]

The note strongly asserts the attack was carried out by the Bostonians opposed to inoculation. There were subsequent threats that a second attempt should "do the Business more effectually."[3] This incident occurred in the midst of one of the most lethal smallpox epidemics ever to hit Boston. Cotton Mather had tried to prevent further contagion by initiating a smallpox inoculation project with his surgeon friend, Zabdiel Boylston. Boylston also suffered death threats and, according to one report, a similar attack on his home.[4] The report on an incendiary attack on Boylston's house has been in doubt according to another author, although Dr. James Thacher mentioned it in his biography of American medical figures in 1828.[5] Even after the initial fury had settled down, the surgeon was often forced "to visit his patients at midnight and in disguise."[6]

Unlike in England, smallpox was not endemic in the Boston colony. Epidemics occurred about every 12–20 years. Outbreaks had taken place throughout the 1600s and again in 1702. Since survivors of the last epidemic were immune to the disease, there had been relief from the dreaded

DOI: 10.4324/9781003312369-1

pox for about 19 years.[7] But when the British ship, the HMS Seahorse, sailed into Boston harbor from Barbados in April 1721, a crew member developed smallpox symptoms a day after the ship had passed inspection at Spectacle Island and received permission to enter the port. The crew member was quarantined, but by early May nine more crewmen had signs of smallpox, and soon Bostonians developed symptoms of the disease.[8]

The epidemic would last from the early spring of 1721 until the winter of 1722. October 1721 saw over 400 deaths as the disease waxed, seemed to have reached a hiatus and then returned in several waves. In this outbreak between 5000 and 6000 contracted the disease out of over 10,000 inhabitants. Deaths

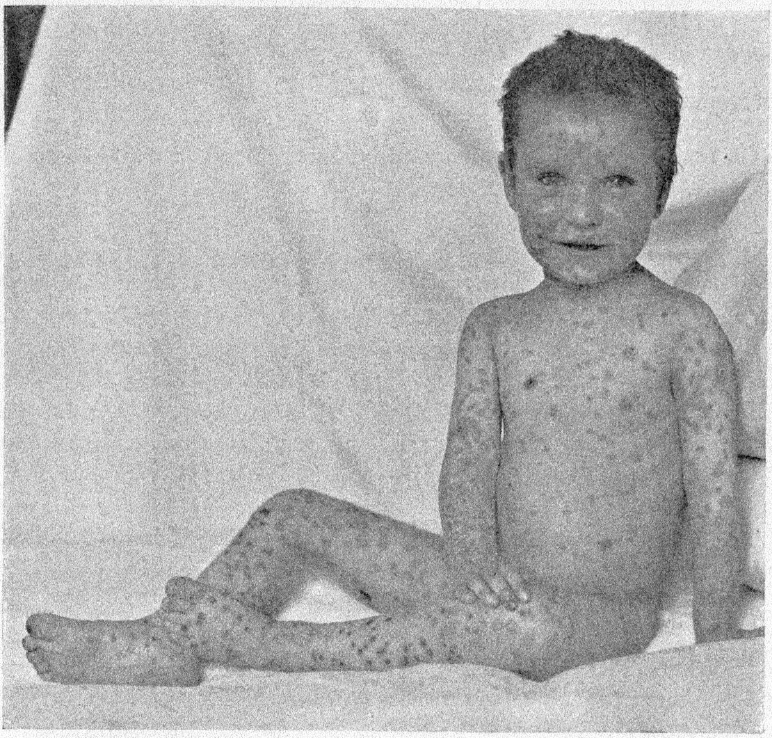

PLATE XV.

The eruption in this case was obsolescent. The scabs had fallen from the upper part of the body, their former position being marked out by pigment-splashes on the surface. The scabs still lingered on the legs. Distribution was characteristic. The rash was most dense on the face and forearms. On the upper extremities there was a distinct gradation in density from the wrists upwards. On the lower extremities the gradation was similar but less obvious. The rash was most scanty on the front part of the trunk, but was thicker on the chest than on the abdomen.

Figure 0.1 Small Boy with Smallpox, Wellcome Collection.

numbered at least 850, and many survivors were left with numerous disfigurements and chronic illnesses contracted during the immune-deficient phases of the disease.[9] In Boston at the time there was only one degreed doctor, William Douglass, although altogether there were ten practitioners of *Physick*[10] (physicians), surgeons, apothecaries, who dispensed drugs, herbalists, and midwives.[11]

Because smallpox has been eradicated, this horrible disease and its manifestations are unfamiliar. The virus exists today only at a lab at the Center for Disease Control in Atlanta in the United States and in a lab in Russia. In 2014 vials of the virus were discovered at the NIH in Bethesda, Maryland, flown to the CDC, and destroyed.[12] From an account written in the 1820s, smallpox is described as: "The head is swollen to a monstrous size, the eyes are swollen closed, the lips swollen and of a livid color, and the face and surface of the whole body are covered with maturated pustules, from which issue purulent matter; the miserable being has the appearance of a putrid mass, and scarcely the semblance of a human form remains."[13] Dr. Zabdiel Boylston in his 1726 book, which was a careful report of his inoculations during this controversy, gives an even more detailed account of smallpox:

> Purple spots, the bloody and parchment Pox, Hemorahages of Blood at the Mouth, Nose, Fundament, and Privities: Ravings and Deliriums; Convulsions, and other Fits; violent Inflammations and Swellings in the Eyes and Throats; so that they cannot see, or scarcely breathe, or swallow any thing, to keep them from starving. Some looking as black as the Stock, others as white as a Sheet; in some, the Pock runs into Blisters, and the Skin Stripping off, leaves the Flesh raw, like Creaturs flea'd. Some have a burning, others a smarting Pain, as if in the Fire, or scalded with boiling Water; Some have insatiable Thirsts, others greedy Appetites, and will crave Food when dying. Some have been fill'd with loathsome Ulcers; others have had deep, and fistulous Ulcers in their Bodies, or in their Limbs or Joints, with Rotteness of Ligaments and Bones: Some who live are Cripples, others Idiots, and many blind all their Days; besides the other Deformities it brings upon many in their Faces; Limbs, or Body, … .[14]

Bostonians frantically searched for deliverance from this scourge, beseeching their religious leaders, health practitioners, and others. Antidotes ranged from traditional medicines to more prayers and heightened shows of faith. Cotton Mather turned to inoculation. Because smallpox was known as Variola, the inoculation was also referred to as variolation. Later the term *vaccination* would be developed, and most vaccines do not use the live virus, although the Measles/Mumps/Rubella and Chicken pox immunizations today are live but weakened or attenuated. The term *vaccination* comes from the Spanish word for cow, *vaca*, because of the early association with cowpox, which was used in some early vaccinations in England. Other vaccines use a killed virus or a different variant of the virus. Variolation used the live virus from a patient with full-blown poxes.[15] Yet this type of treatment, injecting a form of a disease into a patient to achieve a lighter case and then immunity, had not been tried in Boston or documented in the other American colonies before. Treatments in Physick had included foods and liquids to ingest, herbal poultices, plasters or *plaisters,* and bleeding. It was revolutionary indeed to use this early form of vaccination to achieve positive outcomes. Some will object to the use of the term *vaccination* for the primitive procedure and use of live and not weakened form of the disease to inject for immunization. However, a case could be made for crediting Dr. Zabdiel Boylston, Onesimus, and Cotton Mather for first discovering and/or using vaccination in the Americas. Throughout this text, *inoculation, vaccination, and immunization* are used interchangeably when referring to smallpox inoculation. This usage may upset some readers. However, injecting the body with a disease-related liquid was revolutionary, a sea change. The medical practice had previously involved taking fluids and other substances from the patient, not injecting something into them. The only intake that patients experienced was through liquids or solids that were drunk, eaten or applied to the skin of the body. The process of injecting them with a substance similar to, like, or the same as the disease was a distinct departure.

One could also argue that the new mRNA injections for Covid-19 are also revolutionary because they are not formulated in the same way as many vaccines. Unfortunately, some Anti-Inoculators during the Covid pandemic have refused immunizations because they falsely believe such injections will change their DNA. They will not. "mRNA carries the code for the production of the Covid virus capsid protein. It can be made in bulk and encapsulated in a lipid bilayer which protects it from enzymes that could destroy it (RNAases) and allows it to fuse with the lipid bilayer of muscle cells. The muscle cell is then co-opted to make the Covid protein (antigen). This protein is secreted by the muscle cells and reaches immune cells that produce specific anti-Covid capsid protein antibodies or T-cells."[16] In essence, the mRNA vaccine begins with a messenger RNA that enables the muscle cells to signal the body to make antibodies and T-cells to build immunity to Covid-19 should it invade the body as a contagion.

Before 1989, when researchers first started working on mRNA vaccines, most vaccines were referred to as *live* or *non-live* aka *killed* vaccines. Other designations were *active* versus *non-active* or *attenuated.* All of these types used either a replicated strand of the original pathogen or, in the case of killed or non-active, just a component of the pathogen. The difference, then, between those vaccines and the mRNA vaccine for Covid-19 is that the new formulation is a copy of an mRNA molecule found on the spike of the pathogen. Despite the difference, the newest formulation is still referred to as a *vaccine* and the inoculation as *vaccination.*

Most people credit Edward Jenner as first discovering *vaccination* in 1796. Inoculated people were being immunized using the smallpox virus in

1721 in the same way in both America and England as the live virus from cowpox was used by Jenner in 1796. Since then, the idea that Jenner was the first to discover and try this type of immunization has become controversial in some medical circles, but not because the credit was being directed to Cotton Mather, Onesimus, and the inoculating physician, Zabdiel Boylston in Boston or to Dr. Maitland and Lady Mary Wortley Montagu in England.

Others have also discovered that the story of Jenner and the milkmaids was somewhat of a myth.[17] His biographer had written that the beautiful, un-poxed faces of the women must have been so lovely because of their already having had cowpox that kept them from being disfigured by smallpox, all of which was supposed to have led to Jenner's discovery. According to Arthur Boylston, the milkmaid story is a lie invented by Jenner's friend and first biographer, John Baron.[18] Jenner himself never claimed to have discovered vaccination, nor did he ever say, despite a huge volume of correspondence, how he first came across the idea. The myths of the milkmaids as his source of inspiration are just that, myths. To modern eyes, Jenner is revered for preventing some smallpox cases by using cowpox; in his lifetime, however, Edward Jenner faced severe criticism from jealous competitors, anti-vaxxers, and from many ordinary doctors who did not trust his method because, unlike inoculation [with fluid from a live smallpox pustule], it did not give permanent immunity to smallpox. John Baron had also invented the milkmaid story to counteract these criticisms.[19]

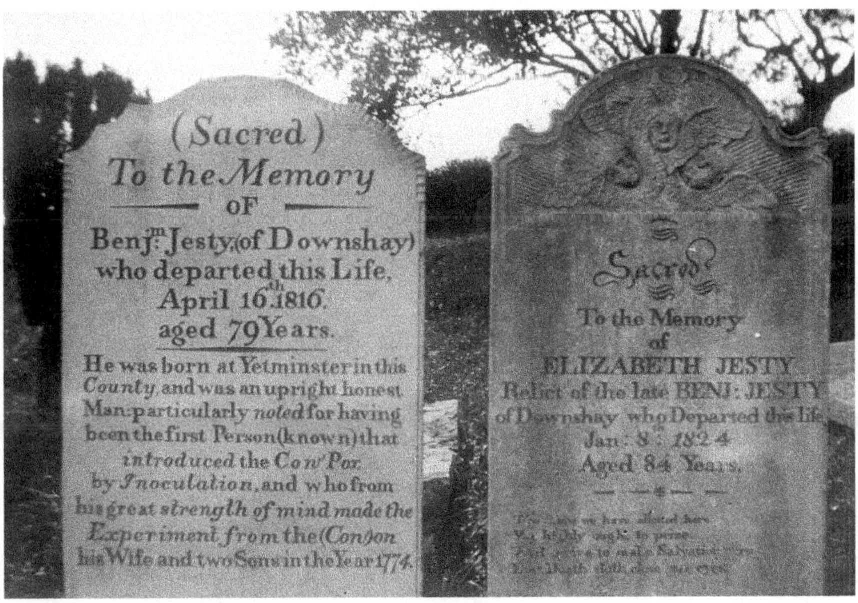

Figure 0.2 Jesty Tombstones, Wellcome Collection.

In 1796 Jenner conducted an experiment after 25 years of untangling a very convoluted web of information. The definition of "cowpox" itself was the main problem. Three different diseases were responsible for ulcers on cow teats that could transfer to human hands and bodies, only one of which was a result of the actual cowpox virus. Jenner had admitted the frustration of this discovery and had written: "this for a while damped, but did not extinguish my ardour."[20] Jenner's real contribution was that he devoted years to untangling true cowpox from the other diseases. For example, there could be a painful problem on the fingers of the milkers, "milker's nodes," caused by bacteria, not a virus, and other staphylococcal infections on the udder that spread beyond the teats.[21]

Others had been connecting cowpox inoculations and smallpox ones during Jenner's years of rumination, Benjamin Jesty among others. According to James Hammarsten, M.D., and William Tattersall, M.D., Jesty, a cattle farmer, had experience with cowpox and its seeming protection against smallpox and had taken both of his young sons and his wife to a neighboring farm where he knew the cows had cowpox. He then used a small, sharp knitting needle to take fluid from a pox on a cow and pushed it into a small wound he had made above the elbows of his family members. He himself had already had cowpox. Jesty performed the inoculations in 1774, and all survived, the two- and three-year-old boys without any symptoms, although his wife had a difficult case of cowpox from which she recovered. The two boys would later be inoculated with smallpox itself in 1789 during a large outbreak of smallpox with the actual smallpox fluid by the surgeon, Mr. Trowbridge. Most of the locals felt that cowpox would not always prevent smallpox itself. The inoculated boys were among the few children who survived the smallpox that year after being vaccinated earlier with cowpox and later with smallpox. Jesty continued his practice on others, and tombstones from that time feature brief accounts of his vaccinations. In 1805 Jesty was invited to the Jennerian Society to have his portrait painted, receive two golden lancets for inoculations, and be honored with a statement signed by members as the known person to have implemented the practice, based on knowledge he had since his boyhood. Still others suggested it was known even before this, but the evidence for Jesty's work had been clearly referenced in several cemeteries.[22]

Jenner most likely had heard of cowpox as a possible defense against smallpox as early as 1768; as a young man of 19, he had been apprenticed to a country surgeon, Daniel Ludlow. There he had attended meetings of local doctors at an area pub and had met John Fewster, another health practitioner who had spread the idea of cowpox possibly resulting in this block against smallpox because he had talked to those who had not had a response to the smallpox inoculations being done in the area after they had been vaccinated. On questioning, many of the farmers and their milkers had already had cowpox but never had smallpox, and because of hearing those testimonials believed perhaps the prior infection had blocked a reaction to a

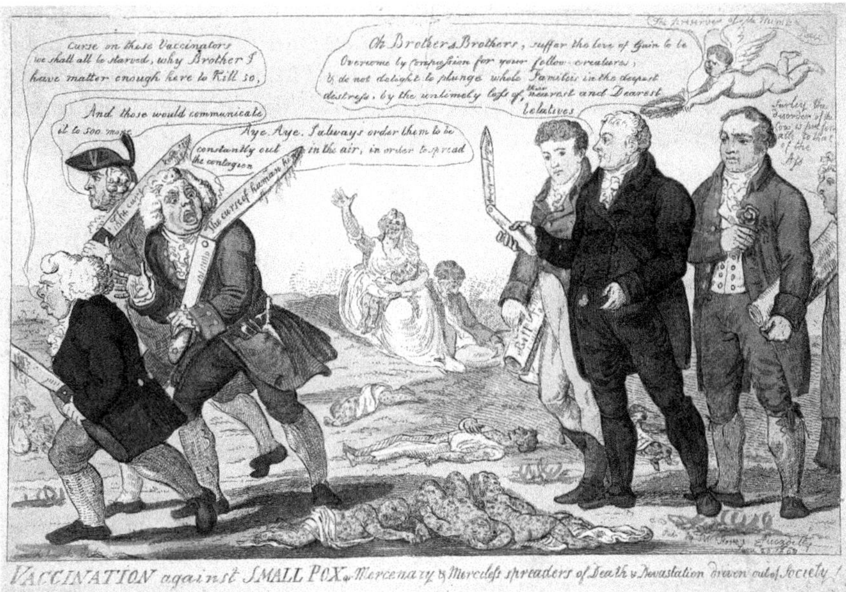
Curse on these Vaccinators we shall all be starved, why Brother I have matter enough here to Kill 50,
And those would communicate it to 500 more
Aye Aye. I always order them to be constantly out in the air, in order to spread the contagion
The curse of human kind
Oh Brothers Brothers, suffer the love of Gain to be Overcome by Compassion for your fellow creatures, & do not delight to plunge whole Families in the deepest distress, by the untimely loss of their nearest and Dearest Relatives
VACCINATION against SMALL POX or Mercenary & Merciless spreaders of Death & Devastation driven out of Society!

Figure 0.3 Cartoon Against Jenner, Wellcome Collection.

smallpox inoculation.[23] Fewster, a country doctor with lengthy experience, had apparently not been interested in pursuing cowpox as an inoculant, as he believed that cowpox was a more serious disease than "inoculated" smallpox. Thus he would not want to bring on a case of cowpox with it.

This belief showed that smallpox vaccinations were already successful in the Chipping Sodbury area of England, and Fewster had met Mr. Sutton, a well-known smallpox inoculator, whose greatly improved method of variolation had made it so popular. His method was not unlike that of the one done earlier in the 1720s, but it did have some cautions. For one thing, patients were not to be bled before or after the inoculation, and would hopefully do some preparation in advance, which meant no bleeding, a good diet based more on vegetables, fresh air, and exercise if possible. In addition, he chose his subjects carefully when and if he could, as those who seemed "temperate" or not alcoholics and otherwise healthy. Most importantly, though, he also stressed the importance of a "very clean" lancet and using the smallpox vitreous matter from a case that was not an extreme one, but milder itself. He published a book on the topic after some 30 years of experience, which clearly laid out what he believed would enable the most success. By the time he published, he estimated having inoculated or heard about inoculated persons in the hundreds of thousands. The book was published in 1796 although he probably had started the procedure in the 1760s.[24]

The method for inoculating with smallpox was identical to that of cowpox, and it was shown that in fact, smallpox inoculations had already had great success in the area in which Jenner had first done his apprenticeship before the completion of his training. He had then moved on to work with a well-renowned surgeon in London. Also, it's clear that others had been inoculated with cowpox decades before he had done so. Perhaps Dr. Zabdiel Boylston, the inoculating surgeon with Cotton Mather, as well as Mather himself should be credited with having brought vaccination to the Americas, and that his enslaved man, Onesimus, and the other Africans should also be recognized and credited. Lady Mary Wortley Montagu could also be named as the first to bring smallpox vaccination to England in the same years as those in America, and her contribution will also be explored in the following chapters.

Mather had first learned about an inoculation procedure from Onesimus and other enslaved West Africans (specifically Coromantee or Guramantee) in 1706.[25] In his medical compendium the clergyman recorded Onesimus's dialect as he described the process of inoculation:[26] "That in their Countrey *grandy-many* dy of the *Small-Pox*: But now they Learn This Way: People take Juice of *Small-Pox*; and cutty-skin, and putt in a Drop; then by'ndby a little *sicky, sicky*: then very few little things like *Small-Pox*; and no body dy of it; and no body have *Small-Pox* any more."[27] In 1716 Mather read narratives in *The Royal Society Philosophical Transactions* that included news of an Inoculatrix in a Turkish city (now Grecian) and Lady Mary Wortley Montagu, a Londoner who had learned of the technique in Turkey. A third source Mather credited was his own microscopic examinations. Although he misidentified what he saw using the instrument, he believed he had discovered the cause of the disease.[28] Most likely he saw bacteria, as microscopic lenses were not fine enough then to see viruses.

In July 1721 Zabdiel Boylston, the first and only Bostonian physician to agree with Mather's suggestion, inoculated one of his own sons, his adult enslaved man, and the man's son.[29] Later another two physicians in nearby towns also followed Boylston's example. These first inoculations ignited a firestorm of response resulting in a pamphlet war that would pit many of Boston's clergy against those practicing medicine. Mather wrote in his diary, "The people rave, rail, they blaspheme; they talk not only like Ideots but also like *Franticks*. And not only the physician who began the experiment, but I also am an Object of their Fury; their furious Obloquies and Invectives."[30]

Lines were drawn and sides taken; area clergy and health practitioners took to their battle stations sending out salvos of tracts, letters, and news articles. Journalists of three newspapers also chose sides and excitedly published the various written attacks. Those favoring inoculation included Cotton Mather (pastor) and his father, Increase (pastor); John Webb of the *Boston Gazette;* Samuel Mather, C. Mather's son; Benjamin Colman (Harvard degreed Congregationalist pastor of Brattle Street Church in

Boston); Thomas Prince (Congregationalist pastor of Old South Church); Nathaniel Williams (Headmaster Boston Public Latin School); Samuel Gerrish (publisher); Isaac Greenwood (student at Harvard); and William Cooper (pastor). Those against inoculation who called themselves the Anti-inoculators included William Douglass (the only European degreed doctor in the colony); most of Boston's physicians except Boylston, John Checkley, John Williams/Mundungus (apothecary and tobacconist); Samuel Grainger (private school headmaster in Boston from 1720 to 1734 and zealous Church of England man); Nicolas Boone (bookseller working with Grainger); James Franklin (publisher of the *New-England Courant)*; Benjamin Franklin (helping publish anti-inoculation editorials in his brother's newspaper), most of the Selectmen (Boston's local government members); Alexander Stuart, John Forland, and others. The Bostonian physicians, most likely led by William Douglass, created an organization called the Society of Physician Anti-Inoculators during this time, *one* of the first if not *the* first physician society in the colonies.

The main writers/spokespersons for the two groups were the Mathers (all three: Increase, Cotton, and Samuel), Z. Boylston, Greenwood, Cooper, and Colman for the Inoculators, and Douglass, John Williams/Mundungus, the Franklins, Grainger, and Checkley for the Anti-Inoculators. Although both Mather and Boylston documented the results of the inoculations, the other physicians with William Douglass at their head, opposed the inoculations on a number of grounds. The invectives flew across the city, keeping the newspapers and printers busy. Again Mather noted that he had never seen "the Devil so let loose upon any occasion. A lying Spirit was gone forth at such a rate, that there was no believing any Thing one had heard … . The People that made the loudest cry … had a very Satanic Fury acting them. They were like the possess'd people in the gospel, exceeding fierce."[31]

The increasing opposition eventually involved Boston's Selectmen. The colony was still under the rule of a British Governor sent by the Crown. The Selectmen were a City Council that could set regulations and rule on day-to-day matters that affected the Bostonians. On July 21, 1721, after much controversy, and as the epidemic had seemed to wane, the Selectmen attempted to shut down the inoculation project. They insisted that Boylston cease the practice of inoculating Bostonians against smallpox. Boylston continued to receive threats and had to hide in his house for 14 days "while men patrolled the town in parties with halters, threatening to hang him from the nearest tree."[32] After a brief delay, he continued the inoculations on August 5, 1721. The epidemic had flared up again shortly after the Selectmen's edict. In all, Boylston, Robie, a physician of Roxbury (with 11 inoculations), and Thompson, a physician of Cambridge (with 28) would inoculate 286 with only six deaths.[33] It would be many decades before variolation continued. Cotton Mather and Zabdiel Boylston were using a substance (not unlike today's vaccines) that used an actual or similar pathogen to help immunize a patient against a more devastating form of the disease. The expectation both with smallpox and later with cowpox was that a much lighter, smaller, and certainly not fatal disease would break out and then, after recovery, the patient would be immune from a much more dangerous and deleterious form of the disease.

A number of articles about the controversy have been published from different disciplinary perspectives, but it has never been closely examined in a full scholarly text that examines all the various arguments of the virulent debate. As John B. Blake pointed out, this project heralded the beginning of public health that organizes and manages the health and diseases of humans in large groups through institutions, regulations, and policies.[34] No longer would health be just a personal matter that was solved through visits by physicians in the wealthier homes and hospitals that were more like pest houses, quarantine stations, and/or almshouses for the poor. The body would become a "social" entity rather than just an "individual" one or even one just under the purview of a religious leader. As societal health norms were established, some individual health agencies eroded in the face of the edicts by the Selectmen, which began to occur under a waning and weakening American religious theocracy. Boston and its surroundings became polarized between pro- and anti-inoculation.

Of the articles and scholarly essays that have examined only one or two reasons that such a controversy was fomented around smallpox immunization, the most popular reason was that the medical practitioners had been against inoculation as they had sought to professionalize themselves. Those making that argument included: James Schmotter, Cristobal Silva, and Matthew Sivils.[35] As Schmotter argued, William Douglass's challenge of ministerial expertise in medical matters "represented [one of] the earliest calls for medical professionalism heard in the colonies."[36] A number of other authors have discussed the controversy historically, but did not find all the factors that were evident in arguments: John B. Blake, E. H. Henry, Shawn Buhr, Ross Rudolph, Stephen Coss, and Daniel M. Musher.[37] Still others have looked briefly at the role race played in the controversy: Kathryn Koo and Margot Minardi.[38] Louise Breen has examined the history through Mather's religious lens.[39] Cristobal Silva argued correctly that very little had been written about this event, and he himself only covers it in his last chapter.[40] Matthew Sivils claimed in a recent article that this inoculation project was indeed a "crucial moment in … medical knowledge-making."[41] This statement is true; however, I do take issue when he assigned motive to Cotton Mather's narratives and arguments promoting vaccination and claimed that Cotton and the other Inoculators were trying to promote a more democratic medicine.[42] That claim was not proven and at best, it is an oversimplification. In fact, more in-depth analyses reveal a rather chaotic and at times contradictory set of cultural tensions at work in the vehement response to the smallpox inoculation project. The original texts of the medical practitioners, editors, ministers, and citizens of Boston show that this controversy was over theology, Cotton Mather's character and history, colonial politics, race, and professionalization, all of which are important factors. Indeed, many key questions remained, and the archival texts of the debate have yielded some surprising answers.

The overarching questions were as follows: Did the controversy over smallpox inoculation represent a major reformulation of power over peoples' bodies in the colony, and why did many oppose, some violently, a life-saving medical intervention? What role might religion have played in the controversy given the emphasis on predestination that was part of the theology of the colony? Could Mather's arguments for inoculation, given his overblown involvement in the witchcraft trials as a much younger man, have impacted the negative reactions of the populace toward such a new medical procedure? Could Mather's first origin of the variolation itself, Onesimus, have caused racist resistance? Also, in this pre-revolutionary time period, would some resistance to the theocracy that the Mathers and other ministers represented and Harvard's role in the education of the ministerial leaders have already existed, ready to ignite? Could such reactions be found in the primary texts? Were there still other reasons as well? Could such an analysis provide a model for understanding the communication and social attitudes that underlie American resistance to medical interventions both then and today?

No medical rhetoricians have yet addressed this important incident in colonial Boston. In this text, I analyze the arguments in the various pamphlets, letters, newspaper articles, and broadsides of the controversy to reveal complex aspects of colonial resistance. This book explores the following: (1) It examines the text theoretically through the multiple lenses. (2) Close attention is given to the rhetoric of both sides. (3) It interrogates as many different exigencies (not just one or two) as can be determined via textual evidence. (4) Understanding underlying issues in their complexity in medical and scientific controversies lends a type of power: the power to communicate effectively to bring life-saving discoveries to fruition in a timely way. This text provides a model for unpacking the communication that underlies American resistance to medical interventions and challenges readers to compare the historic events with current controversies.

Using rhetorical theory implies close readings of texts to understand not just the use of language itself, but also how it persuades and how it reveals various traits, practices, belief systems, and chasms in a culture. In addition to rhetorical and other theoretical lenses, because Foucault had written so extensively about the changes in French medicine brought about as a result of the French Revolution, his concepts were valuable to further analyze the dramatic events of 1720s Boston. At the beginning of this project, it was clear that certain possibilities might exist in such a controversy, but even more questions originated from the documents themselves, which seemed to suggest a wider variety of influences. The specific documents that are rhetorically analyzed here reveal these various cultural factors. In this introduction, the Foucauldian concepts are introduced and highlight what evidence was discovered in the primary texts to document the claims. In the assembled whole, the reader will find that no single or even dominant exigence (except that of the smallpox epidemic itself) existed. Instead, multiple areas of tension must be considered to give the fullest understanding of this historical cultural controversy.

America's First Smallpox Inoculation: The Controversy of 1721–22 explores questions such as these via multiple theoretical lenses, including several different Foucauldian concepts of power, seeking within the various rhetorics to unpack the textured interrelations among the discursive formations found in these early American texts. In a period marked by religious, intellectual, social, racial, and political upheaval, early American medicine in general and an inoculation project in specific reveal some emerging understandings of the diseased body and the volatile body politic in their manifold cultural contexts. While much has been written about the formation of the American character in historical documents, little has been written about the formation of early American attitudes toward medical advances using Foucauldian constructs. These as interpretive lenses will not only be used but also extended.

Foucault saw biopower as the beginning of and continuation of public health, managing humans in large groups through institutions' regulations, and policies. It is that and more. The theorist's argument was that biopower began in the late 17th and early 18th century and underlies the development of Western capitalism.[43] In the American colony, the seeds of change began to impact "social" as well as "individual" bodies. As societal health norms were established, sites of cultural power change, erode, and gain strength. In the realms of health and disease, rather than limiting biopower to a healthy workforce able to serve the demands of a nation-state,[44] it can also be extended to the power and status of societal groups and institutions over less powerful individuals or a tug-of-war over who has the power to change, improve, or degrade medical practice. To put it another way, examining a particular disease outbreak and the resulting controversy over a type of preventative intervention on a granular level enables us to see more deeply into the underpinnings of formations of biopower. It's important to understand how concentrations of power disrupt, resist, and reorganize themselves as a result of such dramatic ruptures. Because much of the inner workings of biopower are hidden by social structures, it's important to expose them to the light through a microscopic examination of the smallpox variolation project of 1721–1722, which could be called America's first vaccination.

In addition, a few words about the field of rhetoric and the uses of rhetorical analyses: Rhetoric reaches back in Greece to the time of Sophists before Aristotle wrote the first book on rhetoric. In Greece and in the Roman Empire, the cultures were heavily dependent on the arguments and debates held in the Greek Assembly and later the Roman forum that led to important decisions for the populace. The spoken word carried much of the weight of governing, thus rhetoric was studied in the schools, especially by those who would be the main leaders of their city-states. In the hundreds of years since that time, rhetoric has been an academic study, although it's followed a pattern much like the systole and diastole of the human heart. There were times when rhetoric was a very narrow, diastolic, contracted study of linguistic figures and tropes, and other times when its course was more systolic, expanded, and fulsome. It was part of the trivium (grammar, rhetoric, and logic), mentioned in Plato's *Dialogues*, and taught in classical times, as well as in Medieval and Renaissance education that wealthy young men were required to study. In recent decades, rhetoric has been in a systolic moment, in which new specialties were added, such as the rhetoric of science, and the rhetoric of health and medicine. Also, many of the scholars of rhetoric now combine rhetorical analysis with cultural analysis or cultural studies in our lenses; many other disciplines also contribute to cultural studies, and there's been some achievement of interdisciplinality. Given the excellent preservation of Bostonian texts and the digitizing of a number of them, the controversy of 1721–1722 is well documented. Each chapter here is grounded on the many archival documents that lent themselves to rhetorical and cultural analyses.

Overview of the Chapters

Chapter 1

Chapter 1 presents a series of contextual analyses so the reader can understand how the issues that arise during the controversy fit into the historical scene of Boston in 1721 and 1722. These include a further explanatory history of Foucauldian theory used here; a brief history of smallpox from 10,000 BCE till the Renaissance; quarantines in Boston and Europe; Puritan interest in science or "natural philosophy"; the reigning medical paradigm; the method of inoculation; Cotton Mather's sources for the idea of variolation; an introduction of the main proponents and opponents of the practice; and the common sense trope. A brief history of smallpox itself is necessary to explore because the disease was eradicated from the globe in the 1970s except for the strains of the virus in heavily protected scientific labs. Today's reader has little knowledge and no memory of this horrific disease. In addition, the last context and first claim unpacked in this chapter concerns the legitimate fears about smallpox itself. It doesn't make sense to Bostonians that their lives could be saved by the introduction into their bodies of the very disease that was currently threatening their lives. Many colonists feared that the actual inoculation itself was counter-intuitive because drops from the pox of a suffering patient were placed in the arm or leg of a person receiving the inoculation. Even though the procedure resulted in very light cases that prevented death, serious disfigurement, and other serious complications in almost all of the almost 300 inoculated, strong counter arguments and misinformation further frightened the populace.

Chapter 2

An important aspect to consider is that the inoculation project was deeply embedded in the religious discourse of the day. Although the Puritans were interested in science, then called Natural Philosophy, their religion was Calvinistic, and predestination was a major tenet. Therefore, a brief explanation of how Calvinism impacted the Puritan religious beliefs is important to understand. Many Bostonians feared that the smallpox inoculation would bring down divine wrath, as colonists were interfering with their God's Will. The rhetoric of this controversy abounds with ironies: for example, those most supportive of Mather's and Zabdiel Boylston's project were the ministers of Boston and its surroundings who centered their beliefs in variolation on science. The majority of physicians were opposed to the practice and were those who most often used religious arguments against the project. While there are no surprises that the reactions, some of which were violent, were influenced by the religious doctrinal practices at the time, the analysis of how the proponents and opponents created their arguments reveals much about the beginnings of our culture and its fixations. Many of the opponents of the inoculation project were practicing doctors, apothecaries, and lay people who articulated religious views and used Biblical texts to support their antagonism toward inoculation, while many of the supporters of smallpox inoculation ironically were those most well-versed in religious doctrine and preached it weekly if not more often. The ministers, especially Cotton Mather himself, used scientific arguments and testimonials from witnesses, although some other ministers for immunization did rebut the religious arguments from the physicians and those against variolation using Biblical interpretations.

Throughout the medical and religious arguments for and against vaccination, there ran a strong thread of legality: the "Law of Physick," the law of Queen Anne, and religious or doctrinal law. In a yet unformed nation, in a land of pestilence and plagues, colonists had little to keep the new settlements in order; thus, they used their religious law, royal strictures and, in medicine, the "Law of Physick," which was the commonly held beliefs and usual medical practices at that time. In reading the original texts, one is struck by how issues of law permeate the thinking of the protagonists and antagonists in this period and influenced the early colonists over many decades.

Chapter 3

Still another aspect in this controversy concerns Cotton Mather's character, reputation, and personal history, especially his role in the witchcraft trials almost thirty years earlier in Salem, Massachusetts. During the smallpox epidemic and inoculation project, the memories of his actions in the earlier times returned to haunt Cotton Mather's seemingly sincere motivation to help the victims of smallpox in Boston. After the witchcraft trials, Massachusetts colonists and many regional clergies realized that their actions had gone far astray of appropriate and civilized behavior. Many recoiled in horror at the mass hysteria in which they had participated and the harm they had done to innocent women and children. Cotton Mather's writings were extensive about witchcraft and his supposed experiences with witches as an eyewitness. At one point as a young man, he had taken a supposed young witch into his home and documented her feats of flight through his house and other bizarre activities. He himself never renounced his actions in print. When he set out to write a text doing so, he had ended up adding further documentation of supernatural incidences of witchcraft and seemed unable to recant his testimonies. There was some reasonable expectation that most Colonists would never again indulge in that same mass hysteria that promulgated the earlier incidents; yet, some of the language Mather used to defend the smallpox project and gain adherents reminded opponents of his language some thirty years earlier, raising alarm and triggering strong, emotional reactions. In his books on witchcraft, he had often referred to invisible cloaks, mice, and other phenomena, and in his discussion of his discovery in his microscope of moving "animalculae" he thought were responsible for smallpox, he wrote about them being *invisible* to the naked eye, visible only under a special lens. A close examination of texts by the opponents revealed the fear that another dubious project being spearheaded by Mather and others was as dangerous and immoral as his previous obsession with witchcraft in the past. Although in many ways, Mather was on the right track in looking for "little live invisible animals" being responsible for disease, his microscope of that time was far too primitive to be able to see viruses. However, such an echo of a previous enthusiastic campaign that included the viability of an invisible power was another trigger for fear among those who heard about and read his descriptions of smallpox observed through a less-than-familiar technology.

To contextualize Mather's use of the microscope, it's important to also look at early germ theory and the role of the development of microscopes from even before the minister's time. His own work as someone interested in science and disease was informed by both his father's and his own well-appointed libraries. The Mather libraries were known as the finest in the colony and are still preserved in Massachusetts. The early texts on germ theory and microscopy can be found there as befitting the strong interest in science on the part of Puritans, especially the Mathers.

Chapter 4

In addition to antagonistic reactions to microscopic and scientific sources of knowledge, anti-intellectualism and class bias or rivalry played a role. The ministers had been the well-established Bostonian intellectuals of the time, and this class or caste included Mather's father, Increase Mather, who was influential in Boston's only institution of higher learning, Harvard. Conversely, anti-intellectualism was personified and well represented by the figure of "Mundungus" or John Williams, an illiterate apothecary and tobacconist who became curiously literate in his ability to attack Mather and the "Inoculators," as they were called. Advocates of immunization suggested that Williams's texts were written by someone else. Possibilities included the most prominent physician in Boston, Douglass, and/or James and Benjamin Franklin, the printers who published his texts. Most of the texts' pro and con variolation were carried in the Franklins' newspaper. While Mundungus/Williams provided some comic relief in this dramatic period, there is nothing funny about contracting, dying from, or being forever hideously marked or immune compromised by smallpox. However, almost like Falstaff in the Shakespeare's plays, although Mundungus does not represent the Puritans per se, he does appear as a comic figure, and he is frequently held up to ridicule by proponents of vaccination. Mundungus's letters in James and Ben Franklin's paper, because the apothecary was not regarded as in the same class as the educated ministers and physicians of the town, were especially effective in rallying the "common folk" and further enraging them against the Mathers and other "Inoculators."

The two Franklin brothers had started their own newspaper in 1721 and were the most involved printers in a fight against the Mathers' hierarchy in Boston, British rule over the colony, and especially to oppose smallpox variolation. Although Ben Franklin was only fifteen, he was capable of pulling his own weight in the battles he and his brother waged. He ran the newspaper when his older brother was jailed at one point, and, unknown to James, young Benjamin penned and printed his own writing: The Silence Dogood letters. Those often ventured opinions on the Mathers and Harvard, although less often on the inoculation project itself. It was clear in the documents, however, that both brothers would be against any project the Mathers (father-Increase, son-Cotton, and grandson-Samuel) would undertake.

Still other texts, such as the *Academics Dialogues*, clearly showed the biases and assumptions between the two classes or between the elite and all the other colonists. Harvard came under attack often during the smallpox controversy. However, the *Academicus* texts were more humorous as the authors took turns mocking each other's education and class.

The inoculation debate, especially as a result of the Franklin brothers' having started their newspaper, also became intertwined with anti-British governmental politics. Although the Massachusetts colony had already sent one Governor packing, the anti-British sentiment had flared up in full force in the issues of the *New-England Courant*. In fact, the early seeds of revolutionary politics among Colonists also shaped the vehemence of 1720s Boston smallpox inoculation controversy. Unease and resentment already permeated the Colonies because of the Crown's dominance and interference in Bostonian lives going back as far as the 1684 revocation of the Massachusetts charter.[45] Cotton Mather himself had particularly complicated relationships with the various Governors of the Colony, as some have argued, because of his overly pious and intimidated filial relationship to his father. This layer problematizes an already extensive ideological map of the controversy of 1721–1722.

The political climate, perhaps like what we have experienced recently, was somewhat of a free-for-all among the men vying for power. Earlier the theocracy had been thoroughly in control, but that control by the Puritan clergy was being challenged. There were opportunities and an exigence to debate the issues of the day, and the print media, especially the *New-England Courant,* appeared every bit as active and involved as today's media in fanning the flames of incendiary discourse.

Chapter 5

Part of the ideological map of the 1720s includes the racist and misogynistic reactions that surfaced in the discourse of the time. As mentioned in the first part of the Introduction, the smallpox inoculation process was first introduced to Cotton Mather by the enslaved man who worked for him, Onesimus. This source of viable knowledge drew intense fire from the opponents of the project. In various documents, we see the Colonists attacking smallpox inoculation on the basis of race or country of origin (Africa), as Mather made it well-known that the enslaved person who worked in his house and other Africans he consulted had intimate knowledge of the practice. A number of documents show that the enslavers, traders, and those who bought and sold slaves for their own homes, plantations, or farms regularly practiced the screening of the captives for a sign of smallpox variolation or a past infection that would render them no longer vulnerable to the disease. Although Southern sale bills mentioned the value of an enslaved person having already had the disease or a scar from such an inoculation, it's not certain that Bostonians were as well acquainted with this practice, or that inoculating former Europeans now living in America would be tolerated. The opponents used misogynistic, xenophobic, and/or racist arguments to dissuade other colonists from believing in and undergoing the variolations offered by Mather and Boylston. Original texts show how Mather both valued the information he got from Onesimus and yet was frustrated with him for his lack of enthusiasm for religious study so that he, too, could adopt the religious beliefs the minister preached. He often asked Onesimus to attend the same religious training that some of his fifteen children received. The added fuel of racist opposition fanned the flames of anger against vaccination even higher and lent the rhetoric some of its most disturbing and angry sentiments.

Chapter 6: Then and Now

In the last chapter, I outline the overarching conclusions gained by examining this important issue of scientific medicine within a hauntingly interesting historical period in our country. In the last two-plus years, the vitriol of the smallpox inoculation controversy seemed strangely very familiar as controversies arose over Covid-19 vaccinations. I explore the similarities and differences between then and now. For example, the new vaccines, both Pfizer and Moderna, have been made using a new technique: mRNA also called a "messenger" RNA. Because this represents a new way of creating a vaccine, some of those declining the vaccination do not trust a "new" scientific development. Others have religious reasons, and sometimes in our country's controversies, just as in colonial times, religion and politics mix. Not only are some reluctant to get the vaccines because their pastor preaches against it, but the politics of the Republican Party have been developing resistance to some aspects of our culture since the development of the Tea Party wing. Others who are against all types of immunizations will not get vaccinated against Covid-19. The lessons drawn from this close examination of one scientific incursion in early America reveals a rich pastiche of possibilities that need to be examined and compared to the various alarming reactions and cultural phenomena we are experiencing in this country today.

Although our current Covid vaccination project was not imported from or based on a practice from Africa and Turkey, we have seen racial, religious, political, scientific, and medical issues rise to the surface again, presenting virulent debates that are similar in many ways to what took place exactly 300 years ago. Inoculation of a person with a substance taken from a live pox to immunize them against a much worse case of the disease was based on a new technology, just as mRNA is a new technology in our panoply of medical immunizations.

Also, looking back 300 years, in many ways an entrenched theocracy and the Harvard University, which had graduated mostly Puritan ministers for a number of years, seemed to be seen by the less educated and less powerful as a "deep state." Those who had not had the privilege of higher education (a much larger percentage than today) were pushing back against the establishment, the Mathers (generations of ministers), and Harvard itself. This resistance was further heightened in a period building up hostile reactions to British rule. The two forms seemed intertwined in the minds of ordinary colonists who followed the anti-intellectual publications and misinformation of Mundungus (aka John Williams). The media itself played a large role, even though in those times of no "social" media, there was still very active print sources, town criers, and local gossip.

The initiator and leader of the immunization project, Cotton Mather, was himself a character of past frightening and lethal ideas that threatened the areas of Boston and Salem; his opponents during the 1720s smallpox epidemic also purveyed lies. Today we have misinformation, conspiracy theories, and leaders with sometimes quite strange ideation. Some aspects of American life seem to still hearken back to the dark times of the witchcraft trials, and today one hears cries of "witchhunt" even from leaders or former leaders of the United States. One could argue that mass hysteria in our country is alive and well. Even though Bostonians and Salemites had mostly eschewed belief in witchcraft after the horror of what they had done became clear to them, the older generation remembered Cotton Mather's role as an enthusiastic, young minister and supporter of the witchcraft trials and persecutions, as well as his immense written testimonies and interviews with "witches." If the public was previously persuaded to trust someone who led them astray, that trust may be difficult to build back. Today there are people who refuse to be immunized because they remember terrible experiments conducted by an earlier version of the Centers for Disease Control. Political and professional rivalries are also difficult to negotiate. Now perhaps there are fewer examples of professional jealousies because ministerial roles and professional medical roles are more clearly established. However, at the same time, there are ministers preaching against Covid vaccinations today, which is the opposite of the 1721 situation, while most but not all doctors are urging vaccinations. Those preachers inveighing against CDC guidelines minister to certain sects and sections of the populace, which is challenging the authority of governmental and medical entities. This tug-of-war shows some convergence with the earlier project. What can also be noted is that here, even within a well-established medical system, in spite of its power and control over the health of individual bodies and public health, a medical intervention can be severely questioned and disrupted by politics and cultural mythology or misinformation in the midst of an extreme health crisis.

Notes

1 Cotton Mather, *Diary, 1709-1724*, Vol. 2 (New York: Frederick Unger, 1957), 658; Michael G. Hall, *The Last Puritan* (Middleton, CT: Wesleyan University Press, 1988), 360.
2 Cotton Mather, *Angel of Bethesda* (Barre, MA: American Antiquarian Society and Barre Publishers, 1972), 113.
3 George L. Kittredge, "Introduction" to Increase Mather's and Anonymous's *Several Reasons or Transplanting the Small Pox, Is a Lawful Practice, and That It Has Been Blessed by God for the Saving of Many a Life, etc.* (Anonymous attributed to Cotton Mather) ... ; Cotton Mather, *Sentiments Written on the Small Pox Inoculated* (Cleveland, OH: 1921), 22–23.
4 James Thacher, *American Medical Biography* (Boston: Richardson and Lord, 1828), 21.
5 Stephen Coss, *The Fever of 1721* (New York: Simon and Schuster, 2016), 171.
6 Thacher, *American Medical Biography*, 21.
7 James B. Blake, *Public Health in the Town of Boston* (Cambridge, MA: Harvard University Press, 1959), 77.

8 James B. Blake, *Public Health,* 54; Ross Rudolph and Daniel M. Musher, "Inoculation in the Boston Smallpox Epidemic" in *Archives of Internal Medicine,* (1965), 692–696.
9 Mark Best, A. Katamba, and Duncan Neuhauser, "Making the Right Decision: Benjamin Franklin's Son Dies of Smallpox in 1736" in *Quality and Safety in Health Care,* 16, no. 6 (2007): 479; Harvard Open Collection, *Contagion: Historic Views of Diseases and Epidemics* (2008-2015). According to Best et al., 4917 people were infected in 1721–22, and according to Harvard OCP, 5889 were infected.
10 *Physick* also *Physic* was that period's word for the practice of pre-modern medicine, generally.
11 Gordon Jones, "Introduction" to *Angel of Bethesda* by Cotton Mather (Barre, MA: American Antiquarian Society and Barre Publishers, 1972), xxxiii.
12 Jocelyn Kaiser, "Six Vials of Smallpox Discovered in U.S. Lab," in *Science,* July 8, 2014. Accessed June 3, 2022. https://www.science.org/content/articlesix-vials-smallpox-discovered-us-lab
13 James Thacher, *American Medical,* 20.
14 Zabdiel Boylston, *An Historical Account of the Small-Pox Inoculated in New England* (London: 1726), 38.
15 Cotton Mather, *Angel,* 108.
16 Interview with Dr. Albert Sullivan, M.D., June 2022. Buffalo, New York.
17 Arthur William Boylston, M.D., "Preface" to *Defying Providence: Smallpox and the Forgotten 18th Century Medical Revolution* (North Charleston, S. Carolina: CreateSpace Independent Platform, 2012).
18 John Baron, *The Life of Edward Jenner* (London: Henry Colburn Publisher, 1838), 351.
19 Arthur W. Boylston, "The Origins of Vaccination: Myths and Reality" in the *Journal of Royal Society of Medicine*, 106, no. 9 (September 2013): 351–354.
20 D. Baxby, *Jenner's Smallpox Vaccine* (London: Heinemann, 1981),134–150.
21 Arthur W. Boylston, "The Origins of Vaccination: Myths and Reality," 353–354.
22 J. F. Hammarsten, W. Tattersall, J. E. Hammarsten, M.D.s, *Transactions of the American Clinical and Climatological Association,* "Who Discovered Vaccination? Edward Jenner or Benjamin Jesty?" 90 (1979).
23 Arthur W. Boylston, "The Origins of Vaccination: Myths and Reality," 354.
24 Daniel Sutton, *The Inoculator; or, the Suttonian System of Inoculation, Fully Set Forth in a Plain and Familiar Manner, by Daniel Sutton, Surgeon. Who Introduced the New Method of Inoculation into This Kingdom in the Year 1763.* Author, 1796.
25 Rudolph and Musher, "Inoculation," 692.
26 Otto T. Beall and Richard Shryock, *Cotton Mather: First Significant Figure in American Medicine* (Baltimore: Johns Hopkins University Press, 1954), 98.
27 Cotton Mather, *Angel,* 107.
28 Mather, *Angel,* 109–110.
29 Kittredge, "Introduction," 9.
30 Cotton Mather, *Diary 1709–1724,* 632.
31 Cotton Mather, "An Account of the Method and Success of Inoculating the Small-Pox, in Boston, in New England" (London: 1722), 16–17.
32 James Thacher, *American Medical,* 187.
33 Thacher, 188.
34 Blake, *American Medical, Public Health,* 78.
35 James W. Schmotter, "African Medical Knowledge, the Plain Style, and Satire in the 1721 Boston Smallpox Controversy" in *Early American Literature* 46, no. 1 (December 2010), 25–50; Cristobal Silva, *Miraculous Plagues: An Epidemiology*

of Early New England Narrative (New York: Oxford University Press, 2011); Matthew Wynn Sivils, "Dissecting the Pamphlet Literature of the Boston Smallpox Controversy" in *Literature and Medicine,* 29, no. 1 (2011): 39–57.

36 Schmotter, "African Medical Knowledge," 23.

37 James B. Blake, *Public Health;* Shawn Buhr, "To Inoculate or Not to Inoculate: The Debate and the Smallpox Epidemic of 1721," *Constructing the Past,* no. 1 (2000), 61–67; E. H. Henry, "Experience in Massachusetts and a Few Other Places with Smallpox and Vaccination" in *Boston Medical Surgical Journal* 185, no. 8 (1921): 221–228; Musher and Rudolph, "Inoculation."

38 Kathryn S. Koo, *Strangers in the House of God: Cotton Mather, Onesimus, and an Experiment in Christian Slaveholding* (Wooster, MA: American Antiquarian Society, 2007); Margot Minardi, "The Boston Inoculation Controversy of 1721–17211: An Incident in the History of Race" in *The William and Mary Quarterly* 61, no. 1 (2004): 47–76.

39 Louise Breen, "Cotton Mather, the 'Angelic Ministry' and 'Inoculation'" in *Journal of the History of Medicine and Allied Sciences* 46, no. 3 (July 1991): 333–357.

40 Cristobal Silva, *Miraculous Plagues.* Robert Tindol, "Getting the Pox Off All Their Houses: Cotton Mather and the Rhetoric of Puritan Science," in *Early American Literature* 46, no. 1(March 2011), 1–23. Sivils, Schmotter, and Tindol, all of whom were in literature, had written about this event.

41 Matthew Wynn Sivils, "Dissecting the Pamphlet Literature of the Boston Smallpox Controversy," in *Literature and Medicine,* 29, no.1 (2011): 39.

42 Sivils, "Dissecting," 40.

43 Amadeo Policante, "War Against Biopower: Reflection on an Historicist Foucault" in *Theory and Event* 13, no. 1 (2010).

44 Michel Foucault, *Security, Territory, Population,* trans. Graham Burchell (New York: Picador, 2009), 1–4.

45 Stephen Coss, *The Fever of 1721* (New York: Simon and Schuster, 2016), 14.

Bibliography

Baron, John. *The Life of Edward Jenner.* London: Henry Colburn Publisher, 1838.

Baxby, D. *Jenner's Smallpox Vaccine.* London: Heinemann, 1981.

Beall, Otto T. and Richard Shryock. *Cotton Mather: First Significant Figure in American Medicine.* Baltimore: Johns Hopkins University Press, 1954.

Best, Mark, A. Katamba, and Duncan Neuhauser, "Making the Right Decision: Benjamin Franklin's Son Dies of Smallpox in 1736" in *Quality and Safety in Health Care,* 16, no. 6 (2007).

Blake, James B. *Public Health in the Town of Boston.* Cambridge, MA: Harvard University Press, 1959.

Boylston, Arthur William, M.D. *"Preface" to Defying Providence: Smallpox and the Forgotten 18th Century Medical Revolution.* North Charleston, S. Carolina: CreateSpace Independent Platform, 2012.

Boylston, Arthur William, M.D. "The Origins of Vaccination: Myths and Reality" in *The Journal of Royal Society of Medicine,* 106, no. 9 (September 2013).

Boylston, Zabdiel. An Historical Account of the Small-Pox Inoculated in New England. London: 1726.

Breen, Louise. "Cotton Mather, the 'Angelic Ministry' and 'Inoculation'" in *Journal of the History of Medicine and Allied Sciences,* 46, no. 3 (July 1991).

Buhr, Shawn. "To Inoculate or Not to Inoculate: The Debate and the Smallpox Epidemic of 1721" in *Constructing the Past*, no. 1 (2000).

Coss, Stephen. *The Fever of 1721*. New York: Simon and Schuster, 2016.

Foucault, Michel. *Security, Territory, Population*, trans. Graham Burchell. New York: Picador, 2009.

Hall, Michael G. *The Last Puritan*. Middleton, CT: Wesleyan University Press, 1988.

Hammarsten, J. F., W. Tattersall, and J. E. Hammarsten, M.D.s, "Transactions of the American Clinical and Climatological Association" in *Who Discovered Vaccination? Edward Jenner or Benjamin Jesty?* 90 (1979).

Harvard Open Collection, Contagion: Historic Views of Diseases and Epidemics (2008–2015).

Henry, E. H. "Experience in Massachusetts and a Few Other Places with Smallpox and Vaccination" in *Boston Medical Surgical Journal*, 185, no. 8 (1921).

Jones, Gordon. *Introduction to Angel of Bethesda*. Barre, MA: American Antiquarian Society and Barre Publishers, 1972.

Kaiser, Jocelyn. "Six Vials of Smallpox Discovered in U.S. Lab" in *Science*, July 8, 2014. Accessed June 3, 2022, https://www.science.org/content/article/six-vials-smallpox-discovered-us-lab

Kittredge, George L. "Introduction" to Increase Mather's and Anonymous's [Cotton Mather] Several Reasons or Transplanting the Small Pox, Is a Lawful Practice, and That It Has Been Blessed by God for the Saving of Many a *Life. etc.* and Cotton Mather's *Sentiments Written on the Small Pox Inoculated*, Cleveland, OH: 1921.

Koo, *Strangers in the House of God: Cotton Mather, Onesimus, and an Experiment in Christian Slaveholding*. Wooster, MA: American Antiquarian Society, 2007.

Mather, Cotton. *Angel of Bethesda*. Barre, MA: American Antiquarian Society and Barre Publishers, 1972.

Mather, Cotton. *Diary, 1709–1724*, Vol. 2. New York: Frederick Unger, 1957.

Margot Minardi, "The Boston Inoculation Controversy of 1721–17211: An Incident in the History of Race" in *The William and Mary Quarterly*, 61, no. 1 (2004).

Policante, Amadeo. "War Against Biopower: In Reflection on an Historicist Foucault" in *Theory and Event*, 13, no. 1 (2010).

Rudolph, R. and Musher, G. M. "Inoculation in the Boston Smallpox Epidemic" in *Archives of Internal Medicine*, 1965.

Schmotter, James W., "African Medical Knowledge, the Plain Style, and Satire in the 1721 Boston Smallpox Controversy" in *Early American Literature*, 46, no. 1 (December 2010).

Silva, Cristobal. *Miraculous Plagues: An Epidemiology of Early New England Narrative*. New York: Oxford University Press, 2011.

Sivils, Matthew Wynn. "Dissecting the Pamphlet Literature of the Boston Smallpox Controversy" in *Literature and Medicine*, 29, no. 1, 39–57 (2011).

Sutton, Daniel. The Inoculator; or, The Suttonian System of Inoculation, Fully Set Forth in a Plain and Familiar Manner, by Daniel Sutton, Surgeon. Who Introduced the New Method of Inoculation Into This Kingdom in the Year 1763. Author, 1796.

Thacher, James. *American Medical Biography*. Boston: Richardson and Lord, 1828.

Tindol, Robert. "Getting the Pox Off All Their Houses: Cotton Mather and the Rhetoric of Puritan Science" in *Early American Literature* 46, no. 1 (March 2011).

1 Contextualizing the Smallpox Inoculation of 1721–1722

J. Blake Scott foregrounded both cultural and rhetorical analysis in his claim that scholars who study health and medicine borrow from other disciplines and highlight intertextuality. "At stake in cross-pollinating rhetoric and cultural studies are our very understandings of rhetoric and technoscience."[1] Scott pointed out that the term, *technoscience*: is "Latour's term for science and technology in action."[2] Cotton Mather's smallpox inoculation project in the early 1720s represents a very early use of technoscience in North America, and the practice of the very new technique of smallpox inoculation in this area of the world was certainly "science and technology in action." In this text the arguments for and against the science of variolation were put forward by both the "Inoculators" and "Anti-inoculators." As Kenneth Burke also noted in his concept of terministic screens, the positioning of language determines not only which aspects of a given subject receive attention, but also which aspects do not receive attention.[3] According to Robert M. Entman, the various frames of the debate work through "definitions, explanations, evaluations, and recommendations" that guide audience members, and those can either include or exclude (and certainly shape) the aspects of any "reality."[4] Also, Murray Edelman suggested, " … [A]ny phenomenon becomes radically different as changes are made in what is prominently displayed, what is repressed and especially in how observations are classified … The social world is … a kaleidoscope of potential realities, any of which can be readily evoked by altering the ways in which observations are framed and categorized."[5] Especially when audiences do not know much about possible alternatives and only a few choices (or even only one) are offered in the framing of a particular situation, audiences are more vulnerable to misinformation and manipulation. In the following chapters, the way the Anti-inoculators framed the inoculation debate in 1720s Boston very much persuaded the Bostonians of the dangers of the technique, while they were in the midst of a virulent smallpox epidemic.

Frame analysis theory, first initiated by Erving Goffman, can function as a mixture of older and newer theoretical lenses to achieve a multifocal as well as a multivocal approach. Frames are, like an "apparatus," a construction, but involve more than one aspect of discursive practices, and they

DOI: 10.4324/9781003312369-2

also make no claims regarding "rationality." Frame analyses have typically been used to examine current events or those happenings that have recently occurred. But, because it is possible to have access to a good number of the texts from the actual time of the smallpox vaccination project in 1721 and 1722—newspapers, tracts, pamphlets, as well as diaries, Royal Society *Transactions,* and letters—framing was one important lens through which to view those documents. Entman makes just such a case for framing theory:

> I propose that we ... should identify our mission as bringing together insights and theories that would otherwise remain scattered in other disciplines. Because of the lack of interchange among the disciplines, hypotheses thoroughly discredited in one field may receive wide acceptance in another. Potential research paradigms remain fractured, ... By bringing ideas together in one location, ... [we can] synthesize related theories and concepts ... .[6]

Numerous frames already exist within a given site and time. Culture is made up of "commonly invoked frames; in fact, culture might be defined as the empirically demonstrable set of common frames exhibited in the discourse and thinking of most people in a social grouping."[7] Pre-existing cultural frames can explain why some particular texts have more valence with certain types of audience. The way an argument is framed and provides salience is key to how certain arguments resonate with certain audiences, whether literati, doctors, patients, ministers, shopkeepers, townspeople, or farmers, would determine the success or failure of such a project. Frame analysis is also akin to what rhetoricians call rhetorical analysis, ways we "frame" our arguments for certain audiences in order to appeal to them.

It's useful to consider Foucault's highlighting of "relationships" among and between the elements of an apparatus such as the one constructed during the Boston smallpox inoculation project. So, for example, the discussions of law in the time period of Mather's and Boylston's variolations exhibit a strong relationship between medicine and law. Arguments sought to evaluate such things as the legality of the project (legal in many senses as Chapter 2 will show) and, ironically, to prescribe certain courses of action, some of which were violent and illegal. Also, framing the medical arguments in legal terms resonated with or had salience for the colonials of this time period. More on Foucault's definition of the apparatus is useful here.

Foucault's "Apparatus" as Lens

In *Power/Knowledge,* during an interview Michel Foucault had with members of the Quel Corps,[8] "What I'm trying to pick out with this term [*apparatus*] is, firstly, a thoroughly heterogeneous ensemble consisting of discourses, institutions, architectural forms, regulatory decisions, laws, administrative measures, scientific statements, philosophical, moral and philanthropic propositions,—in short, the said as much as the unsaid. Such are the elements of the apparatus." [9] By institution, Foucault later qualified, he meant " ... every kind of more-or-less constrained learned behavior. Everything which functions in a society as a system of constraint and which isn't an utterance, in short, all the field of the non-discursive social, is an institution."[10] Even this definition, though, he later changed when challenged by J. A. Miller, who insisted that of course the institution is also discursive, and Foucault acknowledged that notion as valid, but suggested he was just emphasizing the other aspects as well at that point.[11] One can see in the event of the introduction of the smallpox inoculation into 1721 Boston, some of the elements of an apparatus beginning to assemble themselves, one of numerous re-organizations that led to the paradigm shift that occurred later in Western European medicine as documented in *The Birth of the Clinic*. At the same time, other cultural traditions and elements are also being reorganized or disorganized in the same years as the epidemic.

In addition to discourses, it is also important to consider such institutions as Harvard, the Royal Society and the predominant church; regulatory laws handed down from the Selectmen of Boston, as well as the Governor from Britain; laws, such as the "Law of Physik" and liturgical laws and doctrines; administrators in Boston, such as the Selectmen; scientific statements from the Royal Society *Philosophical Transactions*; and philosophic and moral propositions from the Church as part of the "apparatus." These institutions prescribed, proscribed, and initiated what could be said at the time, and they also came under some serious critique, correction, challenge, and threat themselves. As in the biological science of medicine, the struggle over who and what discipline had the power/knowledge began to change. In short, who owns the body? The discursive practices of these various institutions were instrumental in enabling and disabling the actions of a community in a time of crisis. In effect, the institutions and the actors initiated and/or reinforced the frames and attempted to set up new ones, which/who then framed, dictated and/or initiated certain discursive practices, while disassembling others.

The institutions themselves were also a part of what Foucault maintained were the "elements" that make up such an "apparatus," but he further defined the term, that it "itself is the system of relations that can be established between these elements."[12] In this text, these broadly defined institutions are showcased in the various discursive practices of the time and the interactions (or "relations") among them. "Thus a particular discourse can figure at one time as the programme of an institution and at another it can function as a means of justifying or making a practice, which itself remains silent, or as a secondary re-interpretation of this practice, opening out for it, a new field of rationality."[13] Because the inoculation practice in 1721 occurred on the cusp of "New Science" both in the colonies and in Europe, the discourse seemed to exhibit the struggles that this "new field of rationality" was undergoing.

In the American colonies, an inoculation project had not been tried before, especially on this scale (or there is no written record of it being tried in the past that could be discovered). The exigence presented itself in the form of yet another smallpox epidemic making its appearance in Boston.[14] Given the experience of Bostonians with smallpox in the past, the appearance of this disease heralded a true crisis. And as Foucault suggested, " ..., I understand by the term 'apparatus' a sort of – shall we say – formation which has as its major function at a given historical moment that of responding to an *urgent need*,"[15] echoing here Lloyd Bitzer's sense of the rhetorical situation. A smallpox epidemic, after the experience of previous, devastating epidemics in Boston, provided such a need. In addition to an exigence, the French theorist made clear that it was necessary to understand that the apparatus was intimately connected to power, was indeed a type of "power analytic .... In reality power means relations, a more or less organized, hierarchical, coordinated structure of relations;" the structure of relations at times in an event can also be ill-coordinated.[16] This power analytic, Foucault maintained, gives us a tool for analysis of events and relationships between knowledge and power. This particular event is partly a story of the conflict between religion and science, not an unusual or unstudied conflict in the U.S., but one which needs further historicizing and explicating in terms of the power relations at this particular juncture in colonial history and within medical rhetoric.

Foucault's Genealogical Lens

Before proceeding further, it's important to situate the inoculation project within Foucault's interest in the biological sciences, medicine, and epistemology in general. Colin Gordon, who edited the theorist's *Power/Knowledge* interviews and other writings, contextualized the groundbreaking text in a retrospective afterword. Foucault was drawn to working in the "human sciences" or in the biological sciences, such as his archaeology of perception in *The Birth of the Clinic,* because of his very strong interest in the work of Georges Canguilhem, his thesis advisor, who wrote in the 1940s. Foucault eschewed working on histories of the disciplines of physics and mathematics because of Canguilhem's example. Here is the rationale for his choice: "What this work has shown is that the philosophically recalcitrant aspects of the development of these sciences imposes [sic] on the historian certain methodological reflections which yield a series of novel philosophical insights."[17] Foucault could then use his study of the development of the hospital, in *Birth of the Clinic*, to yield more information on his study of rationality and particularly to lay a sort of foundation for his work in power/knowledge.

> Precisely because the biological sciences do not emerge out of discoveries validated through the adequacy and rigor of their mathematical formalization, it becomes unsatisfactory and inadequate for their historian to assume the present standpoint of the more-or-less definitive scientific truth and to reconstruct their development as the immanent logic of a series of transformations through which that truth is attained or revealed.[18]

In short, one cannot apply the same analytic tool to biology and the human sciences that one can to those based in math, although this concept applied more to their historical development, because today there is much more measurement possible through technological changes and developments in biology and even in psychology. In addition, a simple chronological history is also not appropriate. Or as Foucault believed: "The history of biology does not thus transparently unfold itself before the gaze of present truth. But neither can it be made intelligible through a simple descriptive sociology of the beliefs and practices of successive generations of savants. Nor does the solution lie in an amalgamation of the two approaches."[19] Instead the theorist posited that biology must and does subject itself to periodic reevaluation: an "open-ended and provisional critique of its own progress."[20] Applying a Foucauldian analysis to the Boston inoculation project helps us get beyond a positivist (as well as sexist) ideology. Instead it examines the rhetorical situation from an "open-ended" standpoint and through the use of a series of interactions between and among the elements of a newly forming and formed apparatus and between and among certain contexts, audiences, and speakers/writers within the rhetorical situation. In addition, it puts into play Canguilhem's *historical epistemology*, which could be defined as "a history of the production of knowledge or as a line of questioning that considers the history of concepts and *often opposed scientific approaches* as developing systems of knowledge" (emphasis added).[21]

The Galenic system of medicine had been in place for centuries, and, like the scientific method today, was thought to be unquestionable and carried strong and seemingly indisputable truth claims, making it difficult for breakthroughs or paradigm shifts. Foucault's project was to formulate history in such a way to disrupt the idea of history as a regime of truth but instead see it more as a network of relations. Rhetorically analyzing the texts of an historical debate constituting a challenge to the reigning regime of truth in 1720s Boston reveals the power relations at the time. The relations reflected in the discursive practices of various institutions and groups of individuals (in 1721 Boston: ministers and physicians) suggested numerous factors that appeared at the time representing both attempts to institute new practices and to resist them. These attempts were not just in the medical realm; other challenges in government, politics, and religion were also taking place. While this approach was part of Foucault's "genealogical" approach, *The Birth of the Clinic* included the theorist's further development of the "archaeological" lens as part of his "analytic." Both of these theoretical developments in the history of Foucault's thinking led to this reformulated power, with its recognition of how politics, government, and control over populations works. Power moves from one locus at the beginning of the inoculation period into other social bodies as a result of the controversy. Ruptures change the sites of operation, and biopower gains new agents for its functioning. The term *rupture is* often associated with Foucault who used it in many of his works and often uses the term in historical analyses of disruptions in long-standing social divisions. In addition, it can apply to changes in disciplinary structures, such as that of medicine. This text uses the above lenses to examine a culture from three hundred years ago, an ethnography of the past. Fortunately, the archives from that time and place are intact, well preserved, and richly revealing so that many factors in the debate can be studied.

To understand the movement taking place during a "rupture," it's important to understand the other contexts, which include: a brief history of the disease of smallpox; an overview of the already developed quarantine system and social "gaze" or surveillance system; an explanation of colonial medicine and science in the 1720s and their history; a clear definition of the procedure that initiated the debate; the sources Cotton Mather relied on that impelled him to initiate an immunization program; thumbnail sketches of the main antagonists: a clergyman and surgeon versus a Scottish physician and printers; and the common sense trope.

Brief History of Smallpox

Epidemiologists think the disease itself originated in northeast Africa in approximately 10,000 BCE.[22] Many believe that descriptions in Egyptian papyri that date from 1350 BCE are of smallpox. Sometimes, however, smallpox, measles, and chickenpox were confused in recorded history as aggressive scratching of measles and chicken pox can also lead to scarring, and all three illnesses can lead to death, although smallpox was the most lethal. Egyptologists thought the lesions on the face of the mummy of Pharaoh Ramses V, who died about 1156 or 1157 BCE, were caused by smallpox.[23] Europeans brought smallpox, aka "the red death," "the red plague," and the "speckled monster," across the ocean to the Americas, specifically to the island of Hispaniola in the Caribbean in 1507.[24] Smallpox killed kings of Siam and Burma, two Japanese emperors, the first Abbasid Caliph, the last Aztecan ruler, a Hapsburgian king, and perhaps Marcus Aurelius. Some believe it contributed to the downfall of Athens, and some also believe it paved the way for colonizers to use ethnic cleansing against the native peoples in the Americas.[25] Queen Elizabeth I contracted smallpox in 1562 and survived it with light scarring. The rumor that she had become bald and wore wigs as a result of the illness was false.[26] As a result of nursing the queen, Lady Mary Sidney contracted the disease, survived, but was terribly disfigured. She never appeared in court again.[27] Queen Mary II of England suffered and died of Variola hemorrhagica at age 32 in 1694. That form of smallpox was one in which a victim experienced internal bleeding, and bleeding also took place inside the pustules themselves, as well as from other body surfaces. Thomas Macaulay wrote that:

> The havoc of the plague had been far more rapid: but the plague had visited our shores only once or twice within living memory; and the smallpox was always present, filling the church-yards with corpses, tormenting with constant fears all whom it had not yet stricken, leaving on those whose lives it spared the hideous traces of its power, turning the babe into a changeling at which the mother shuddered, and making the eyes and cheeks of the betrothed maiden objects of horror to the lover. Toward the end of the year 1694, this pestilence was more than usually severe. At length the infection spread to the palace, and reached the young and blooming Queen [Mary].[28]

In the American colonies, tremendous epidemics swept through on a regular basis, although it was endemic in England and other European countries. Between 1619 and 1698, Boston itself suffered at least six smallpox epidemics. Native American tribes were especially vulnerable to smallpox infections because unlike the British and Europeans who arrived from locales where the disease was endemic, they had no natural immunity. Known and documented epidemics included the one in 1617–1619 that wiped out 90% of the Massachusetts Bay natives.[29] In 1689 French courtier Count de Frontenac Louis de Buade, describing the effects of smallpox on the Iroquois, termed it the "Indian Plague:" "The Small Pox desolates them to such a degree that they think no longer of Meeting nor of Wars, but only of bewailing the dead, of whom there is already an immense number."[30] Other smallpox epidemics among the Native Americans continued to severely impact the tribes across the country for many years as soon as contact with Europeans took place. Epidemics continued to hit Boston throughout the 1700s with the repeated outbreaks of 1702, 1721, 1752, 1764, and 1775 that were especially severe and accompanied with high death rates among colonists as well as native peoples.[31]

As recently as 1967 the disease sickened between ten and fifteen million people each year in 43 countries and caused two million deaths.[32] Donald R. Hopkins suggested that over three millennia, smallpox most likely killed more people than the plague.[33] It would be impossible to calculate how many smallpox victims there were over that time, but in the 20th century alone, it's thought to have killed between 300 and 500 million people.[34] D. A. Henderson, former C.D.C. Director for Disease Surveillance, wrote that smallpox killed more people than World Wars I and II combined.[35]

Inoculation against smallpox was reported in China as early as 1000 BCE through the same method Mather recorded: injecting fluid from a full-blown

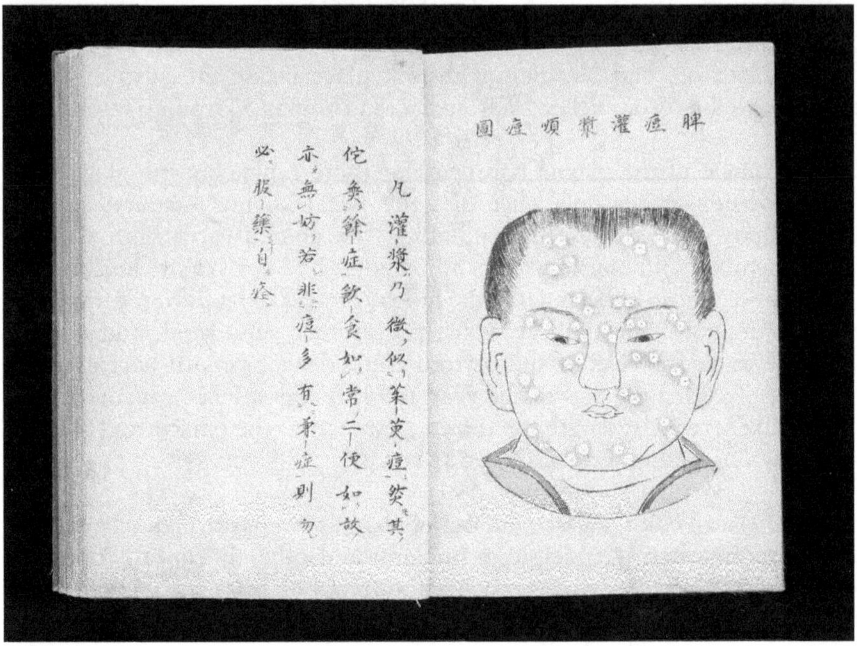

Figure 1.1 Asian Smallpox Illustration, Wellcome Collection.

pox into a person's skin. In China a second method was also used: a tube to blow dried powder from smallpox scabs into the nostrils of a healthy person. While both methods could work to protect the patient, those inoculated were infectious to others during the period that his or her antibodies were forming and were quarantined. Keekok Lee reports,[36] based on a text written during the Tang Dynasty in China (618–907 CE) by Sun Simiao, a very similar procedure to the one Mather and Boylston was used for prevention of a more severe case of the disease.[37] The traditions continued and were documented, too, during the Song Dynasty (960–1279 CE) in *Discourse Definitive on Smallpox* by Zhu Chunjia, who related that a Chancellor Wang Dan had arranged for a famous medical practitioner he called a "miracle physician" from Sichuan Province to inoculate his son to protect him from the disease.[38] By the 1500s, during the Qing dynasty and under the reign of emperor Ming Longqing (1567–1572), inoculations and inoculators were much more frequent.[39] It wasn't until 1682 that the emperor Qing Kangxi, based on his own experience, mandated variolation for every part of his empire, especially among a tribe known as Manchu Banners.[40] In addition to the two methods used in China mentioned above, a third method had been reported in the 1600s: have healthy children wear under garments of infected children; a fourth: to use the fluid from a pox, gather it on a piece of cotton wool, and insert it into the nose of a child and remove it after 12 hours; and a fifth: to grind the scabs and add a little water or breastmilk for the child to ingest.[41]

According to Keekok Lee, Russian doctors were sent to China to learn the various ways to protect people from smallpox in 1688. In the 1700s such knowledge migrated to Japan and Korea. Russians took the method of using the fluid from the pox and putting it into a cut on the body to Turkey where Lady Montagu observed it in 1716. While Western medicine is aware of the Mather project and that of Lady Montagu in England (from Turkish practices), Mather's initial knowledge was not from either source. Western medicine in general has only recently acknowledged the role that China played in vaccination, inoculation, and variolation.[42]

The smallpox virus extant in this early history was always the *Variola Major*, the most virulent and deadly form of the disease. Later versions, such as *Variola Minor*, did not appear until the late 1800s in the U.S. *Variola Major* killed at least 25% if not 30% of its victims, while *V. Minor*'s toll was about 1%.[43] Over the centuries, various natural philosophers, the early term for those interested in science, and those practicing *Physick*, *Physik*, or *Physic*, the early term for medicine, found different causes for the dread disease. Even before Christianity began, Egyptians and Indians subscribed to certain theurgical beliefs that their gods were punishing them for evil behavior. Christians expanded the theory of punishment by including redemption if one repented of wicked practices.[44] Greek humoral theory developed by Hippocrates and enhanced by Galen (129 CE to c. 216 CE) held that an imbalance of the elements based on earth/air/water/fire or the four fluids of the body were to blame, while later natural philosophers suggested tiny seeds, worms, and little animals invisible to the naked eye caused smallpox. The miasma theory of bad air as infectious was held by still others who moved to different locales to minimize illness, consequently often moving away from contagion.

In the 6th- and 7th-century Europe, the rapid spread of leprosy helped introduce quarantine as a means of control. Local and provincial governments were often charged with enforcing a quarantine. Reactions to plagues from the 6th century to the 14th also meant putting new quarantines in place. Isolation hospitals were set up, not so much to treat patients, but to keep them separate from the general population.[45]

Quarantines in Boston and Earlier

A system of quarantines was already part of Boston's colonial history. The convergence of a growing city and a very active port increasingly made Boston and its surroundings a scene of significant epidemics of which the smallpox contagion in the 1720s was only one incidence. That epidemic provided a viable setting for the inoculation drama. This factor meant it became more and more incumbent on the inhabitants, but especially on the leaders and administrative bodies of the urban center to begin more actively constructing and policing laws and policies relating to public health and addressing the public as a whole. Previously, health and quarantines centered solely on individual patients within a family or parish or on ships in port towns. Emphasis had begun to shift from families, small neighborhoods, and ships to a larger venue.

Foucault noted that ports, ships, prisons, and hospitals were the sites for institution of some of the earliest public medical interventions. "A port, and a military port is—with its circulation of goods, men signed up willingly or by force, sailors embarking and disembarking, diseases and epidemics — a place of desertion, smuggling, contagion: it is a crossroads for dangerous mixtures, a meeting-place" for disease.[46] Maritime laws in Boston mandated that ships coming into port were to be quarantined, and any passengers or crew already ill were to be taken off the ships to be housed in a quarantine hospital on Spectacle Island.[47] Not until 1720 was the hospital fully staffed and operational. By 1729, all Irish ships were to be quarantined to Spectacle Island, and all their passengers and crew were discharged onto the island because colonists assumed Irish ships always carried smallpox.[48] This singling out of Irish ships maps onto one of the well-known biases of the British and former British toward the Irish.

Although some sailors and passengers from Irish ships died of smallpox on the island, many were later brought into town.[49] The earliest quarantines in the Boston area had been enacted by the General Court in 1647, repealed in 1649; brought against the plague in 1665, repealed in 1667; and brought against smallpox as ordered by the Selectmen in 1678 for Salem.[50] The Colony quarantine law passed in 1700 was disallowed and then passed again in 1701.[51] So this arena of social control had already been established in Boston (and in other colonies besides the ones in Massachusetts) in the last half of the 17th and early 18th centuries, but it was usually done on an *ad hoc* basis depending on epidemics.

Quarantines were early sites of the "gaze" in medicine or surveillance. Because Cotton Mather specifically cited his discovery of "animalculae" in the vitreous matter of a smallpox pustule in his medical compendium, the gaze also shifted from the outer body to the inner body. Such a discovery served as one of the exigencies for the paradigm shift that would occur several decades later, but clearly quarantine had already begun in Western history, and was not an American invention. When the gaze had been employed, for example during a French plague in the 1600s, a whole town was closed off; no one could leave "on pain of death;" and all stray animals were killed.[52] The town would be divided into areas, and a supervisor would be chosen to oversee each area. Another person would be appointed to keep each street under surveillance; if the surveillance officer left the street, he would be killed. Citizens were ordered to stay indoors or be executed. The street supervisor would lock the door of each house from the outside, and then he collected all the keys and gave them to the area supervisor, who kept them until the end of the quarantine.[53] In addition, long, drawn-out, thorough rules dictated the ways the family would receive rations and provisions without any contact with other people. "Canals" were set up between the streets and the interior of homes, and baskets to receive supplies were let out of windows and pulled up by ropes. Corpses were to be pushed outside the house to be collected by "people of little substance."[54]

Such rules and segmentation seem a rather horrific model of the early quarantine measures in Europe in which individuals were quarantined in their homes or rooms, and no one was allowed to visit. Today we still see "quarantine" (now called "isolation") enacted in medical centers with extensive gowning, masking, hand-washing, gloving, and covering of shoes by those health professionals who must enter the room and treat the contagious or immune-compromised patient. The entire globe has experienced a form of quarantine and masking during the last two-plus years in homes and public places, and some countries are still in lockdown or in lockdown again in the SARS-CoV-2 (Covid-19) pandemic. While our quarantines are often more individualized, and those who are known to be contagious must be isolated, most citizens in the West are not overly surveilled or certainly not locked into their homes. However, before the Beijing Olympics, China's 2020s quarantines were much stricter and more akin to the French 1600s and other former more stringent European quarantines. In Beijing, all 13 million residents had been forced to remain in their homes and could not leave their domiciles to buy food or other supplies. While free speech is widely discouraged by the government there, citizens still used social media to complain. Authorities were said to be providing free food to households, but some had not received much needed aid as their supplies ran very low. A number of citizens had been forcibly removed and bussed to a quarantine facility during the late hours of the night. In addition, the city continued to quickly build hospitals for those who were most ill.[55] In more recent quarantines in Shanghai, Hong Kong, and Jilin Province in China, the same stringent enforcement of quarantine had been taking place. People were being locked in their homes and buildings and also had mandatory testing. Those infected continued to be sent to quarantine centers until those filled up.[56]

According to Foucault, quarantine then and now engendered a "segmented, immobile, frozen space. Each individual is fixed in his place. And, if he moves, he does so at the risk of … contagion, or punishment. Inspection functions ceaselessly. The gaze is alert everywhere."[57] Many men had or have to be available to enforce such a system. However, our Western quarantines have not been enforced as in the 1600s France. In Europe then and now in China, so many men had to be available to enforce such a system, often the militia was used. As part of this surveillance, there was also a type of roll call on each street, and if someone did not appear at once at windows and doors, there must be either a corpse or an ill person produced at a window for the count.[58]

In Britain, the smallpox and quarantine situation was somewhat different, because the disease was endemic there, rather than epidemic as it was in some parts of Europe and in the American colonies. Because it was endemic in the population, a complete quarantine would be much less effective with the intermittent cases. Ships were quarantined, much as they were in the colonies, but not usually whole towns. At times a particular town or village that might be hard hit with many smallpox cases would be advertised as off limits and to be avoided if possible.[59]

In the 1720s Boston epidemic, patients were expected to adhere to quarantine laws and stay in their homes; however, access to active cases was not completely limited, and practitioners of medicine or Physick could come and go. Yet life and disease would be regulated; the Selectmen would rule whether quarantine could be used or not, and those going up against the law would be subject to jail. But in 1721–1722, this surveillance fixed on those who were vaccinating as well as those who were not following quarantine regulations.

Although certainly the role of medicine in the 1720s American colonies was not yet organized or as important a part of the "machinery of power" as it eventually would be, there was a hint toward medicine's future place in the administrative system.[60] This role would become somewhat broader and stronger throughout the 1700s, as physicians and local government would begin to gain more importance and garner social power.[61] Eventually physicians, pharmaceutical and health insurance companies, and medical researchers would be the impetus for medical discoveries and advancement while at the same time developing tremendous political power or a "medico-administrative system" that would become a major force within American culture.[62] As will be seen in the Mather project, the merging of medicine with the local governmental, political, and eventual public health systems had some of its early beginnings in this country during the smallpox epidemic of 1721–1722. What began as laws and regulations made for passengers and crew on ships arriving in port would soon be extended to active cases in an epidemic, including what treatments or preventatives could be used, and by whom they could be administered, including whether or not citizens would be allowed to be immunized against the terrible disease.

Puritan Interest in Science or "Natural Philosophy"

The Puritans were heavily influenced by the Calvinistic religious frame, and the next chapter offers a more in-depth analysis of the role of religion in the controversy. That does not mean they were not interested in science; in fact, their embrace of science and the "natural world" was indeed prodigious. Cotton Mather was particularly fascinated with scientific inquiry, precisely *because* such wonders of nature demonstrated a phenomenal proof of what Puritans believed was the natural law in the universe.[63] Susan Scott Parrish argues in her *American Curiosity: Cultures of Natural History in the Colonial British Atlantic World* that this wide interest in science, particularly botany, biology, and medicine, both shaped and was shaped by colonial relations among those in the British Atlantic world between the 1600s and the revolutionary war era. In addition, this interest was not limited to just the elite and educated, as, for instance, those members of the Royal Society in London. Instead, it also included colonial naturalism, African magic, Native American healing, and the practical lore the enslaved brought with them.[64]

Part of this interest could be said to be a result of the early move toward modernity and also of Enlightenment philosophy toward natural science.[65] The European countries competed to explore, collect, catalogue, and analyze the flora and fauna of the Americas, attempting to understand the new natural phenomena of the landscape as well as the cultural knowledge that developed as a result of colonial experience.[66] In fact, Europeans in general saw the Americas as a vast treasure trove of riches, novelties, and fascinations. Robert K. Merton had long ago pointed to the Puritans as avid purveyors of the sciences and maintained that if the inscrutable actions of their deity had not occasioned scientific investigation, human behaviors in reaction to these actions did.[67] There were contingent movements and changes that tended to merge Puritan culture with those in science. Some of those included: the changing social structure with the rise of the Puritan mercantile class, the strong belief in the value of work or the Protestant ethic, and their positivistic confidence in human progress.[68] Merton also conceded that even their religion partly inspired its followers to a profound interest in science, as was the case for Cotton Mather.[69]

Cotton's father, Increase, had founded a Philosophical Society in Boston in 1683 to discuss new scientific discoveries and issues of interest, but this early group of which his son was a member dissolved over religious and political differences.[70] As Cotton Mather had written in his epideictic text in memory of his father, he had "... formed a *Philosophic Society* of Agreeable Gentlemen, who met regularly once a fortnight for a Conference upon Improvements in *Philosophy* and Additions to the Stores of *Natural History;* ... But the Calamity of the Times, anon gave a total and fateful Interruption to this *Generous Undertaking.*"[71]

Mather would later use the lists of natural curiosities assembled by the disbanded group for his *Curiosa Americana,* a series of letters to the Royal Society between 1712 and 1724.[72] Many of these letters have been lost, but a few are still in archives on the East coast. One such letter, for example, was one he sent to the editor of the Royal Society *Philosophical Transactions* about a large, fossilized tooth that had been found in the Hudson Valley. Mather had claimed this tooth proved the existence of human giants. The acerbic editor had replied that Mather "had sent neither drawings nor explained his reasons for considering these bones and grinders to be human."[73] Such "curiosities" and fantastic interpretations were not uncommon among letters sent to the Royal Society, although Mather's contribution of such missives had been unusually prodigious.

The Reigning Medical Paradigm

Mather's exposure to the latest developments from The Royal Society coupled with his microscope and some other Puritans' interest in science began to interrupt the more traditional religious paradigm of Colonial America vis-à-vis medicine and healing. Because of Mather's well-read scientific interest, he was able at times to see beyond the lens of humoral medicine to the beginnings of modern disease theory. That is not to say his medical compendium, *Angel of Bethesda,* he was working on in the early 1720s was modern in any sense of the word. Several competing notions of disease existed side-by-side in Mather's text. This text embodied the cusp of the confrontation between two competing paradigms; the rhetoric of science was starting to compete with the dominant rhetoric of religion in America. However, the "science" of medicine then was still primarily based on ancient models.

An analysis of Mather's medical text showed that most of the practice was based on the humors: blood, yellow bile, phlegm, and black bile. This Western system of balancing these elements and the four fluids begun by Hippocrates and Galen was known not just throughout the Mediterranean world but also in Europe and the Middle East, even attributed to the Prophet Muhammed in Islam as late as the mid-9th century.[74] The system centered not only around the elements and bodily fluids, but also around qualities and elements such as hot and moist, cold and dry; the four seasons; the four ages of man; fire, earth, water, and air; and three planets along with the moon. The Greek philosophers also linked the elements to one another, and even applied them to temperaments or human characteristics. In *On the Temperaments*, Galen emphasized that the best personality would reflect a well-balanced mixture of the four qualities. Those that are out of balance are named according to their fluid appearances: sanguine (blood), choleric (yellow bile), melancholic (black bile), and phlegmatic (phlegm). Not only were these emotional and behavioral types, but they were also types that led to certain types of diseases and health problems. If all of these qualities and elements then are combined, these are the results the humoral system relied on: *Sanguine* = Humor: Blood, Element: Air, Season: Spring, Age: Adolescence, Qualities: Hot & Moist, Organ: Heart, Planet: Jupiter. *Choleric* = Humor: Yellow Bile, Element: Fire, Season: Summer, Age: Childhood, Qualities: Hot & Dry, Organ: Gall Bladder and Kidneys, Planet: Mars. *Melancholic* = Humor: Black Bile, Element: Earth, Season: Winter, Age: Old Age, Qualities: Cold & Dry, Organ: Spleen, Planet: Saturn. *Phlegmatic* = Humor: Phlegm, Element: Water, Season: Autumn, Age: Maturity, Qualities: Cold & Moist, Organ: Brain, Planet: Moon.[75]

In Shakespeare's time, the bard referred to humors in at least three plays: "The Taming of the Shrew," "Hamlet," and "The Merchant of Venice." In "The Taming of the Shrew," Both Petruchio and Kate are possessed by choleric natures. The husband, Petruchio, recognizes Kate's characteristics but not his own as similar. His goal, then, in the taming of his wife to a more compliant and suitable housewife, is to address her choleric nature by changing her humor. To do this he attempts to change her diet and lifestyle suggesting at dinner that roasted meat is much too hot and dry for her. In his mind, he is denying her dinner in order to better balance her humors. In addition, he tries to withhold from her the comfort of women friends and new clothes. Eventually she is so exhausted and deprived that she submits to his wishes for her compliance.[76] In "Hamlet," it is clear that Ophelia is the character exhibiting a melancholic nature. She grieves the death of her father, is missing someone who might offer her comfort in the court, and whose hoped for lover is denying her much attention. She feels cast out and isolated; the Globe's audience would recognize her depression as a problem of an overabundance of a melancholic humor, an imbalance of the brain. Her suicide is not unexpected. Shylock in "The Merchant of Venice," too, is supposed to be an old man who is, along with unrequited virgins and widows, also melancholic in the last stages of his life. Certain features of melancholia figure here as clues for audiences well-versed in humors. His lack of willingness to enjoy the feast to which he has been, his "retentiveness" or an inability to let go of a debt, and his deep anger against the anti-Semitism of Venetians were thought to be the markers of an unresolved depression and the overabundance of black bile.[77]

Fluids of the body were observed carefully by those who sought to help and cure the sick. Bloodletting was frequently practiced especially in fevers and in the "hot" humors. Either a lancet or what was called a *fleam* was used, which looked much like a Swiss army knife with multiple blades. Cupping was another practice used; a small fire was lit in a special cup with a little alcohol in it, and the mouth of the cup was slapped onto the skin. If a blister was raised, that could then be lanced and a decent amount of blood might flow. Leeches were also used. Barbers or "surgeons" more typically used these practices once a physician had suggested such a treatment. Part of the purpose was simply to "cool" the body by evacuating some blood near the organ that was associated with the humoral imbalance or the body part most affected. Some barbers advertised their occupations as blood letters by putting a bowl of blood in the shop window.[78]

Other fluids and body products were of course also observed, be they sputum, urine, or stool. The 1994 film "The Madness of King George" features a scene at the bedside of the mad King with several physicians, including the King's Physician, standing around discussing the poor man's madness. They dare not touch the King's body, but they are examining his urine and all the contents of his chamber pot. Often there were urine wheels or linear charts available with 20 or more choices in terms of color. The doctors not only compared the color, but the odor, and sometimes the taste. It was particularly germane when the urine had a sweet taste, indicating of course spillage of glucose into the urine or diabetes. Rumor had it that King George's urine was purplish in color. The charts

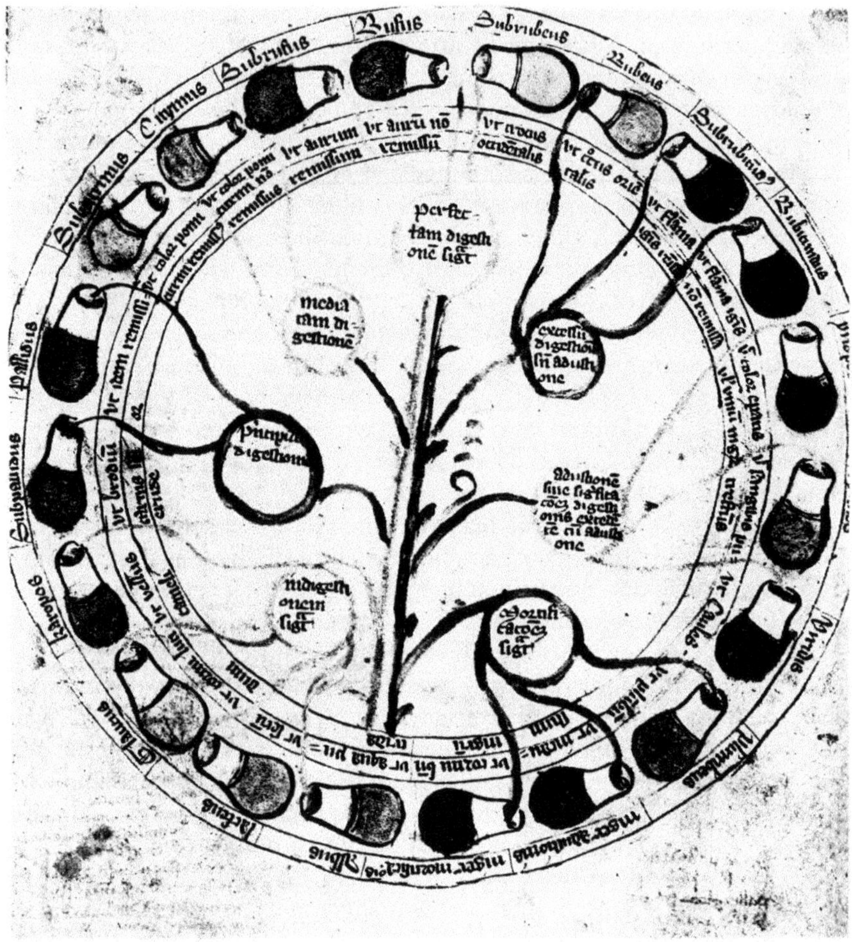

Figure 1.2 Urine Chart, Wellcome Collection.

were in common usage and physicians were more likely to work with the fluids for the most helpful diagnostic evidence.

One example of the humoral paradigm in Mather's medical compendium, *Angel of Bethesda* is the following: "The Grand Secret, and Sole Method for Long Life, is To keep the Blood and Juices, in a due State of Fluidity … . It is a Mistake, that Thin Blood is Poor Blood. There is nothing under Sun, that can render the Blood and Juices, Thin, and Sweet, and Right and constantly in a Flowing State, but keeping to a Spare, Lean, Fluid sort of Diet."[79] Humoral theory, the balanced body, and moderation were also illustrations of common sense and rationalism. The discourse in *Angel* shows how application of these beliefs played out in medical practices through purgatives, emetics, evacuants, and bloodletting. Typically, prayers and religious exhortations were combined with one or more of these types of treatments. An inner balance was attempted by evacuating some of the excess, changing the quality, or moderating the speed with which the humors moved through the body. Humoral practitioners worked not only with the easily observable fluids constituting more concrete, tangible evidences of the body, but the notion of achieving inner balance and connecting humors not only with "passions," but like Mather, writers in the 16th, 17th, and early 18th century also linked emotions and humors with religion.[80] Timothy Bright, a physician, argued in the late 1500s that "a balance between states was optimal not only medically, but also morally."[81] Thomas Wright, an English Jesuit arrested in the reign of Elizabeth I, wrote that passions were dangerous and bestial, "because when these affections are stirring in our minds they alter the humours of our bodies, causing some passion or alteration in them … ."[82] The early American colonialists saw a strong link between body and soul or humors and morals, but the precise interactions were more complex and also subject to much revision.[83] There were large differences between Wright's ideas and those of Lemnius.[84] Thus, there were not always consistent views of the humors when it came to specifics. Before wider and more accurate use of the microscope, which had limited ability in the 1720s, and before the discovery over a century later of cells, fluids "wrote the body" for the physician/minister to read. Humors rendered the invisible and mysterious world of illnesses of minds, bodies, and spirits somewhat more understandable and visible, just as prayers and readings of scripture attempted to communicate with the invisible Puritan deity.

In Mather's compendium, the mixture of religion and humoral medicine is very obvious. The religious exhortations regularly punctuate the panoply of possible treatments for each disease. Here's an example of the frequent combination of both in Chapter 24, which is titled "Bethlem' Visited or The Cure of Madness." His reference to Bethlem was based on the monastery founded in 1247 CE called St. Mary's of Bethlehem in Bishopsgate, London that was converted to a hospital for the insane in the mid-16th century; it was more commonly referred to as "Bedlam." He began the chapter with:

> Oh Sober Spectator of the *Mad*, Think [and so prove thyself to be *Sober-minded.*] "How Thankful to my Gracious God, ought I to be, for *Powers of Reason*, in the free Exercise thereof, Conferred upon me, and Continued unto me! *The Unreasonable Things* that I have done in *Denying the God that is above,* while I have also been prostituting of my *Reason* to mean and base Purposes, render me worthy to be *Smitten with Madness, and Blindness, and Astonishment of Heart,* and be like the *Chaldean* Emperour, *driven from among Men,* and *have my Dwelling with Beasts of the Field,* O my SAVIOUR, Tis Thou, who doest *Enlighten Every Man that Comes into the World;* and unto thee

> am I Endebted for my Use of *Reason,* wherewith I am *Enlightened.* And it is owing to thy Compassionate Mediation for me, that my forfeited *Reason* is not utterly taken from me.[85]

The minister/healer continues in this vein for at least another page before he starts listing various treatments for madness including fasting, purging, blood-letting, spare diet, St. John's Wort, opiates, donkey blood, etc.

Another aspect of Mather's concept of disease found in colonial Boston and in his compendium was the confusion between disease and symptoms. For example, Chapter 41 in *Angel of Bethesda* was called "Icterus Looked Upon, or the Jaundice Cured."[86] This discussion also illustrates the way humoral medicine was used in practice. In Mather's text, this term *jaundice* had the same taxonomical status of a disease in the compendium and was associated with yellow bile, even though it was a symptom not a disease in itself. Jaundice is characterized by the yellowing of skin and eyeballs combined with weight loss, lethargy, and weakness. It's symptomatic of many different diseases: hepatitis, cirrhosis of the liver, over-abundance of bilirubin shortly after birth (because the liver is not yet fully functional in newborns), and drug use, to name a few.

In his chapter on jaundice, Mather made many literary and Biblical allusions to gold (yellow) and suggested the jaundice sufferer was bound "in *Icteritrous Chains,*" and needed to hear the voice of St. John Chrysostom (a golden-mouthed father of the church) to heal.[87] The cures for jaundice were manifold as was typical for each supposed disease in Mather's text. The first treatment was to examine the soul. The physician/minister suggested that jaundice was always accompanied by "*Sadness*" that indicated a "*Repentance which is not to be Repented of.*"[88] His first prescription was for the patient to pour his soul out to the "SAVIOR," and thus to lose his sadness. His other treatments of jaundice that a patient or physician could choose from included the following: a wine concoction with juniper berries; a white-wine/orange/saffron mix; a "gentle Vomit;" infusion of turmeric, celandine, gentian, centaury, saffron, and rhubarb; a syrup of horehound and honey; various roots boiled together with earthworms; while fasting, the urine of a healthy lad with sugar in it; sheep-dung infused in wine; castile soap dissolved in milk; hempseed and new milk; and others. Such treatments were very typical of those Mather gave for each disease, which stood in somewhat stark contrast to the smallpox inoculation chapter in the compendium that was clearly informed by Onesimus, his enslaved man; Royal Society sources; and his own microscope.

The Method of Inoculation

Mather wrote at length on smallpox; it was the largest chapter in his text. In addition to detailing the actual procedure for carrying out the inoculation or variolation, his text included an argument that was well supported, a review of the literature, persuasive statistics, and a voice at times filled with *pathos* as he described the horrific disease.[89]

In *Angel,* when he credited the enslaved Onesimus as his first source for how a smallpox inoculation was accomplished and used his vernacular, he produced one of the earliest transcriptions of African American dialect in the American Colonies, as was quoted in the Introduction. Mather wrote in a diary entry for December 13, 1706 that members of his congregation purchased for him "a very likely Slave; a young Man who is a Negro of a promising aspect of temper."[90] Mather gave him the name *Onesimus* after a Biblical enslaved man who escaped from his master, an early Christian named Philemon.[91] Onesimus's description of variolation showed that a person with an active smallpox case must be found to inoculate a person with no symptoms of the disease. This process usually resulted in the variolated person then having a very mild case of smallpox, and within a couple of weeks, the patient had immunity to the disease and was usually fully recovered. Mather suggested that the person who had the active pox useful for inoculating others (the donor) should be an "[otherwise] Healthy a Young Person as they can find, that has the Small-Pox of the best Sort upon him."[92] It was advantageous if the "donor" was in his or her 12th or 13th day of the disease (well developed, in other words). The "Matter" coming out of "Larger Pustules" should be collected in a small glass bottle with a stopper for it. Mather suggested that the person who collected the fluid from the live pox should not be the same as the person who had come into contact with the recipient because the garment of the collector might have the pox on it. The glass should be handed off to someone else who put the bottle in his or her breast pocket to keep warm as it was conveyed to the recipient. He recommended the recipient have a surgeon make at least three wounds with a three-sided needle till there were some blood droplets.[93] The Matter (more liquid than pus) should be dropped on each of the three wounds and the whole covered with a half walnut shell and bound into place, so that it wouldn't be rubbed off by the clothes. The recipient should stay home, keep warm, and follow a careful diet (perhaps refrain from meat and meat broth).[94] Usually patients developed fewer pustules than those found in a natural case; some had a maximum of one hundred compared with many hundreds of pustules in acute cases of smallpox. The pustules usually scabbed and fell off sooner in inoculated patients, leaving no pits or terrible scars or any other problematic results like in cases incurred in "the common way."[95] Boylston, Mather's friend and supporter, did most of the inoculations in and around Boston at this time. His method was slightly different, using cabbage leaves rather than a walnut as bandage at first but changing to a walnut shell later. Mather recorded the inoculation, unlike his other reports, in a procedural list of 14 very detailed steps rather than in prose, most likely hoping it might be followed as steps for future variolations by others.[96] He had hoped for a timely publication of the book, but that did not happen.

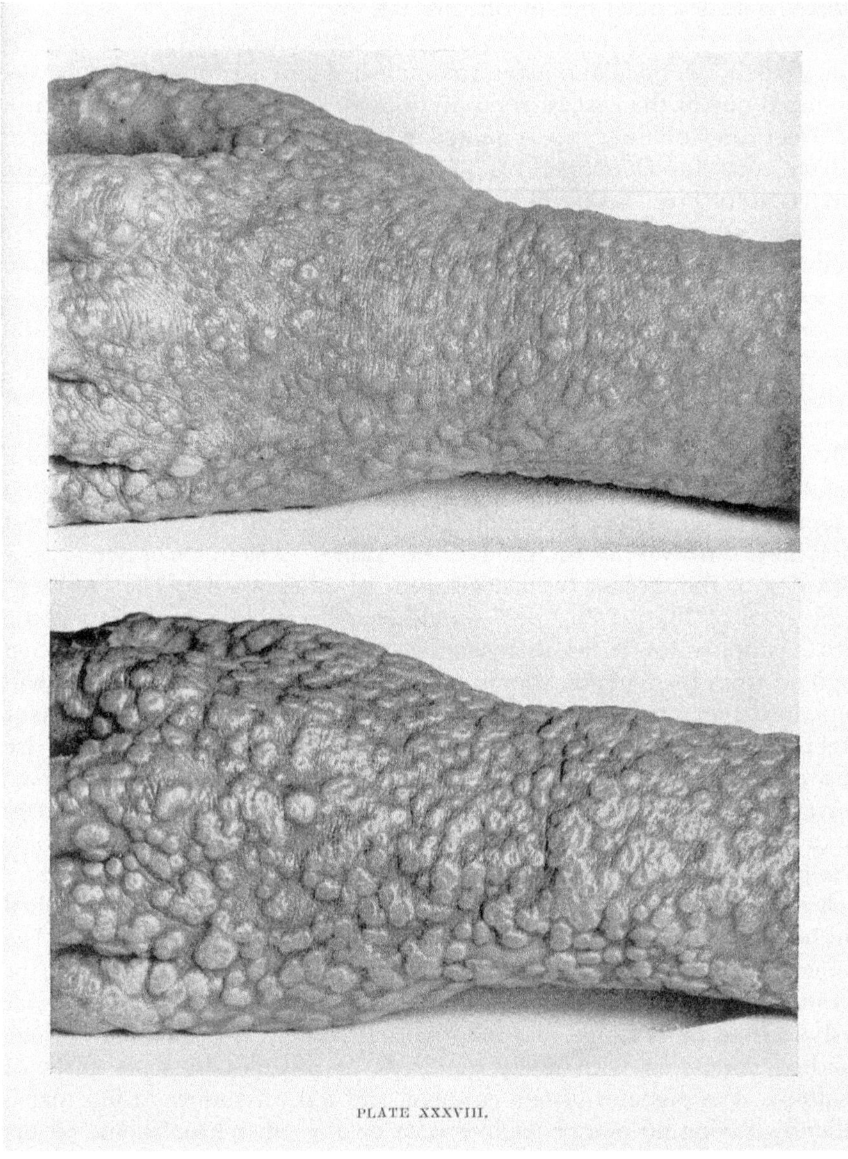

Figure 1.3 Smallpox on Arms/Hands, Wellcome Collection.

In the smallpox vaccinations used in much later times here and abroad, no active smallpox virus was used; instead a live virus referred to as *vaccinia* was used, which produced effective antibodies against the more virulent smallpox virus. Often there has been confusion as to its origin, but smallpox vaccine is still studied. One of the most current insights about vaccinia is that it's now much more related to horsepox, and even the pox suffered by camels, rather than cowpox.[97] Leslie Collier developed the freeze-dried vaccine most useful for inoculating in tropical areas.[98] There has been no active case of smallpox in the United States since 1949 and no active case in other countries since one in Somalia in 1977.[99] Today the virus exists only in laboratories, but would be most dangerous in the hands of bio-terrorists, one of the scenarios the U. S. Department of Homeland Security has hypothesized and for which it has prepared. Monkeypox is a current relative of smallpox, but not nearly as dangerous, nor is it as easily transmitted.

Mather's Sources and Possible Purposes

As to Mather (1663–1728) himself, the initiator of this project, he has often been called one of the high priests of New England Puritanism. He was one of the youngest graduates of Harvard University, of which his father, Increase Mather, was a president for a time. Mather was a prolific writer whose own bibliography fills three volumes.[100] That copiousness would produce its own problems. At least 100 of his 468 publications were books not articles, although his sermons, like many of that time, were long, predictable, and forgettable. Mather was known for writing a dozen words when one would do, and like many clergies of his time, was known for quoting or writing extensively in Hebrew, Greek, and Latin. His medical compendium follows this pattern, too, but even in modern Western medical texts, many Latin and Greek terms are still used as names of diseases, organs, and procedures.

Among his many works, his 1702 ecclesiastical history of New England *Magnalia Christi Americana* is a major contribution to early American literature.[101] Mather's *Bonifacius* had a large influence on Benjamin Franklin's life, and their two lives intertwined in ways often quite surprising and largely unmentioned in either's history, which I address later in the book. Mather's text, *Christian Philosopher*, printed in 1721, contained many descriptions of his work in microscopy; he had already examined much flora and fauna through the primitive lenses. His *Angel of Bethesda* was "the only large, inclusive medical work of the entire American Colonial period" according to Gordon W. Jones.[102] However, although Jones was correct in stating it was the only "large, inclusive medical work," there were several, more modest, and less comprehensive medical texts from this period.

The first work discussing medicine in colonial America was written in 1643, probably by Dr. Stafford.[103] The first American colonial work published on a specific disease, smallpox, was a pamphlet written by a Reverend Thomas Thatcher in 1677, who conflated measles and "small pocks." This was one of the difficulties among early colonists not only in this culture at this time but in other historical and cultural contexts. Mather also wrote on measles in 1713, after the disease had decimated his family with the deaths of a wife and four of his children, but at that point he was seemingly able to distinguish between the two. He had had much tragic experience with the loss of children to both smallpox and measles.[104] In his medical compendium, when Mather had written on measles, he had given a clear clinical description of the disease, warning against excessive treatment and later immune deficiencies.[105] In 1710, *The Husbandman's Guide* was printed in Boston (originally in England in 1707), and its second chapter has some remedies for human illnesses, although much of the text serves as more of a veterinary guide and overall husbandry compendium. There were other medical texts as well, including a reprint done in 1720 in Boston from an English author, Nicholas Culpeper: *Pharmacopoeia Londinensis*, written during the 1600s.

What Mather's medical compendium does provide is a rich source for scholars interested in exploring the particular historic medicine of colonial culture. What could appear to be a monologic voice of early America was in fact a multi-layered one. Mather's text includes the voices least often heard in any retrospective look at these times, such as Onesimus's words and Native Americans' contribution of cinchona bark to use in the treatment of malaria. We also see evidence of early germ theory in the compendium long before Pasteur, credited with the discovery, conducted his research and published his works. Mather writes in the smallpox chapter how he saw in his microscope small, moving "animalculae" in the vitreous matter from an active pox. He wrongly thought at the time he was seeing the living cause of the disease, even if it couldn't have been the virus because of the limits of his microscope. However, he had the right general idea about the cause of some diseases.

Mather acknowledged inoculation as a "Wonderful Practice" and wrote that Onesimus and other Africans "all agree in one Story."[106] He later cited other sources for the procedure in *Angel of Bethesda*, but it is significant that he situated the African American lore first in support of the technique. Mather articulated his purpose in *Angel:* "This is the Story, which I have now to tell you. And hundreds of Thousands of Lives will be soon Saved if my Story be harken'd to."[107] However, his opponents found him at best a meddler, perhaps sometimes misguided, and among the Anti-Inoculators' texts, there are accusations of other motivations, too.

In addition to Onesimus, Mather had sought out and read other sources about smallpox inoculation in writings of the Royal Society of London he had received from abroad. Mather had read an account of an Italian surgeon's observations of the inoculation method in *The Royal Society Transactions* and reported it in his compendium and elsewhere:

> But our Advice of this Matter, as it comes from Superior Persons in the *Levant*, is what may have most Attention given to it. Our first Communication comes from Dr. *Emanuel Timoni* R.S.S.[108] who writes from *Constantinople*, in December, 1713. To this effect. The Practice

> of Procuring the *Small-Pox*, by a Sort of *Inoculation*, has been introduced among the *Constantinopolitans*, [and] the *Circassians* and *Georgians*, and other *Asiaticks;* for about Fourty Years.[109]

Mather's interest in reading accounts that backed up the African testimonials he had heard from Onesimus and others in the previous decade was keen. We know that he had found the text by Timoni significant almost five years before the 1721 smallpox epidemic in Boston. He sent a letter to John Woodward, M.D. (distinguished English paleontologist of Gresham College, the original college meeting place of the Royal Society) on July 12, 1716. In that letter, Mather stated that he had read the April–June 1714 *Philosophical Transactions of the Royal Society* account by Timoni of the inoculation practice in Constantinople. The Colonial minister had then commented on the history of smallpox epidemics in New England and mentioned the measles epidemic in 1713.[110] Mather also wrote Woodward that he "had gotten the same information from Onesimus, who is a 'pretty intelligent fellow.'"[111] When Mather had inquired whether he had ever had smallpox, Onesimus had answered, "Yes and no."[112] The enslaved explained that he had had the operation [variolation], as had most all Guramantees, which protected them from smallpox. The slave had also shown Mather the scar on his arm.

Since Mather learned from Timoni that the practice of variolation had been in existence in Constantinople since the 1660s or 1670s, the earliest discoveries of a preventative from China could have been disseminated along the various trade routes west into Mesopotamia, Egypt, and on to West Africa or vice versa. Mather documented what he read or extrapolated from the Royal Society texts in support of African narratives, but he had clearly also corroborated the information by writing directly to Woodward. In that letter, he also asked him if he had tried inoculation.

In *Angel,* in addition to Onesimus and Timoni, Mather cited two other sources from The Royal Society to enhance his credibility. Both documented and reinforced the process Africans described. Giocomo Pilarino's "Nova et Tuta Variolas Excitandi per Transplantationem Methodus" featured the narrative of a Grecian woman, a well-known "Inoculatrix," who took mercy on a poor Grecian man fretting about the fates of his four young sons (age eight and under) during a smallpox epidemic there. She vaccinated all four sons and they lived, although the eight-year-old, a child in poor health already, had a difficult time for a while, contracting a fever with very few pustules, leading Mather to surmise the fever had been from some other source.[113]

Still another Royal Society source was Peter Kennedy, a London surgeon who had been in Constantinople and had himself observed inoculation in Turkey. His text, "An Essay on External Remedies," was published in the *Transactions* in 1715. Jones, who wrote the introduction to *Angel*, speculated that the minister had a copy of the Kennedy essay,[114] because Mather had written that Kennedy claimed to have been assured in Turkey that some two thousand had been inoculated, and only two had died because they had already contracted the disease before the inoculation.[115] Mather featured proofs of successful inoculations from enslaved Africans, Italians writing from the Levant, Turks, and Greeks, but these sources provided another avenue of attack for the Anti-Inoculators.

A word about the source for the three Royal Society citations that Mather used: The Royal Society had met regularly since 1645 in London, when a group of scientists got together to share their empirical knowledge and study what they called "Natural Philosophy" and later "New Philosophy" or "Experimental Philosophy." Alan Gross describes the history of The Royal Society as a mixture of both talented natural philosophers (scientists) and very curious people interested in the natural world.[116] Most of funding for the group came from members' dues and contributions, but Charles the 2nd, on the throne at the founding, had also contributed.[117] Equally important to the meetings and even more important to later colonists, were the *Philosophical Transactions,* which reported on various curiosities and scientific news through letters that were assembled and edited. Henry Oldenburg, the Royal Society secretary and founder of the *Philosophical Transactions,* initiated the edition in 1665 as a private enterprise.[118] By the time of Mather's and Boylston's inoculation project in the 1720s, the Society had changed from a place of experimentation and discussion to mostly the gathering and reading of letters and reports.[119] Over time, the group functioned as a clearinghouse and then distributor, including for those observations and curiosities gathered from the "New World."

In addition to his conversations with West Africans and the Royal Society texts, Mather's own observations made up his third set of evidence for his claim. Although he misrecognized these *animalculae* as the cause of smallpox, this mistake still put him squarely in the conversation regarding early germ (animalculae) theory at the time. Instead, he most likely saw bacteria.[120] Although Mather relied heavily on the conversations and texts, the microscope was especially important because in his mind, with the scope as well as with autopsy, the "invisible [had become] visible."[121] Because he and his family had access to the Royal Society *Transactions* and the largest personal libraries of the colonies, he also knew of Robert Hooke's work as well as other microscopists. Mather's observation of the "invisible" to the naked eye also became a key aspect of one of the many claims by opponents against the inoculation project. It's not known if other "natural philosophers" or doctors in Boston also had microscopes. There's a record of Harvard getting a microscope in 1732, a "Wilson screw-type microscope," that Frederick Lewis claimed had arrived as a gift to the school with a hint that it should be used.[122] Isaac Greenwood, a Harvard student and supporter of Mather's inoculation process, had become a Professor there in 1727 and along with another Professor later used the microscope frequently in research and classes. They eventually ordered a larger one, and microscopes were in much greater use in that colony.[123]

The Main Antagonists: Mather (the Minister), Boylston (the Surgeon) vs. Douglass (the Doctor) and the Franklins

In turning over all the stones to discover the many strands of argument within this controversy, it's worth briefly examining the main characters of this drama: Cotton Mather, the leader of the inoculation project, and Dr. William Douglass, the leader of the Anti-Inoculators. They were the driving force behind the debates, although both sides had supporters.

The Mather family had been most prominent in the Puritan theocracy within Boston for several generations. Their vision for the country, and Cotton Mather's oft repeated view of the "New Jerusalem" in his many religious writings, serves as a standpoint from which the minister took on many fights. For example, his quarrel with Solomon Stoddard was "symptomatic of the shift from Puritan to Yankee culture."[124] He and his father saw the Congregationalist minster's version of Calvinism as moving away from the grand vision of America and the orthodoxy of Puritanism as represented by the Boston dynasty. Stoddard was the main voice of religion in Western Massachusetts at the time. The Mathers, especially Cotton, were driven by the necessity to keep the "Old Guard" in place in order to fulfill a spiritual ideal.[125] The irony is that along with this firmly rooted religious fervor, the interest in science "flourished" in the creative mind of the Puritans, as previously noted. This fact was often obscured by anti-cleric sentiments in the 1700 and 1800s, while the myth that science started later with Benjamin Franklin's experiments thrived.[126]

As a child Cotton had been a source of pride for a very strict father, Increase, who noticed his son's precocious and pious nature. By age 11 he had read the classic Greeks, learned the Greek language, and had started on Hebrew. He was not a popular child, as he chastised his playmates by citing religious doctrine to discipline their wicked ways. Cotton entered Harvard at 11 and a half; he had also developed a stammer. He despaired for a time about following his father into the ministry because of the speech problem and thought about being a physician instead.[127] Most young physicians were trained by an experienced one in the practice itself and not in school courses. However, the curriculum at the school was varied, even though at that time mostly young men seeking the ministry attended. Harvard's goal was to train both religious and civic leaders, offering in the first two years: Greek, Hebrew, and Logic, in the third and fourth: Ethics, Literature, Arts, Sciences, Metaphysics, Theology, Mathematics, Rhetoric, and Oratory.[128] At that time Harvard was floundering with run-down buildings, a total student population of 20, with only four students in Cotton's class.[129] The pious youngster still managed to focus his attention on his studies and read voraciously. Over time Mather worked on his stammer while keeping the career of physician as a back-up plan, but he eventually overcame the speech problem and joined his line of predecessors as a Puritan minister.

As a young man he was often at the center of efforts for developing good citizens in the Boston area, as well as stirring up controversies over various issues. To say he was well-known would be an understatement. Cotton made many efforts to please and court the Crown's various governors, seeming to have some of the same cringing loyalty as he demonstrated toward his parent, Increase. On other occasions, he helped organize revolts against a governor, Andros, while his father was back in England for a time.[130] Just as during the witchcraft time when Robert Calef called the young minister "ambidexter," Mather was often seen as holding two contradictory views at the same time. In his text, Calef was referring to the witchcraft trials, when Cotton seemed to be playing a full advocacy role, urging the prosecution and testing of so-called witches, while at the same time he cautioned against such leanings.[131] At this time he was in his 20s and especially as a young man could be overly exuberant.

In his late 50s and early 60s, Mather had had a very active but not financially successful life as well as been visited often by personal tragedies. He married three times, and was outlived by his third wife. His first wife, Abigail Philips, bore him nine children; his second, Elizabeth Hubbard had six; and his third wife, Lydia George, had one daughter from her previous marriage. Of the wives, only Lydia was wealthy, but her pre-nuptial agreement prevented Mather, who had great difficulty financially, from improving his money problems. Only six of his 15 children lived to adulthood. He lost his wife, Elizabeth, a newborn, and two other children when they had all succumbed to a measles outbreak. The only offspring of his that was involved in the vaccination controversy was his son, Samuel, who was attacked in print by the Anti-Inoculators along with his father and grandfather. Samuel had made attempts in print to defend his father, causing more anger among the Anti-Inoculators and the Franklins. Of the 15 children, only two were left after their father's death. However, the continual tragedies in Cotton's life and his fears of being jailed because of his debts occurred during the smallpox epidemic of 1721 and 1722, which increased the concerns and weight of the controversy on the minister himself.[132]

As for the volume of his written works, Kenneth Silverman wrote that "beginning in his youth, Cotton probably hand-wrote as much as any human being ever has." Before becoming a minister, himself, he would sit in church and write down every word his father preached. Between the ages of 13 and 32, in his sermon notebooks of 250-words per page, it is estimated that they contain about 7000 pages.[133] As a religiously precocious child, Cotton was able to write down what he remembered of sermons and compose prayers on his own. By 11 or 12, he had already read all of Ovid, Cato, Tully, and Virgil, and read and wrote fluently in Greek. Hebrew and Latin were other languages he also quickly absorbed, and could simultaneously write a sermon he was listening to in Latin, while hearing it in English.[134] He owned two to three thousand books, and by the end of his life had what was considered the best library in Boston and other colonial cities.[135] C. Mather's writings influenced everyone from Nathaniel Hawthorne to Herman Melville among others.

Mather's life and the regard in which he was held were often interrupted by numerous battles and skirmishes regarding church doctrines, local politics, and reports of his being two-faced and hypocritical. Silverman cites many different occasions in which he was in trouble with the citizenry and even his own congregation at times. His financial and familial problems were also causing him to lose patience with others. His congregation had deserted him more than once already when new and finer churches were built in Boston.

> Acknowledging that this new, very large, and nearby church was the finest in New England, while his own was in 'crazy condition,' he drafted a set of subscriptions [that his parishioners were expected to pay] toward building a new meetinghouse for his congregation ... How many left Mather's ministry is unknown, but must have been substantial.[136]

Given Mather's need for support and praise, he did recognize the invaluable service of the one surgeon he had recruited for the variolations, Zabdiel Boylston. As Coss wrote: "Cotton Mather had introduced inoculation to Boston hoping to please God, earn the gratitude of people, and expiate the sins of Salem." His initiation of variolation had eventually been recognized by the Royal Society.

Zabdiel Boylston, the main Inoculator at this time, was the only surgeon or health practitioner of any kind to have joined the minister. He had been more willing to try new procedures to help his many patients such as the first mastectomy and taking out bladder stones from children. His patients had better survival rates, and one author suggested that Boylston's emphasis on cleanliness might also have been the reason for his success. Both Zabdiel and his wife, Jerusha, had suffered from severe cases of smallpox as young people. Zabdiel had the disease at age 22 during the 1702 epidemic. Both husband and wife had nearly died, and the pockmarks that marred their faces and bodies testified to their having barely survived. They had been eager to make sure their children did not succumb to the infection, so Jerusha and four of their children had left Boston for a rural village. Two boys remained with the surgeon.[137]

It's not known if his having experienced the disease and concern for his children motivated Boylston to separate from his fellow health practitioners and take on the inoculations. It was a difficult and courageous task that Mather had reached out to him to undertake, and under the onslaught of anger and invective responses, a dangerous one. Mather at first, the ambidexter that he was, withheld any mention or praise for the Inoculator he had recruited, and even took a long time to have his own son, Samuel, a student and roommate of a smallpox victim at Harvard, vaccinated. However, at the end of 1724, before Boylston sailed to London with his data on the inoculations and "be celebrated" for his success, Cotton had given him an introductory letter for Dr. Jurin of the Royal Society. He had written: "This is the Gentleman who first brought the way of saving Lives by the Inoculation of the Small-Pox, into the *American* world."[138]

Boylston's book, *An Historical Account of the Small-Pox Inoculated in New England*, was first published in 1726 in England. In the book, he not only kept track of those whom he inoculated and the dates, but he also used the actual patients' names and described how their disease manifested itself. One such example is:

> I inoculated Mrs. Jane Colman of about 14, and Mr. Grafton Feveryear of about 30 Years old; on both these the Small-Pox came out at the usual Time, of a kind distinct Sort, the Symptoms friendly, they soon grew well. Mrs. Jane had about 50 or 60, Mr. Feveryear a good handsome sprinkling; he had lived in an infected House about a Month before inoculated.[139]

In his book, Boylston apologized to the people he had inoculated, because he had used their names, ages, and cases without asking their permission. He had sought the pardon of those whose lives he had saved, and especially of "the young ladies." It was important to include the data, especially ages and cases, but he had been polite and considerate to make such an apology. The surgeon had also used charts of the numbers of those inoculated by month and by age in his thorough account of his work. Boylston's book represents "one of the first times quantitative analysis [had been] applied to a medical problem."[140] Toward the end of his text, he also gives very detailed instructions for caring for those inoculated afterwards. For those six who had lost their lives, he had opined that it would be best not to inoculate in the cold months, as that seemed to have had adverse effects for those.[141] Also, in 1726 the physician was voted a Fellow of the Royal Society; he was the first full-time physician to gain such an honor and the eighth New Englander.[142]

William Douglass (1691–1752), on the other hand, was a relative newcomer to Boston from Scotland. Douglass had been born in Gifford, in the Scottish county of Haddington. His father, George, had been the proprietor or manager of an estate under a local Marquis, and possibly owned his own small piece of land.[143] Mather himself credits Douglass for giving him a copy of the *Royal Society* in which Pylarino and Timoni, two of Mather's sources for the project, were featured. The Scot was practicing in Bristol when he discovered a friend might become Governor of the Colony of Massachusetts. He quickly readied himself and set sail for the city of Boston. Douglass was disappointed to learn on his arrival that in fact his friend had not been chosen governor and that he did not have an immediate and powerful supporter within the colony and port town.[144] When he first came to Boston in 1718, he brought letters of introduction to both Increase and Cotton Mather, as well as to Benjamin Colman, another well-known

Boston minister. Douglass was known in the community for being patronizing toward others; he was also an "outsider." The young 25-year-old William often touted his European university training as a physician. In 1718 Boston, as well as in the rest of the colonies, where most physicians had served in local apprenticeships, Douglass had trained under Pitcairne at Edinburgh, and also studied at Leyden and Paris.[145] During the smallpox epidemic three years later, the Scot claimed that he was the "only regulated practitioner in that city."[146] Some of his later detractors thought that he may have even been jealous of the Mathers, as they had been part of the elite of Boston society. Still he could have so begrudged the forays into his field that resentment took on a valence of its own.[147] Silverman points out the Scottish physician had an avaricious nature, and perhaps that was why he had come to Boston and had hoped to quickly make his fortune through his acquaintance with and acceptance by the Governor. He had earlier written to a friend that his early years were not as prosperous as he hoped, but he was very entrepreneurial and would ultimately become a wealthy landowner. It's easy to see that he may have envied the Mather family because of their status and would become deeply offended and angry that Cotton, particularly, was on his professional territory by initiating the vaccination project.

Douglass for a time was not remembered kindly by some biographers such as William Allen:

> He was a skilful physician. His prejudices were very strong, and in his language he was frequently intemperate. His notions of religion were very loose. In his history of the American colonies, he is often incorrect in point of fact, and it was his foible to measure the worth of men by his personal friendship for them. A town of Massachusetts, of which he was a proprietor and benefactor, bears his name.[148]

However, on the other hand, Douglass contributed much to medicine in Boston after the controversy in the first years of his arrival. He wrote on both medicine and financial matters between the 1720s and 1750s. In later years, after Douglass's death, Bullock pointed out the various views of the physician both the positive and negative ones. W. Allen in the *American Biographical Dictionary* and J. Eliot in the *Biographical Dictionary* both denigrated the Scot and emphasized his flaws and foibles. Then in 1828, J. Thacher combined both their views in the later version of the *American Biographical Dictionary*.[149] In contrast to these three, Dr. Oliver Wendell Holmes had lauded Douglass and said that Boston had probably "owed the reform of its Materia Medica largely to William Douglass."[150] After Mather had died, Douglass went on to write many significant works according to later physicians. He had been widely praised for his documentation of an epidemic in New England of miliary fever in 1735. Miliary fever is an archaic term meaning any infectious disease with acute fever and a rash. It was called *miliary* because cases could evidence a rash with a grain-like appearance like the small seeds of millet. Douglass had studied the cases he saw and kept extensive notes for a publication: "Practical History of a New Epidemic Eruptive Miliary Fever" published in 1736. This essay was reprinted in *The New England Journal of Medicine* in 1825 with an editorial note that said "it has been pronounced by competent judges one of the best works extant upon the subject of which it treats."[151]

Douglass also initiated the first real physicians' medical club or society in Boston. Douglass had initiated this group in 1721, and it was frequently thought to have been in response to the Mather and Boylston inoculation effort. Because of the bitter controversy in 1721, some suggested that had been the motivation for the group's initiation and perhaps had served as a body founded to work against the Mathers, Boylston, and the clergy who advocated for variolation. An item appeared in the *Boston Gazette* of August 28–September 4, 1721 concerning the group:

> To the Author of the *Boston Gazette*
>
> Sir,
>
> I read lately in the Boston News-Letter, a heinous charge against a Club of Physicians in Town, ... The Society are only accountable for their own pieces, and not for other matters inserted by the Publishers of News-Papers ... The members of the Society of Physicians Anti-Inoculators do not conceal themselves, I am Yours Etc.
>
> W. Anti-Inoculator [William Douglass].

This letter showed the "Club of Physicians" had been started possibly between June 6 and September 4, 1721, the first of its kind in Boston as far as any record can be found.[152]

The Scottish physician, like Cotton and his father, was interested in other topics such as the weather, botany, economics, business, land ownership, and others. He, like the Mathers, was a prodigious writer on medicine and many of his other interests.[153]

Even before initiating inoculations with Boylston, Cotton attempted to gather up all the physicians in town for a meeting to propose vaccinations during the 1720s smallpox epidemic. Douglass said he had never been invited, while the minister claimed he *had* invited him. The invitation was by a letter written on June 6, 1721.[154] In an earlier diary entry on April 26, 1721 and in his compendium, Mather had written, "The Grievous Calamity of the Small-Pox has now entered the town. The practice of conveying and suffering the Small-Pox by Inoculation has never been used in America, or indeed in our nation. But how many lives might be saved by it, if it were practiced."[155] Although the letter was well circulated, it was never printed by a Boston printer (that can be discovered). Mather mentioned his appeal in *Angel of Bethesda* in the smallpox chapter and lamented the lack of support from all but two physicians.[156]

> About the Month of May 1721, the *Small-Pox* being admitted into the City of Boston, I proposed unto the Physicians of the Town, the unfailing Method of preventing Death, and many other grievous miseries, from a tremendous Distemper, by Receiving and Managing the *Small-Pox,* in the Way of *Inoculation.* One of the Physicians had the Courage to begin the Practice upon his own Children and Servants [Zabdiel Boylston]. And another Expressed his Good Will unto it. But The rest of the Practitioners treated the Proposal with an Incivility and an Inhumanity not well to be accounted for. Fresh Occasion I saw, for the Complaint of a Great Physician: '*Heus, quanto Dolore auger, dum video Naturae ministrum Medicum, Hostem eius devenisse!*'[157]
>
> [Translation: Behold how when I glimpse a natural cure he should become its enemy!]

In the appeal that was circulated, he also included the two abstracts of Timoni's and Pilarino's works that he had used in addition to his own sources and closed with this sentence "Gentlemen, my request is, that you would meet for a Consultation upon this occasion, and so deliberate upon it [the operation], that whoever first begins the practice (if you Approve that it should be begun at all) may have the countenance of his worthy brethren to fortify him in it."[158] Although Douglass had loaned Mather the article from Timoni and Pylarino, before others, including Boylston, could read it in its entirety, Douglass had sent a message to Mather demanding the piece in the Royal Society's *Transactions* be returned to him immediately.[159]

Having been convinced of the efficacy of the prevention method, when that epidemic threatened Boston in 1721, even though his attempt to recruit all the local practicing physicians to try the inoculation method had failed, he and Boylston kept meticulous records of the inoculations; when Boylston traveled to London to report his success a few years later, he was very well received there. William Douglass was not convinced of the value of the variolation until years later, although it had been accepted by many by that time before his own admission as to its effectiveness.[160] The hostility surrounding the inoculation project had come from the physicians and the populace, not from clergy in Boston.[161]

While Mather, Boylston, and Douglass appear to be the main combatants in the 1721–1722 controversy, James and Benjamin Franklin also played key roles. When they appeared on the scene, it was via a third Bostonian newspaper, *The New-England Courant.* Both were very young, but their print media played a large role in attacking the Smallpox Inoculation project. James at 21 had returned to Boston after a number of years as a printer's apprentice in England and had been eager to start a new press, while his younger brother, Benjamin, had an indenture to his father as candle-maker but was uninterested in the work. Although he had been forced to leave school at 11, the 15-year-old Ben was an avid reader and writer and could relish the work as a printer's apprentice. However, he chafed under a long apprenticeship with a brother who had been away and whom he barely knew. The younger brother was to be indentured for nine years to James and would be free from indenture and poor wages at age 21.

Before starting his own newspaper, James had taken on the printer's position at *The Boston Gazette,* bringing Benjamin with him. Covering a very dramatic shipwreck near shore, James, who had cut his teeth on Grubs' Street doggerel, thought to print a story about it to attract attention in Boston. He had his younger brother, Benjamin, who had written poetry in the past and was up to the task, write a ballad about the wreck. James printed it, and it was sold on the street to an appreciative audience. After a couple of years, the printer was forced out of the job at the *Gazette,* and in early August 1721 set up his own press and initiated *The New-England Courant.*[162] The brothers' paper needed to earn them profits in order to keep it and them going. They knew successful sales would be guaranteed if James, a friend of Douglass, could print a newspaper against inoculation and against the Mathers, Boylston, and also the British government. The new paper flourished. Benjamin Franklin, especially when his brother went to jail for his anti-government newspaper articles, not only ran the press, printing issues on June 18 and July 2, but at age 16 had already begun writing his own anti-government and anti-elitist views in the *Courant.*[163] Although both Franklin brothers had sponsored so many of Douglass's diatribes against Boylston, later the Franklins had reached out to the physician for help. One request took place after James had been jailed in a dark, hot, damp, and airless room, and, in his already poor constitution, had become ill. His family pleaded with authorities at least to let him have some fresh air in the yard. Also, they asked Boylston to examine James, and he had not only done so, but he also pressured the government members who had put him in jail to let him have access to fresh air, which was then granted. A couple of years later when Boylston was in London, Ben Franklin had also gone there but ended up stranded without funds. When he found out the surgeon was there, he reached out to him for help, and Boylston rescued him.[164]

The Common Sense Trope

It's important to acknowledge the legitimate fears that would necessarily attend the inoculation project itself. Certainly a number of arguments against variolation could be made just using common sense. One would have thought that an understanding of sympathies would have been helpful in contemplating how injecting a small amount of the disease directly into the skin could ward off a more acute case of the same disease. Both sympathies and antipathies were a part of humoral medicine at this time. Some Colonial Bostonians would have had an understanding of sympathetic medicine; Mather certainly did. He advised in the compendium that when a pregnant woman had a "White Jaundice," which was also known as the

"Green Sickness" indicating too much gall in the system, she was to take an agreeable wine and add to it "a dram of the Galls and Livers of *Eels* dried and powdered."[165] Thus one is using a substance sympathetic to, the same, or similar to the overabundant matter in the body to bring balance. But such an understanding did not seem to help many of the citizens accept a technique that injected smallpox into a healthy individual, although almost 300 had been persuaded. Antipathies were also used, just as when Petruchio withheld roasted meats from Kate because of its association with her choleric overabundance.

The beginning of the 1721 epidemic invoked a relatively recent memory (the last large smallpox epidemic in Boston had been in 1702); fear loomed large. While some Colonists could anticipate not getting smallpox a second time because they had had smallpox in the previous epidemic and survived, all those who had not had smallpox in 1702 or who had been born since then were vulnerable. Infant mortality, childhood and even adult malnutrition, substandard sanitation, and crowded living quarters particularly among the poor all contributed to legitimate fears of another massive smallpox epidemic. Those who had been through earlier epidemics knew that many would be infected, at least 15–30% would die, and the rest would be left with disfiguring scars, maiming, chronic illness, and/or compromised immune systems. Parishioners understood and practiced what was most obvious to their eyes and experiences. Thus, vaccination made no logical sense to many Bostonians, yet many other issues against the practice also surfaced during the controversy.

Notes

1 J. Blake Scott, *Risky Rhetoric: AIDS and the Cultural Practices of HIV Testing* (Carbondale, IL: Southern Illinois University Press, 2003), 16.
2 Scott, *Risky Rhetoric*, 16.
3 Kenneth Burke, *Language as Symbolic Action: Essays on Life, Literature, and Method* (Berkeley: U of California P, 1966), 44.
4 Robert M. Entman, "Framing: Toward Clarification of a Fractured Paradigm." *Journal of Communication* 43.4 (1993): 54.
5 Murray Edelman, "Contestable Categories and Public Opinion." *Political Communication* 10.3 (1993), 232.
6 Entman, "Framing," 51.
7 Entman, "Framing," 53.
8 Alain Grosrichard, Gerald Wajeman, Jacques-Alain Miller, Guy Le Gaufey, Dominique Celas, Gerard Miller, Catherine Millot, Jocelyne Livi and Judith Miller.
9 Michel Foucault, *Power/Knowledge, Selected Interviews & Other Writings, 1972–1977*. Ed. Colin Gordon (New York: Pantheon, 1981), 194.
10 Michel Foucault, *Power/Knowledge,* 197.
11 Foucault, *Power/Knowledge*, 198.
12 Foucault, *Power/Knowledge*, 194.
13 Foucault, *Power/Knowledge*, 194–195.

14 Lloyd Bitzer, "The Rhetorical Situation" in *Philosophy of Rhetoric,* 1 (1968). Lloyd Bitzer defined exigence as "an imperfection marked by urgency; it is a defect, an obstacle, something waiting to be done, a thing which is other than it should be" (6).
15 Foucault, *Power/Knowledge*, 195.
16 Foucault, *Power/Knowledge*, 198–199.
17 Colin Gordon, "Afterword" in Michel Foucault's *Power/Knowledge* (New York: Pantheon, 1980), 240.
18 Gordon, "Afterword," 240.
19 Gordon, "Afterword," 240.
20 Gordon, "Afterword," 240.
21 Georges Canguilhem. *Writings on Medicine* (New York: Fordham University Press, 2012), 12.
22 Nicolau Barquet and Pere Domingo, "The Triumph Over the Most Terrible of the Ministers of Death," in *Annals of Internal Medicine,* 127 (1997): 635.
23 Stefan Reidel, "Edward Jenner and the History of Smallpox and Vaccination," in *Baylor University Medical Center Proceedings* (Dallas, TX: Baylor University Medical Center, 2005), 21.
24 Stanley M. Aronson and Lucile Newman, "God Have Mercy on this House: Being a Brief Chronicle of Smallpox in Colonial New England," in *Smallpox in the Americas 1492 to 1815: Contagion and Controversy* (John Carter Brown Library of Brown University Exhibition, 2002), n.p.; Barquet and Domingo, 636; D. Stetten, Jr. "Victory Over Variola," in American Society for Microbiology's ASM News 44 (1978), 640.
25 Donald R. Hopkins, *Princes and Peasants: Smallpox in History* (Chicago: University of Chicago Press, 1984), 3.
26 Hopkins, *Princes and Peasants*, 2.
27 Hopkins, *Princes and Peasants*, 3.
28 Thomas Babington Macaulay, *The History of England from the Accession of James the Second* (Philadelphia: Porter and Coates, 1848 and in Project Gutenberg, 2008). Vol. 4, Ch. XX.
29 John H. Blake, "Smallpox Inoculation in Colonial Boston." *Journal of the History of Medicine.* 3 (1938), 284–300.
30 The College of Physicians of Philadelphia. *The History of Vaccines.* Accessed January 10, 2022. https://www.historyofvaccines.org/timeline#EVT_9.
31 Blake, "Smallpox in Colonial Boston," 284–300.
32 Jonathan B. Tucker, *Scourge: The Once and Future Threat of Smallpox* (New York: Grove Press, 2001), 3.
33 Hopkins, *Princes and Peasants,* xi.
34 Kelsey Piper, "Smallpox Used to Kill Millions of People Every Year. Here's How Humans Beat It." *Vox* (February 5, 2021).
35 D. A. Henderson, *Smallpox: The Death of a Disease* (Amherst, NY: Prometheus, 2009.) as cited in Piper, "Smallpox Used," (February 5, 2021).
36 Keekok Lee, "Towards a More Comprehensive Assessment of Medical Achievements: Smallpox as A Case Study." *Academia Letters,* pre-print. 2021.
37 Sun Simao, *Essential Prescriptions Worth a Thousand Gold* (China: Tang Dynasty). 600s CE.
38 Zhu Chunjia, *Discourse Definitive on Smallpox* (China: Song Dynasty). n.d.
39 Yu Mao kun, *Variolation* (China: Qing Dynasty). n.d.
40 Lee, "Towards."
41 Zhang Lu, *Clarifying Medicine* (China). Mid 1600s). n.p.
42 Lee, "Towards."
43 Hopkins, *Princes and Peasants,* 32.

44 Hopkins, *Princes and Peasants*, 9.
45 George Rosen, *A History of Public Health* (Baltimore: John Hopkins University Press, 2015), 59.
46 Michel Foucault, *Discipline and Punish: The Birth of the Prison (*New York: Random House, 1979), 144; "The Politics of Health in the 18th Century," in *The Foucault Reader,* ed. Paul Rabinow (New York: Pantheon, 1984), 175.
47 City of Boston, "History of Boston's Harbor Islands" (Boston: City of Boston, 2011), n.p.; Nathaniel Bradstreet Shurtleff, *A Topographical and Historical Description of Boston, Part I* (Boston: City Council, 1871), 516; David Kales, *The Boston Harbor Islands: A History of an Urban Wilderness* (Charleston, SC: The History Press, 2007), 36–37.
48 Kales, *The Boston Harbor,* 37.
49 Kales, *The Boston Harbor,* 37.
50 Edward G. Huber, "Control of Communicable Disease Prevalent in Massachusetts" in *Boston Medical Surgery* (Boston: Massachusetts Medical Society, 1926), 169.
51 Huber, "Control," 169.
52 Foucault, *Discipline*, 195.
53 Foucault, *Discipline*, 195.
54 Foucault, *Discipline*, 195.
55 *BBC News*. Accessed January 10, 2022. https://www.bbc.com/news/world-asia-china-59855689.
56 Robin Brant, "Shanghai Lockdown: Whole Communities Relocated in Anti-Covid Drive in BBC News," Shanghai (April 21, 2022). Accessed April 26, 2022. https://www.bbc.com/news/world-asia-china-61160210
57 Foucault, *Discipline,* 195–196.
58 Foucault, *Discipline*, 196.
59 F. Fenner, Donald A. Henderson, Isao Arita, Zedenek Jeznek, and Ivan Danilovich Ladyni, *Smallpox and Its Eradication* (Geneva: World Health Organization-IRIS, 1988), 274.
60 Foucault, "Politics of Health," 176.
61 Foucault, "Politics of Health," 176.
62 Foucault, "Politics of Health," 176.
63 Thomas H. Johnson and Perry Miller, eds. *The Puritans: A Sourcebook on their Writings* (New York: Harper Collins, 1963), 730.
64 Tomami Kinukawa, review of *American Curiosity: Culture of Natural History in the Colonial British Atlantic* by Susan Scott Parrish, *New England Quarterly* 80, no. 2 (June 2007), 323.
65 Susan Scott Parrish, *American Curiosity: Culture of Natural History in the Colonial British Atlantic* (Chapel Hill, NC: University of North Carolina Press, 2006), 6.
66 Parrish, *American Curiosity*, 6.
67 Robert K. Merton, *Science, Technology, and Society in Seventeenth Century England* (Bruges, Belgium: St. Catherine's Press, 1938), 235.
68 This chapter from Merton was originally published in 1938 as Chapter 5 in his *Science, Technology and Society in Seventeen-Century England.* Bruges, Belgium: St. Catherine's Press.
69 Merton, *Science, Technology, and Society,* 229.
70 Otto T. Beall, Jr., "Cotton Mather's *Curiosa Americana* and the Boston's Philosophical Society of 1683." *The William and Mary Quarterly* 18, no. 3 (July 1961), 361.
71 Cotton Mather, *Parentator: Memoirs of Remarkables in the Life and Death of the Ever-Remarkable Dr. Increase Mather* (Boston: 1724), 86.

72 Beall, "Cotton Mather's Curiosa," 363.
73 Rhoda Rappaport, *When Geologists Were Historians 1665–1750* (Cornell, NY: Cornell University Press, 1997), 115.
74 Emilie Savage-Smith, "Fundamental to Islamic Medieval Medical Practice? *The Body in Balance: Humoral Medicines in Practice,* eds. Peregrine Horden and Elisabeth Hsu (Oxford, NY: Berghahn Books, 2015), 89.
75 National Institutes of Health. "History of Medicine. Accessed January 11, 2022. https://www.nlm.nih.gov/exhibition/shakespeare/fourhumors.html.
76 National Library of Medicine, "Medical History Collection," accessed April 2, 2019. https://www.nlm.nih.gov/exhibition/shakespeare/fourhumors.html.
77 National Library of Medicine, "Medical History Collection."
78 Wellcome Collection. "Blood-letting at the Barber-surgeons." Accessed January 11, 2022. https://wellcomecollection.org/articles/XKyzchIAAPeWNq1l
79 Cotton Mather. *Angel of Bethesda* (Barre, MA: American Antiquarian Society and Barre Publishers, 1972), 17.
80 Noga Arikha, *Passions and Tempers: A History of the Humors* (New York: Harper Perennial, 2008), 219.
81 Timothy Bright, *A Treatise on Meloncholy* (London: 1586), 84ff.
82 Thomas Wright, *The Passions of the Mind in Generalle* (London: T. Thorpe, 1608), 64.
83 Stephen Pender, "Subventing Disease: Anger, Passions, and the Non-Naturals" *Rhetorics of Bodily Medicine and Health in Medieval and Early Modern England*, ed. Jennifer Vaught (Surrey, UK: Ashgate, 2013), 210.
84 Levinus Lemnius, *The Touchstone of Complexions* (London: Thomas Marsh, 1576), 62.
85 C. Mather, *Angel,* 130.
86 C. Mather, *Angel*, 191.
87 C. Mather, *Angel*, 191.
88 C. Mather, 192.
89 Barbara Heifferon, "The New Smallpox: An Epidemic of Words?" in *Rhetoric Review* 25, no. 1 (2006): 84.
90 C. Mather, *Diary* (New York: Frederick Ungar Publishing, 1911), 1, 579.
91 Stephen J. Niven, "Onesimus." *African American National Biography*, ed. Henry Louis Gates and Evelyn Brooks Higginbotham (London: Oxford University Press, 2008), accessed April 3, 2019. https://sites.fas.harvard.edu/~aanb/SHTML/SHTML/sampleEntries.shtml.
92 Cotton Mather, *Angel*, 108.
93 Cotton Mather, *Angel*, 108.
94 Cotton Mather, *Angel*, 108.
95 Cotton Mather, *Angel*, 108.
96 Cotton Mather, *Angel,* 113–115.
97 Darin S. Carroll, Ginny L. Emerson, and Yu Li, et al. "Chasing Jenner's Vaccine: Revisiting *Cowpox Virus* Classification" in *PLoS One,* 6.8 (2011), e23086.
98 Leslie H. Collier, "The Development of a Stable Smallpox Vaccine." *The Journal of Hygiene,* 53, no. 1 (1955), 76.
99 I was fortunate to have met one of the last Africans to have had smallpox. She had it as a child, had come to the U.S. to get her Doctor of Pharmacy degree and was the pharmacist at an American drug store where I had my prescriptions filled.
100 Thomas James Holmes, *Cotton Mather, A Bibliography of His Work* (Cambridge, MA: Harvard University Press, 1940).
101 Kenneth B. Murdock and Elizabeth W. Miller, "Introduction" to *Magnalia Christi Americana* (Cambridge, MA: Harvard University Press, 1977), 89.

102 Gordon W. Jones, "Introduction" to *Angel of Bethesda* by Cotton Mather (Barre, MA: American Antiquarian Society and Barre Publishers, 1972), xxxvi.
103 Michael Flannery, "Building A Retrospective Collection in Pharmacy: A Brief History of the Literature with Some Considerations for U. S. Health Sciences Library Professionals." *Bulletin of the Medical Library Association,* 89.2 (April 2001), 215.
104 Kenneth Silverman, *The Life and Times of Cotton Mather* (New York: Columbia University Press, 1985), 271–272.
105 John Duffy, *From Humors to Medical Science* (Urbana, IL: University of Illinois Press, 1993), 20.
106 C. Mather, *Angel*, 107.
107 C. Mather, *Angel*, 107.
108 RSS = Royal Society Surgeon.
109 C. Mather, *Angel*, 107.
110 Kittredge, "Introduction," 3.
111 Kittredge, "Introduction," 3.
112 Kittredge, "Introduction," 4.
113 Quoted in Cotton Mather's *Angel*, 109–110.
114 C. Mather, *Angel,* 359.
115 Cotton Mather, *Angel,* 111; Peter Kennedy, "An Essay on External Remedies, Wherein It Is Considered, Whether All the Curable Distempers Incident to Human Bodies, May Not Be Cured by Means" (London: A. Bell, 1715), 12.
116 Alan G. Gross, Joseph E. Harmon, and Michael S. Brody, *Communicating Science: The Scientific Article from the 17th Century to the Present* (New York: Oxford University Press, 2002), 32.
117 Gross, Harmon, and Brody, *Communicating Science,* 32.
118 Gross, Harmon, and Brody, *Communicating Science,* 32.
119 Marie Boas Hall, *Promoting Experimental Learning: Experiment and the Royal Society: 1660–1727* (London: Cambridge University Press, 2002), 2.
120 Seymour Stanton Block, *Disinfection, Sterilization, and Preservation* (Philadelphia: Lippincott, Williams, and Wilkins, 2001), 6.
121 Michel Foucault, *The Birth of the Clinic: An Archaeology of Medical Perception* (New York: Vintage, 1975), 242.
122 Frederick Lewis, "The Advent of Microscopes in America: With Notes on Their Earlier History in *The Scientific Monthly* 57.3 (September 1943), 258. http://www.jstor.org/stable/17981
123 Archana Kapoor, *Making Connections: Microscopy and Scientific Practice in Colonial America and the Wider Trans-Atlantic World*, Thesis: University of Leeds, 2013, 28, 30.
124 Sacvan Bercovitch, *The Puritan Origins of the American Self* (New Haven, CT: Yale University Press, 1975), 96.
125 Bercovitch, *The Puritan Origins,* 95–97.
126 Quoted in Perry Miller, *The Life of the Mind in America* (New York: Harcourt, Brace, and World, 1965), 272.
127 Silverman, *The Life and Times,* 13–15.
128 Silverman, *The Life and Times,* 21.
129 Silverman, *The Life and Times*, 17.
130 Silverman, *The Life and Times*, 69.
131 Robert Calef, *More Wonders of the Invisible World or the Wonders of the World Displayed in Five Parts* (Salem, MA: Reprinted by John D. and T. C. Cushing, Jr., 1823), 303.
132 Virginia Bernhard, "Cotton Mather's 'Most Unhappy Wife': Reflections on the Uses of Historical Evidence. In *The New England Quarterly* 60, no. 3 (September 1987), 341–362.

133 Silverman, *The Life and Times*, 37.
134 Silverman, *The Life and Times,* 14.
135 Silverman, *Cotton Mather*.
136 Silverman. *The Life and Times*, 334.
137 Jennifer Lee Carrell, *The Speckled Monster: A Historical Tale of Battling Smallpox* (New York: Penguin, 2004), 411, 428.
138 Rusnock, Andrea. *The Correspondence of James Jurin, 1684–1750* (Atlanta: Rodopi B. V., 1996), 284.
139 Zabdiel Boylston, *An Historical Account of the Small-Pox Inoculated in New England* (London: S. Chandler, 1726), 13.
140 Gerald Mager, *Zabdiel Boylston: Medical Pioneer of Colonial Boston* (Urbana-Champagne, IL.: U of Illinois P, 1975), 133.
141 Zabdiel Boylston, *An Historical Account,* 50.
142 Stephen Coss, *The Fever of 1721* (New York: Simon and Schuster, 2016), 269.
143 Charles Bullock, ed. of William Douglass's *Discourse Concerning the Currencies of British Plantations in America* (New York: Macmillan Co, 1897), 265.
144 Reginald Heber Fitz, *Zabdiel Boylston: Inoculator and the Epidemic of Smallpox in Boston in 1721,* reprint in *Johns Hopkins Hospital Bulletin* 22, no. 247 (Sept. 1911), 6.
145 William Douglass, *Summary of British Settlements II* (Boston: Printed, Reprinted London: R. Baldwin, 1755), 21. T. L. Jennison, *Memoir of William Douglass* (*Medical Communications of the Massachusetts Medical Society* V), 195–196.
146 Bullock, *Discourse,* 266.
147 Fitz, *Zabdiel Boylston,* 6.
148 William Allen, *American Biographical Dictionary* (Cambridge, MA: William Hilliard, 1809), 255–256.
149 Bullock, *Discourse,* 265 Note 1. W. Allen, *American Biographical Dictionary,* 255–256; J. Eliot, *Biographical Dictionary* (Salem and Boston: 1809), 153–154; J. Thacher, *American Biographical Dictionary* (Boston: 1828), 255–257.
150 Oliver Wendell Holmes, in *Memorial History of Boston,* IV, 558–559.
151 Bullock, *Discourse,* 267. *New England Journal of Medicine,* XIV: 1–13, 1825.
152 Weld, Stanley B. "Boston's First Medical Society." *Yale Journal of Biology and Medicine,* July 1946, 19.6, 924.
153 Weld, "Boston's … ," 927.
154 Kittredge, "Introduction," 8.
155 C. Mather, *Angel,* 112–113.
156 C. Mather, *Angel,* 112–113.
157 C. Mather, *Angel,* 113.
158 Kittredge, "Introduction," 8.
159 Coss, *The Fever of 1721*, 83.
160 Kittredge, "Introduction," 12.
161 G. Jones, "Introduction," xxxiv.
162 Coss, *The Fever,* 27, 31–32.
163 Coss, *The Fever*, 232–233.
164 Coss, *The Fever*, 228–229.
165 C. Mather, *Angel,* 235.

Bibliography

Allen, William. *American Biographical Dictionary*. Cambridge, MA: William Hilliard, 1809.

Arikha, Noga. *Passions and Tempers: A History of the Humors*. New York: Harper Perennial, 2008.

Aronson, Stanley M. and Lucile Newman. "God Have Mercy on this House: Being a Brief Chronicle of Smallpox in Colonial New England" In *Smallpox in the Americas 1492 to 1815: Contagion Controversy*, John Carter Brown Library of Brown University Exhibition, 2002.

Barquet, Nicolau and Pere Domingo. "The Triumph Over the Most Terrible of the Ministers of Death" In *Annals of Internal Medicine*, 127 (1997).

BBC News. Accessed January 10, 2022. https://www.bbc.com/news/world-asia-china-59855689

Beall, Jr., Otto T. "Cotton Mather's *Curiosa Americana* and the Boston's Philosophical Society of 1683" *The William and Mary Quarterly*, 18, no. 3 (July 1961).

Bercovitch, Sacvan. *The Puritan Origins of the American Self*. New Haven, CT: Yale University Press, 1975.

Bernhard, Virginia. "Cotton Mather's 'Most Unhappy Wife': Reflections on the Uses of Historical Evidence" In *The New England Quarterly*, 60, no. 3 (September 1987).

Bitzer, Lloyd. "The Rhetorical Situation" In *Philosophy of Rhetoric*, 1 (1968).

Blake, John H. "Smallpox Inoculation in Colonial Boston" *Journal of the History of Medicine*, 3 (1938).

Block, Seymour Stanton. *Disinfection, Sterilization, and Preservation*. Philadelphia: Lippincott, Williams, and Wilkins, 2001.

Boylston, Zabdiel. *An Historical Account of the Small-Pox Inoculated in New England*. London: S. Chandler, 1726.

Brant, Robin. "Shanghai Lockdown: Whole Communities Relocated in Anti-Covid Drive in BBC News, Shanghai" (April 21, 2022). Accessed April 26, 2022. https://www.bbc.com/news/world-asia-china-1160210

Bright, Timothy. *A Treatise on Meloncholy*. London, 1586.

Bullock, Charles. ed. of William Douglass's *Discourse Concerning the Currencies of British Plantations in America*. New York: Macmillan Co, 1897.

Burke, Kenneth. *Language as Symbolic Action: Essays on Life, Literature, and Method*. Berkeley: University of California Press, 1966.

Calef, Robert. *More Wonders of the Invisible World or the Wonders of the World Displayed in Five Parts*. Salem, MA: Reprinted by John D. and T. C. Cushing, Jr., 1823.

Canguilhem, Georges. *Writings on Medicine*. New York: Fordham University Press, 2012.

Carrell, Jennifer Lee. *The Speckled Monster: A Historical Tale of Battling Smallpox*. New York: Penguin, 2004.

Carroll, Darin S., Ginny L. Emerson, and Yu Li, et al. "Chasing Jenner's Vaccine: Revisiting *Cowpox Virus* Classification" In *PLoS One*, 6, no. 8 (2011).

City of Boston, "History of Boston's Harbor Islands." (Boston: City of Boston, 2011). The College of Physicians of Philadelphia. *The History of Vaccines*. Accessed January 10, 2022. https://www.historyofvaccines.org/timeline#EVT_9.

Collier, Leslie H. "The Development of a Stable Smallpox Vaccine" In *The Journal of Hygiene*, 53, no. 1 (1955).

Coss, Stephen. *The Fever of 1721*. New York: Simon and Schuster, 2016.

Douglass, William. *Summary of British Settlements II*. Boston: Printed; Reprinted London: R. Baldwin, 1755.

Duffy, John. *From Humors to Medical Science*. Urbana, IL: University of Illinois Press, 1993.

Edelman, Murray. "Contestable Categories and Public Opinion" In *Political Communication* 10, no. 3 (1993).

Eliot, J. *Biographical Dictionary*. Salem and Boston, MA.: 1809.

Entman, Robert M. "Framing: Toward Clarification of a Fractured Paradigm" In *Journal of Communication* 43, no. 4 (1993).

Fenner, F., Donald A. Henderson, Isao Arita, Zedenek Jeznek, and Ivan Danilovich Ladyni. *Smallpox and Its Eradication*. Geneva: World Health Organization-IRIS, 1988.

Fitz, Reginald Heber. *Zabdiel Boylston: Inoculator and the Epidemic of Smallpox in Boston in 1721*, reprint in *Johns Hopkins Hospital Bulletin* 22, no. 247 (September 1911).

Flannery, Michael. "Building a Retrospective Collection in Pharmacy: A Brief History of the Literature with Some Considerations for U. S. Health Sciences Library Professionals" In *Bulletin of the Medical Library Association*, 89.2 (April 2001).

Foucault, Michel. *The Birth of the Clinic: An Archaeology of Medical Perception*. New York: Vintage, 1975.

Foucault, Michel. *Discipline and Punish: The Birth of the Prison*. New York: Random House, 1979.

Foucault, Michel. "The Politics of Health in the 18th Century" In *The Foucault Reader*, ed. Paul Rabinow. New York: Pantheon, 1984.

Foucault, Michel. *Power/Knowledge, Selected Interviews & Other Writings, 1972–1977*, ed. Colin Gordon. New York: Pantheon, 1981.

Gordon, Colin. "Afterword" In Michel Foucault's *Power/Knowledge*. New York: Pantheon, 1980.

Gross, Alan G., Joseph E. Harmon, and Michael S. Brody, *Communicating Science: The Scientific Article from the 17th Century to the Present*. New York: Oxford University Press, 2002.

Hall, Marie Boas. *Promoting Experimental Learning: Experiment and the Royal Society: 1660–1727*. London: Cambridge University Press, 2002.

Heifferon, Barbara. "The New Smallpox: An Epidemic of Words?" In *Rhetoric Review*, 25, no. 1 (2006).

Henderson, D. A. *Smallpox: The Death of a Disease*. Amherst, NY: Prometheus, 2009 in Piper, "Smallpox Used," (February 5, 2021).

Holmes, Oliver Wendell in *Memorial History of Boston*, IV.

Holmes, Thomas James. *Cotton Mather, A Bibliography of His Work*. Cambridge, MA: Harvard University Press, 1940.

Hopkins, Donald R. *Princes and Peasants: Smallpox in History*. Chicago: University of Chicago Press, 1984.

Huber, Edward G. "Control of Communicable Disease Prevalent in Massachusetts" In *Boston Medical Surgery*. Boston: Massachusetts Medical Society, 1926.

Johnson, Thomas H. and Perry Miller, eds. *The Puritans: A Sourcebook on Their Writings*. New York: Harper Collins, 1963.

Jones, Gordon W. "Introduction" to *Angel of Bethesda* by Cotton Mather. Barre, MA: American Antiquarian Society and Barre Publishers, 1972.

Kales, David. *The Boston Harbor Islands: A History of an Urban Wilderness*. Charleston, SC: The History Press.

Kapoor, Archana, *Making Connections: Microscopy and Scientific Practice in Colonial America and the Wider Trans-Atlantic World*, Thesis: University of Leeds, 2013.

Kennedy, Peter. "An Essay on External Remedies, Wherein It Is Considered, Whether All the Curable Distempers Incident to Human Bodies, May Not Be Cured by Means." London: A. Bell, 1715.

Kinukawa, Tomami. "Review of *American Curiosity: Culture of Natural History in the Colonial British Atlantic* by Susan Scott Parrish" *New England Quarterly* 80, no. 2 (June 2007).

Kittredge, George L. "Introduction" to Increase Mather's and Anonymous's [Cotton Mather] *Several Reasons for Transplanting the Small Pox, Is a Lawful Practice, and That It Has Been Blessed by God for the Saving of Many a Life. Etc.* and Cotton Mather's *Sentiments Written on the Small Pox Inoculated*. Cleveland, OH: 1921.

Lee, Keekok. "Towards a More Comprehensive Assessment of Medical Achievements: Smallpox as a Case Study" In *Academia Letters*, pre-print. (2021).

Lemnius, Levinus. *The Touchstone of Complexions*. London: Thomas Marsh, 1576.

Lewis, Frederick. "The Advent of Microscopes in America: With Notes on Their Earlier History" In *The Scientific Monthly* 57, no. 3 (September 1943). http://www.jstor.org/stable/17981

Macaulay, Thomas Babington. *The History of England from the Accession of James the Second*. Philadelphia: Porter and Coates, 1848 and in Project Gutenberg.

Mager, Gerald. *Zabdiel Boylston: Medical Pioneer of Colonial Boston*. Urbana-Champagne, IL.: University of Illinois Press, 1975.

Mather, Cotton. *Angel of Bethesda*. Barre, MA: American Antiquarian Society and Barre Publishers, 1972.

Mather, Cotton. *Diary*. New York: Frederick Ungar Publishing, 1911.

Mather, Cotton. *Parentator: Memoirs of Remarkables in the Life and Death of the Ever-Remarkable Dr. Increase Mather*. Boston: 1724.

Merton, Robert K. *Science, Technology, and Society in Seventeenth Century England*. Bruges, Belgium: St. Catherine's Press, 1938.

Miller, Perry. *The Life of the Mind in America*. New York: Harcourt, Brace, and World, 1965.

Murdock, Kenneth B. and Elizabeth W. Miller. "Introduction" to *Magnalia Christi Americana*. Cambridge, MA: Harvard University Press, 1977.

National Institutes of Health. "History of Medicine. Accessed January 11, 2022. https://www.nlm.nih.gov/exhibition/shakespeare/fourhumors.html

National Library of Medicine, "Medical History Collection." Accessed April 2, 2019. https://www.nlm.nih.gov/exhibition/shakespeare/fourhumors.html

New England Journal of Medicine, XIV: 1–13, 1825.

Niven, Stephen J. "Onesimus" In *African American National Biography*, ed. Henry Louis Gates and Evelyn Brooks Higginbotham. London: Oxford University Press, 2008. Accessed April 3, 2019. https://sites.fas.harvard.edu/~aanb/SHTML/SHTML/sampleEntries.shtml

Parrish, Susan Scott. *American Curiosity: Culture of Natural History in the Colonial British Atlantic*. Chapel Hill, NC: University of North Carolina Press, 2006.

Pender, Stephen. "Subventing Disease: Anger, Passions, and the Non-Naturals" In *Rhetorics of Bodily Medicine and Health in Medieval and Early Modern England*, ed. Jennifer Vaught. Surrey, UK: Ashgate, 2013.

Piper, Kelsey. "Smallpox Used to Kill Millions of People Every Year. Here's How Humans Beat It. *Vox*. (February 5, 2021).

Rappaport, Rhoda. *When Geologists Were Historians 1665–1750*. Cornell, NY: Cornell University Press, 1997.

Reidel, Stefan. "Edward Jenner and the History of Smallpox and Vaccination" In *Baylor University Medical Center Proceedings*. Dallas, TX: Baylor University Medical Center, 2005.

Rosen, George. *A History of Public Health*. Baltimore: John Hopkins University Press, 2015.

Rusnock, Andrea. *The Correspondence of James Jurin, 1684–1750*. Atlanta: Rodopi B. V., 1996.

Savage-Smith, Emilie. "Fundamental to Islamic Medieval Medical Practice?" In *The Body in Balance: Humoral Medicines in Practice*, eds. Peregrine Horden and Elisabeth Hsu. Oxford, NY: Berghahn Books, 2015.

Scott, J. Blake. *Risky Rhetoric: AIDS and the Cultural Practices of HIV Testing*. Carbondale, IL: Southern Illinois University Press, 2003.

Shurtleff, Nathaniel Bradstreet. *A Topographical and Historical Description of Boston, Part I*. Boston: City Council, 1871.

Silverman, Kenneth. *The Life and Times of Cotton Mather*. New York: Columbia University Press, 1985.

Stetten, D., Jr. "Victory Over Variola" In American Society for Microbiology's *ASM News*, 44 (1978).

Sun, Simao. *Essential Prescriptions Worth a Thousand Gold*. China: Tang Dynasty, 600s C.E.

Thacher, J. *American Biographical Dictionary*. Boston, MA.: 1828.

Tucker, Jonathan B. *Scourge: The Once and Future Threat of Smallpox*. New York: Grove Press, 2001.

Weld, Stanley B. "Boston's First Medical Society" In *Yale Journal of Biology and Medicine*, 19, no.6 (July 1946).

Wellcome Collection. "Blood-letting at the Barber-surgeons." Accessed January 11, 2022. https://wellcomecollection.org/articles/XKyzchIAAPeWNq1l

Wright, Thomas. *The Passions of the Mind in Generalle*. London: T. Thorpe, 1608.

Yu, Mao Kun. *Variolation*. China: Qing Dynasty, n.d.

Zhang, Lu. *Clarifying Medicine*. China: Mid, 1600s.

Zhu, Chunjia. *Discourse Definitive on Smallpox*. China: Song Dynasty, n.d.

2 The Religious and Legal Frames of the Debate: Who Controls the Body?

Infectious Testimonials

The letters and tracts, starting with John Williams's tract below, are often addressed to the Selectmen of Boston, who were the local authorities in that then current structure of government under the British governor's authority that were elected to serve for six months.[1] They were answerable to the citizenry of Boston. Besides being addressed by the various publications of both Anti-Inoculators and Inoculators as well as other Bostonians about local issues, the Selectmen often held what today we might call "hearings," and individuals in the community were called upon to testify. One of those who was first called upon to speak before the council on July 21, 1721 was Lawrence Dalhonde, who had served as a surgeon in the French service. He testified "that he knew of 'horrible sequelae' [terrible results] from inoculation."[2] Because of his credibility as a surgeon (although considered a lesser professional than a physician or degreed doctor), the Frenchman was given authority to speak by the townspeople and by the Selectmen, whom Bostonians had elected and trusted to protect them.[3] Others reported similar terrible and inflammatory narratives supposedly from outbreaks and attempts at inoculation in Italy, Spain, and Flanders.[4] Almost from the beginning of the actual procedures that Boylston performed, the inoculation project had been framed within these very negative testimonials.

Even though such accounts, like those of the French surgeon, were exaggerations, and most likely misinformation, they were published officially by the Selectmen (often in the *News-Letter* or in *The Courant,* James and Ben Franklin's newspaper) "intensify[ing] the people's terror."[5] In addition, these reports that served as evidence of the dangers of inoculation were embedded in a report published in *The New-England Courant* by the Selectmen in August 1721 that also suggested that the smallpox epidemic, then barely two months old, was waning and not so serious. That information was incorrect; the epidemic would rage on until December 1722, claiming many more lives. Their reasoning was that because the inoculation process itself could cause deleterious effects, and, in addition, the epidemic

DOI: 10.4324/9781003312369-3

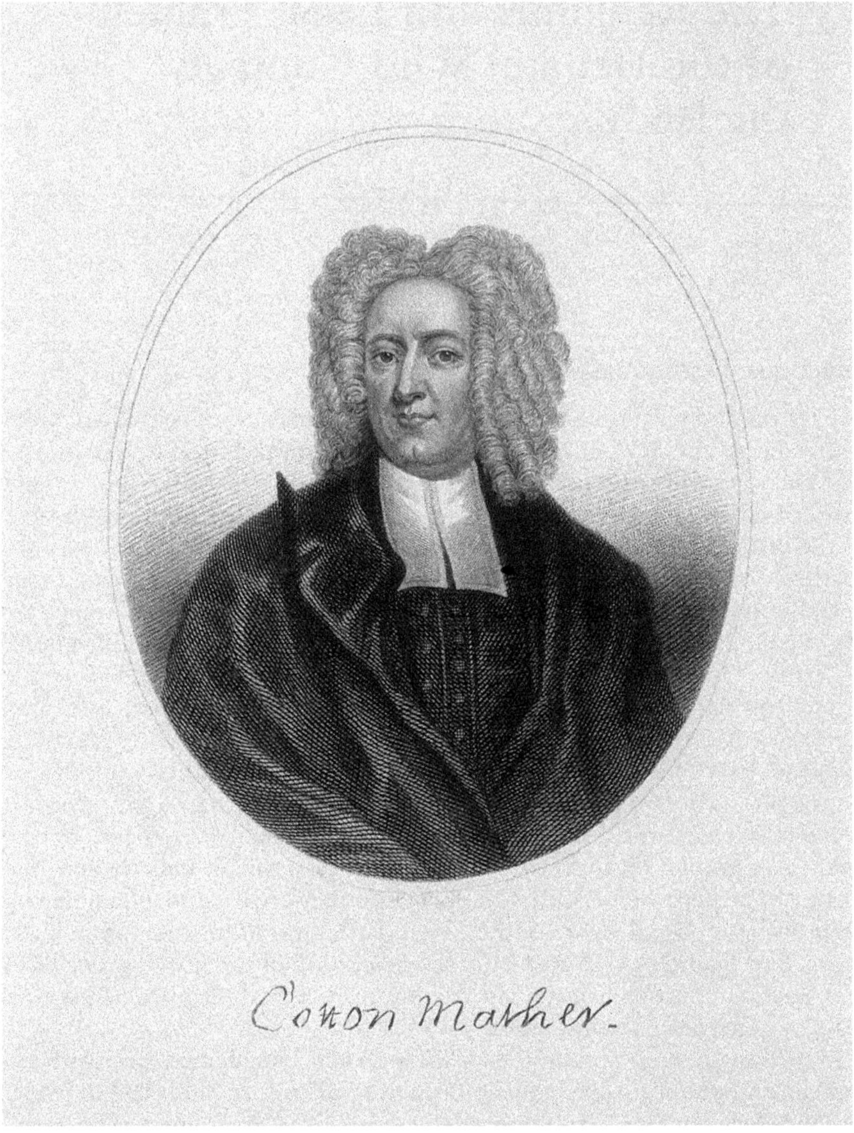

Figure 2.1 Cotton Mather, Wellcome Collection.

was a mild one and almost over, it would be unwise and ill-advised to go forward with such an unproven and perhaps even unnecessary procedure.[6]

The same Selectmen's publication also included a pronouncement by a number of the ten physicians of Boston (minus at least Dr. Boylston) declaring that, "it appears by numerous Instances, That it [i.e. inoculation] has prov'd the death of many persons soon after the operation, and brought distempers upon many others which have in the End prov'd deadly to them." This statement had no basis in fact.[7] Boylston documented all his inoculations and out of 246, only six died. However, it can be noted that the Selectmen attempted to offer a degree of balanced testimony of the two sides of the debate by bringing in both groups: the Anti-Inoculators led by Douglass and the Inoculators led by Mather and Boylston, in order to hear their evidence. However, the Selectmen, as far as it can be determined, also did not publish testimonials (or encourage publishing) of testimonials published in the *Transactions of the Royal Society,* which clearly presented a case for vaccination. It's not known how many or if any of the Selectmen had read Mather's tracts or investigated the matter beyond what the physicians and the Inoculators were telling them in public meetings. It could have been that Dr. William Douglass's *ethos* and that of the other physicians were strong enough to drown out any contradictory opinion before the Selectmen, especially a claim made by religious leaders about medical treatments, although as mentioned above, Mather and other ministers had exercised much control over the individual and body politic in the past. The following chapter that includes some reflections on the witchcraft trials' relation to the inoculation project illustrates the type of control over minds and bodies that had still been in the hands of ministers such as Cotton and Increase Mather 30 years before. However, their power over parishioners' bodies and minds had begun to be challenged in Boston.

Even though in general Puritans propagated an avid interest in science, reading scientific tracts did not seem to filter down to the largely literate population. Books other than the *Bible* or prayer books were rare in poorer Colonial households; however, all three of the newspapers seemed to have been thriving during the controversy.[8] "Although not exclusively an upper-class recreational activity, reading did require the ability to read, some wealth to purchase books, and leisure time to read them – all qualities held most by the well-to-do. The subject matter of books read by the urban gentry was overwhelmingly utilitarian in nature."[9] Also, although literacy levels were as high as 70% in Boston by 1710, there was no desire for books speculative in nature.[10] What was most popular then were religious, legal, agricultural, and navigational texts, along with primers.[11] If many citizens had been reading the proceedings of the Royal Society from London, then the inoculation project perhaps would not have seemed so radically counter-intuitive in the midst of an epidemic. It is doubtful that the *Royal Society Transactions* had been particularly popular or widely disseminated reading materials. They had been avidly read, however, by the Mathers and some of the other literati before Dr. Douglass had confiscated the copy he had loaned the minister.

The parishioners of Boston were very well informed about their own traditional, religious doctrines, so the framing of the discourse had fit neatly into their well-developed schema. Thus arguments from the standpoint of religious dogma and its attendant rhetorics were used successfully by physicians, the "common people," including some of those in Mather's own congregation, as well as by the editors of two of the three newspapers in Boston against the ministers. Of course *The New-England Courant* was the most effective medium for the Anti-Inoculators.[12] This reversal in rhetoric with the ministers' arguments based on current and developing medical science and the doctors and their adherents' arguments based on religious rhetoric began almost immediately after Boylston began the first inoculations on June 26, 1721 on his son and two of his own enslaved Africans. Both religion and Physick (medicine) had both been seen as and framed verbally as "law," whether doctrinal law or law of Physick, and in colonial, theocratic Boston, the law and Christianity had often been fused together.[13]

As Thomas Kuhn said, to move from "normal" to "revolutionary" science, enough events or incidents, speeches, publications, etc. have had to occur to effect a qualitative change.[14] As protectors of the public good, then, the Selectmen "had to resist the ignorant and often knavish quackery of all sorts of waifs and strays among the practitioners of medical folk-lore, — white witches, cunning men, strokers,[15] exorcists, inspired healers, sham astrologers, — to a degree to which modern physicians can hardly appreciate."[16] In other words, many different "practitioners" claimed to have the authority to speak in matters of health and disease, making the situation even more difficult for the citizenry to determine who was telling the truth about inoculation. When so many had authority to speak, and the "professionals" were not yet constituted *as* professionals nor was medicine instituted *as* a profession in today's sense, anyone with any claim of authority, whether true or not, could speak on the smallpox epidemic and did so. However, the Selectmen had seemed to listen and give most credence to the testimonies of Douglass and his group of physicians. As Foucault wrote in "The Politics of Health in the Eighteenth Century": "Medicine … assumes an increasingly important place in the administrative system and the machinery of power, a role which is constantly widened and strengthened throughout the eighteenth century. The doctor wins a footing within the different instances of social power."[17] As is seen in the Mather project, it can be argued that phenomenon also appeared during the smallpox epidemic of 1721–1722 with the Selectmen ruling on the medical intervention of variolation.

Unfortunately, even the best authorities on medical history in America don't often work with the field before 1800. Charles E. Rosenberg assumed nothing much happened till 1800, while this text examines earlier times to see the seeds being sown and to understand why new initiatives such as the smallpox inoculation did not flourish and failed, even though in 1721–1722 it proved a successful preventative for the few people willing to undergo it. Perhaps it is in the times of "rupture," such as an epidemic, that the emergence of new discoveries and professions can send up exploratory shoots. "The power of the Norm appears through the disciplines. Is this the new law of modern society?"[18] At this point, the professionals were in the way of a life-saving technique, and the chaos of an epidemic had caused much upheaval. According to Kuhn, "All crises begin with the blurring of a paradigm and the consequent loosening of the rules for normal research."[19] Also, he suggests there are several possible outcomes: an incursion of a new solution to a crisis and recurring problem can result in it being capable of being handled within normal science of the time (which did not happen with smallpox), otherwise, it could simply mean the paradigm had been too resistant and no new solution would have been accepted at that time, or a new "candidate" would have to vie in a long "battle" for acceptance.[20] It was this last possibility that involved brand new "modes of solution" that would ultimately be successful.[21] A battle for acceptance best describes the smallpox inoculation project in 1721–1722.

In the paradigm shift within the medical practitioners themselves, it's true that actual medical professionalization in the U.S. does not occur until the 1800s, although small, local groups had begun to form as early as the smallpox controversy in 1721, but these were more informal groupings. "Between 1797 and 1850, 117 American medical journals appeared; at the end of the century, 275 periodicals were published in the United States. By 1830, nearly all states in the Union possessed a medical society, and these were supplemented by many local societies."[22] One of the most important developments was the organization of the AMA (American Medical Association) in 1847, in effect giving the societies national status and power. In medical education, chaotic and varying criteria could be found up until the 1870s.[23]

The Selectmen's role in reigning in this "solution" to the current crisis was a conservative and cautious one that tended to enforce current norms and framed the debate using negative narratives, not only in the report mentioned above, but also in another publication on the 31st of July in 1721. This testimonial had been signed by John Forland and featured the following narrative that had taken place on the Greek Island of Milo. Forland had supposedly asked a Greek physician what he should do to escape the smallpox. He testified that the Greek doctor told him,

> There was a Project tried amongst the Greeks, at an island called Corfue [sic], where they put into the flesh something that corrupted the blood; but said he, if you should do it, you would never be a sound man as long as you should live: and further said, that some that had practiced the project, lost the use of their limbs, and that others swelled up and dyed [sic] sometime after, and that others had the small pox afterwards.[24]

Boylston refuted this account based on the results he was seeing in his own practice of vaccination and Cotton Mather himself commented on Forland's testimony, naming it a "yarn in a strain of justifiable irony."[25] Mather strongly questioned the credibility of Forland's narrative by suggesting that it amounted to little more than this, "That a man in

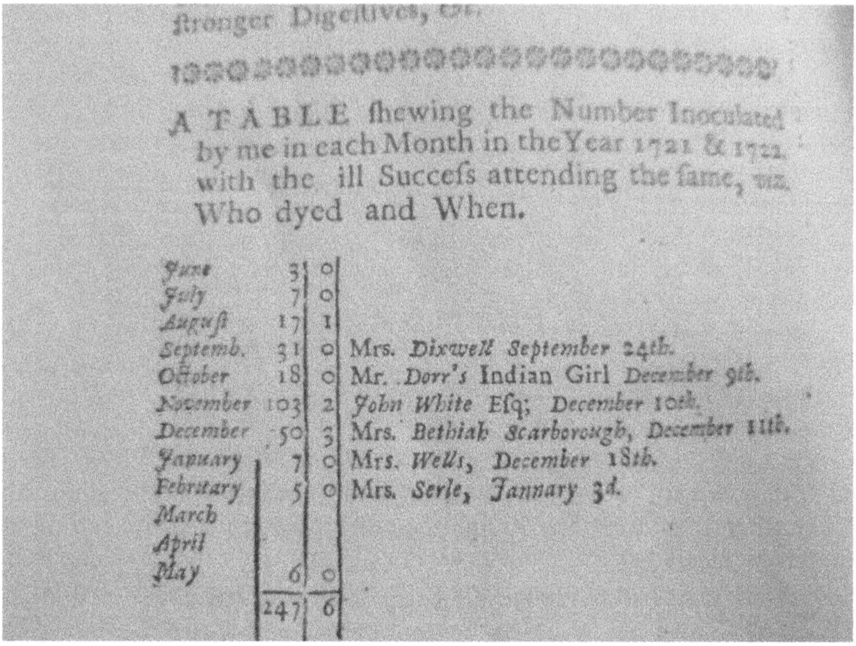
ſtronger Digeſtives, &c.

A TABLE ſhewing the Number Inoculated by me in each Month in the Year 1721 & 1722, with the ill Succeſs attending the ſame, viz. Who dyed and When.

June	3	0	
July	7	0	
August	17	1	
Septemb.	31	0	Mrs. *Dixwell September* 24th.
October	18	0	Mr. *Dorr's* Indian Girl *December* 9th.
November	103	2	*John White* Eſq; *December* 10th.
December	50	3	Mrs. *Bethiah Scarborough*, *December* 11th.
January	7	0	Mrs. *Wells*, *December* 18th.
February	5	0	Mrs. *Serle*, *January* 3d.
March			
April			
May	6	0	
	247	6	

Figure 2.2 Boylston's Record, Public Domain.

the Mediterranean, many years ago, was told by somebody, that somebody told him, that somebody heard, that the Doctors in Archipelago warned people against Inoculation of the small-pox as a dangerous practice."[26] In the various argumentative tracts, writers often held each other and their reports up to ridicule. However, in this particular statement, Mather was clearly questioning Forland's authority to speak, especially since his testimonial arrived through so many other speakers, whose authority could not be known. Although Boylston refuted this narrative in his own text, his refutation was turned on him; by presenting this narrative in his own argument for variolation, he had unwittingly set himself up for further refutation.

The debate was a vigorous one by this time (July 1721) and the newspapers kept the debate current and viable. The *Boston Gazette, The News-Letter,* and *The New-England Courant* were the three main newspapers in Boston. Most scholars agree that the *Gazette* was more sympathetic to the Inoculators and *The News-Letter* more slanted toward the Anti-Inoculators or the recently formed Society of the Physicians. *The New-England Courant*[27] by far used the most *ad hominem* attacks against the Inoculators in its rhetorical repertoire, against both Boylston and Cotton Mather. The paper, run by James Franklin with his younger brother/apprentice, Benjamin, needed funds to compete with the older two newspapers, and had found that being a mouthpiece for one side in a virulent controversy filled the coffers and also excited and matched their own political passions. Perhaps most would assume that at the tender age of 15, young Ben Franklin would have had no real role in the debate that had ensued over smallpox. In fact, the boy was precocious and shortly after the epidemic ended, he began the Silence Dogood letters. But before that time, he edited many tracts attacking the Mathers with great enthusiasm. The *Courant* "was the recognized organ of the anti-inoculators. It had begun ... in 8/7, 1721 when the controversy was in full swing ... . The clergy regarded it as a scandalous and profane rag, published to destroy their influence and debauch the community" and on August 28, 1721, "the *News-Letter* printed a letter declaring that the *Courant*, ... is reported to be written by the 'Practioners [sic] of Physic in Boston,' ... and insinuating that their Society is comparable to the infamous Hellfire Club of London."[28] Douglass answered in the next *Gazette*, under the signature of "w. Anti-Inoculators," protesting the insinuation, but had not denied the connection between the newspaper and the doctors. He had declared, "The Society are only accountable for their own pieces, and not for other Matters inserted by the Publishers of News-papers."[29] Unlike the other newspapers, the Boston *Gazette* accepted advertisements from Boylston, thus spurring Douglass on to dun its publishers.

The opposition led by Douglass had also published a letter on July 24, 1721 in *The News-Letter*. Douglass signed the 7/24 letter not with his real name but with the name *William Philanthropos* (lover of mankind).[30] In the letter he attacked Boylston, the surgeon/physician who was performing the inoculations with Mather, as "'a certain cutter for the Stone' and alleg[ed] that he (and by implication Cotton Mather) had adopted this 'far-fetched and not well vouched method' without 'any serious thought.'"[31] This particular line of argument was addressed in Chapter 1 in the historical background and contextual analysis of the sources of inoculation information documented in *Angel of Bethesda* and the *Transactions of the Royal Society*. Because it's also been documented that Douglass himself called Mather's attention to one of the favorable reports of the success of inoculations in the *Transactions* (and Mather alerted Boylston), we know that the degreed doctor was aware of the readings the Inoculators had studied as well as the fact that Mather had been engaged in this inquiry for at least five years. Most of the Inoculators had shared these Royal Society *Transactions*. Mather had sent a letter to John Woodward, M.D. (distinguished English paleontologist—Gresham College) on July 12, 1716.[32] Douglass's use of "not well vouched" [not well re-searched] was an interesting claim to make. Even if not valid, it was effective rhetorically, as it painted the view that Boylston and Mather had perhaps "gone off half-cocked" or on some wild goose chase; the minister's project was framed as a poorly researched and not carefully examined proposition, which then caused him to lose further authority and credibility with the Bostonians in the face of this accusation.

"Without any serious thought" was a direct challenge to Boylston, too, because the doctor had himself survived smallpox and in addition to researching the method and consulting with Mather, had gathered his own evidence, especially from African Americans, as well as having inoculated his own son and the enslaved members of his household sometime before vaccinating others. On June 26, 1721, he had written: "I inoculated my son, Thomas, of about six, my Negro-Man, Jack, thirty-six, and Jackey, two and a half Years old."[33] He inoculated others in July.[34] Although in that particular letter Douglass or Philanthropos had not attacked Mather directly, Boylston's credibility and authority were thoroughly questioned. At first, with Mather, the opposition was more tangential. In fact, in the beginning of the controversy, the Scot credited the Puritan minister with benevolent intentions and characterized his project as being motivated by "a Pious and charitable design of doing good."[35] This rhetorical maneuver ("Brutus was an honorable man") was a success with his audience of inoculation sceptics. Because Douglass had given some credit to the minister for his intentions, it could also have successfully disarmed part of the opposition. Such a maneuver could have been a successful strategy for dividing one's opponents (in this case the Inoculators) and setting them against each other. However, it did not succeed in dividing Mather and Boylston.

In fact, on July 31st, Mather, outraged at the attack on Boylston, responded with his own letter to the *Gazette*, the only supportive Boston paper willing to publish the minister, defending the only Boston physician agreeing to work directly with him on the vaccination project. This letter was signed by the following: Increase and Cotton Mather, Benjamin Colman, Thomas Prince, John Webb, and William Cooper. Thus, the lines had been clearly drawn, solidifying the two groups into the Inoculators and Defenders versus the Anti-Inoculators and the Attackers, which then included William Douglass, John Williams (Mundungus), the Selectmen, Samuel Grainger, Nicholas Boone, James and Benjamin Franklin, and Alexander Stuart, among others.

The main medical fears of physicians and their followers appeared to be that the smallpox, rather than being arrested, would be spread further. This belief made sense given the constraints outlined above in this chapter under *the Common Sense Trope*. However, Boylston and Mather made sure those inoculated were quarantined until the disease passed. The patients were quarantined usually in their own homes, but sometimes they did so in the Mather or Boylston homes. Boylston's wife and four of his children had been sent to the country to avoid infection. Another fear among the Bostonians had been that inserting the smallpox fluid into the body compromised the blood and the body and could have created terrible fevers (what we would call today infection of the blood or sepsis), and that victims would not only *not* be protected from smallpox, but that such a maneuver could cause either an incurable fever (sepsis) or make those inoculated vulnerable to the plague, also a much feared and dreaded disease.[36]

In the above debate who had been given authority to speak on the topic of smallpox was at issue. The Selectmen, whose status and ethos had been very important in colonial Boston, had entered the fray, but more often seemed to have supported only negative framing of the possibilities of smallpox variolation. Hearsay evidence is admitted as part of "valid" testimony; exaggerations had gone unchallenged by the Selectmen themselves, while being adopted by the Anti-Inoculators. In the recent past, for the Inoculators, who were ministers and literati, their ethos had prevailed. The challenge to their leadership thus became a vital part of the debate. The Selectmen were the legal representatives of the Boston citizenry. As the controversy over vaccination revealed, they no longer saw themselves as obedient subjects in a theocracy.

The Religious Controversy over Inoculation

Religion in colonial America informed almost all discourse. Especially in Boston, Puritanism was part of the societal norms and beliefs that helped people accept a sometimes difficult life to such an extent that there had been instances of young children welcoming their own deaths because they could "go to Jesus" sooner.[37] In their prevailing worldview, they had been predestined to suffer as a test of their faith. In addition to predestination, other Calvinist doctrines the Puritans followed were original sin, grace, and the evil nature of man, which informed not only the discourse, but all aspects of colonial life, including medical practices. However, there were opposing views on how Calvinist doctrine might be applied to illness and its preventatives.

John Calvin developed his most comprehensive theology in his major work, *Institutes of the Christian Religion,* published in 1536, adding new material in 1539, 1543, and 1559.[38] By the last edition of the book, he had completed four volumes of 80 chapters. In addition, he also articulated his theology in sermons, treatises, and Biblical commentaries. Calvin spent his whole life as a reformer after a conversion following his removal from training for the priesthood by his father. The removal had been based on his father's belief that his son should become a lawyer so that he would make more money.[39] Although the young man studied diligently and gained his law degree in Paris, within a few years, he had found religious reformation as his true calling.

Calvin had been a master at organizing churches as representative bodies and assemblies as opposed to top-down autocracies. He attempted to involve the laity in all major decisions.[40] However, until recently, historians did not treat the reformer sympathetically. Instead, he was accused of being a leader who imposed on and cowed helpless parishioners. His version of religion had been seen as a joyless and fearful belief system at the mercy of a God who treated human beings as his puppets, punishing them for the least deviation from his moral code. Recent scholarship is correcting that view.[41] Calvin believed that "human wisdom consists of two parts: knowledge of ourselves and of God." He believed the whole person, mind and body, was in a spiritual relationship with the deity.[42]

Calvinism adheres to scripture and seeks to derive its theology solely from the *Bible*. It focuses on God's sovereignty and the idea that all control of humanity is through the deity.[43] Very briefly, Calvinism was centered on four main points: (1) God's grace can predetermine who is to be saved; (2) Jesus died for those who were predestined by God; (3) God "regenerates" an individual who wants to choose God; and (4) Those who are redeemed will not lose their salvation.[44] At the same time, Calvin stressed that his followers be involved in all aspects of social life, even as he had been. It was natural for the Mathers and other Puritan ministers, in other words, to be interested in natural philosophy (science), politics, government, and education. Although educated colonists read other texts, they did believe, as Calvin had written, that it was through the study of scriptures that humans could know about the Creator and themselves.[45] In addition, Calvin maintained that the deity's ways were mysterious, and humans could not fully understand why certain actions were taken by their God.[46]

The arguments over the role of illness, in this case, smallpox, especially those of the Anti-inoculators, had often been religious in nature, and many had centered on predestination. What actions were parishioners allowed to take to prevent smallpox, and what might their deity expect them to do? Would they be thwarting the will of God and his punishment for their evil by finding a way to avoid contracting smallpox? Some Puritans believed their smallest negative action could bring on certain judgments from their God.[47] In the following texts debating inoculation, it's clear that many colonists had been convinced the smallpox had indeed been brought on by their own evil deeds. Both sides addressed this belief extensively, although the Inoculators often used other topics, only using scriptures to rebut the religious arguments of those against vaccination. This religious exchange became one of the most important reasons that inoculation was opposed. It seemed, then, ironic that the Puritan ministers, the experts in theology, had almost all argued for inoculation. Often the physicians and those siding with them used predestination and the sinful nature of the colonists as their counter arguments against inoculation. That did not mean that some colonists and a few physicians had not changed their minds during the two-year-long debate. Several physicians in Roxbury had joined Boylston and the Inoculators in the variolation of some of their neighbors.

Patricia Roberts-Miller notes that American Puritans' views on predestination were based on their belief in the rationality of both God's mind and the world He created.[48] As we will see in the debates, holding to the doctrine of predestination did not mean that their discussions were without "emotional and intellectual" objections to the idea that out of so many only a very few people should be saved.[49] The parishioners' beliefs had been more nuanced, as were Calvin's, than the written tenets would sometimes indicate. Even Calvin taught that biblical teachings were complex and did not need to be reduced to one central idea; the theologian appreciated the complexity even when various lessons seemed to contradict one another.[50]

Calvin rightly imagined himself a true reformer after having rejected Catholicism, and the famous theologian had also believed civil and religious authorities should be separate. This view was ultimately the origin of the U.S. doctrine of separation of church and state.[51] The irony was that Boston had been a Puritan theocracy, and under the ministerial line of Mathers and others, church and state had been united. That point, too, had become part of the debate over inoculation and was key in the growing opposition to the theocratic leaders. Puritanism, as one of the Protestant denominations heavily influenced by Calvinism, provides the religious context for the following discussion of the pro- and con-arguments regarding the inoculation project. Calvinism adheres to scripture and seeks to derive its theology solely from the *Bible*. It focuses on God's sovereignty and the idea that all control of humanity is through the deity.[52] The interpretation the Puritans adhered to was not only that one could have been predestined to be saved, but also that one's time of death, health, suffering, etc. had been predetermined. Thus, the most grievous charge of illegality in a theocracy would be that the inoculation project went against God's law or Biblical law. In colonial New England, the law and Christianity were fused together.[53] In the newspapers, pamphlets, and arguments this charge of illegality surfaced again and again, resonating strongly with Bostonians, whether they were Puritans or Congregationalists.

Because in early colonial Boston, Puritan ministers had been expected to minister to both the souls *and* bodies of their church members, it was natural for Cotton to have considered himself also a practitioner of Physick. For example, then in a Harvard class, all might have been graduated as clergymen and as such could be called to the mission of caring for the whole person. Some clergy had taken on the physical care and treatment more than others alongside the barbers, physicians, apothecaries, herbalists, and midwives. Foucault wrote that both Quakers and other dissenters from England had played an important role in their own development of health policy. They had set standards for hygiene, exercise, healthy diet as well as care for their ill parishioners and oversee (or surveil) their health habits.[54] Unlike in Europe during this same period, no hospitals or clinics existed in the colonies except for a few almshouse infirmaries in Boston in 1685 and later in Philadelphia in 1732, and the quarantine building on Spectacle Island.[55] In the past, healing had taken place in the Puritan home; there had been no need for another place of healing.

Cotton Mather, partly because of his fascination with science and medicine had embraced dual roles as physician and spiritual leader enthusiastically. Thus, atomism was also not intrusive in Mather's medical compendium, *Angel of Bethesda,* where body/mind/soul were united with none of the separations as in today's medical texts. His description of testimonials for support of inoculation was more straightforward. The body as separate from mind and soul that had developed as a result of Cartesian thought barely influenced the Colonial ministers at this time, although both

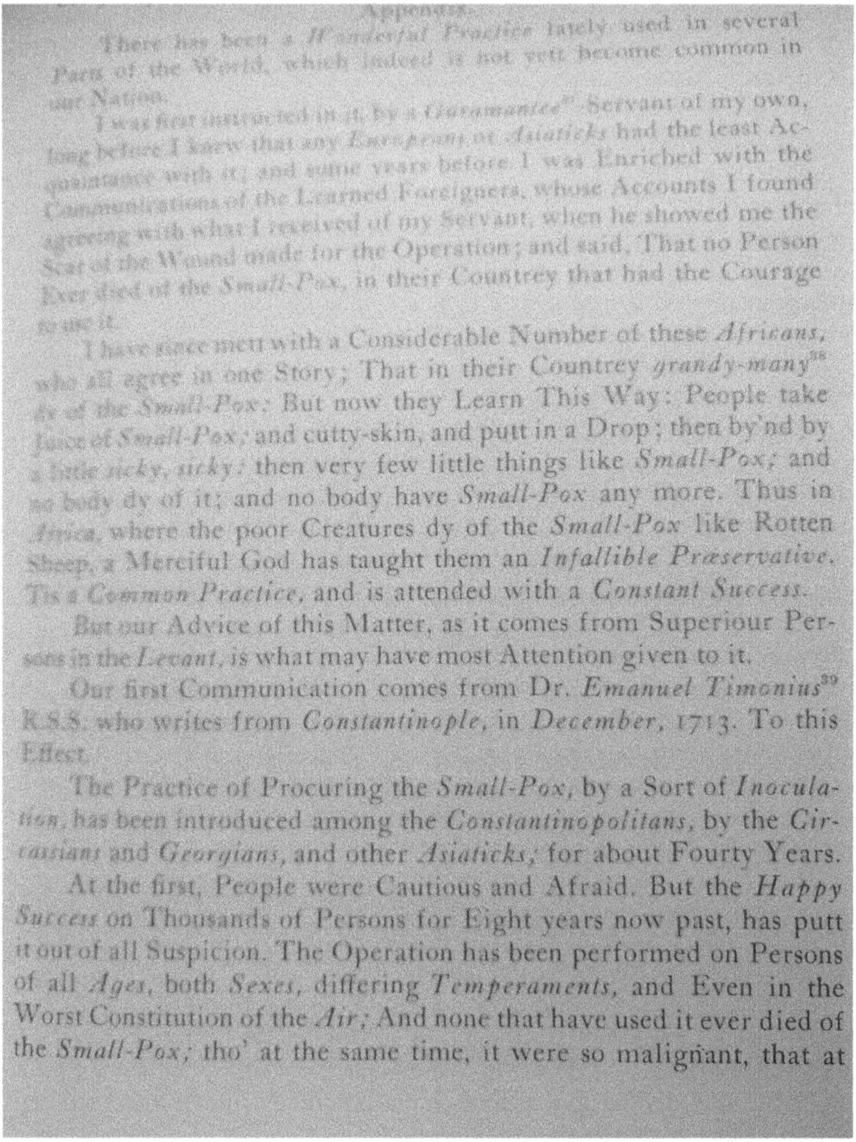

Appendix.

There has been a *Wonderful Practice* lately used in several Parts of the World, which indeed is not yett become common in our Nation.

I was first instructed in it, by a *Guramantee*[37] Servant of my own, long before I knew that any *Europeans* or *Asiaticks* had the least Acquaintance with it; and some years before I was Enriched with the Communications of the Learned Foreigners, whose Accounts I found agreeing with what I received of my Servant, when he showed me the Scar of the Wound made for the Operation; and said, That no Person Ever died of the *Small-Pox*, in their Countrey that had the Courage to use it.

I have since mett with a Considerable Number of these *Africans*, who all agree in one Story; That in their Countrey *grandy-many*[38] dy of the *Small-Pox*: But now they Learn This Way: People take Juice of *Small-Pox*; and cutty-skin, and putt in a Drop; then by'nd by a little *sicky, sicky*: then very few little things like *Small-Pox*; and no body dy of it; and no body have *Small-Pox* any more. Thus in *Africa*, where the poor Creatures dy of the *Small-Pox* like Rotten Sheep, a Merciful God has taught them an *Infallible Præservative*. 'Tis a *Common Practice*, and is attended with a *Constant Success*.

But our Advice of this Matter, as it comes from Superiour Persons in the *Levant*, is what may have most Attention given to it.

Our first Communication comes from Dr. *Emanuel Timonius*[39] R.S.S. who writes from *Constantinople*, in *December*, 1713. To this Effect.

The Practice of Procuring the *Small-Pox*, by a Sort of *Inoculation*, has been introduced among the *Constantinopolitans*, by the *Circassians* and *Georgians*, and other *Asiaticks*; for about Fourty Years.

At the first, People were Cautious and Afraid. But the *Happy Success* on Thousands of Persons for Eight years now past, has putt it out of all Suspicion. The Operation has been performed on Persons of all *Ages*, both *Sexes*, differing *Temperaments*, and Even in the Worst Constitution of the *Air*; And none that have used it ever died of the *Small-Pox*; tho' at the same time, it were so maligñant, that at

Figure 2.3 *Angel of Bethesda*, by Cotton Mather, "Courtesy of American Antiquarian Society".

father and son (Cotton and Increase Mather) were familiar with Descartes' works, as indicated by Cotton's marginalia in the elder Mather library's Descartes collection. Much of Cotton Mather's medical compendium is given to exhortations to mend dissolute ways to protect one's health with overtones of the jeremiads for which the Puritan ministers were well known, for example:

> All that have any Sense in them, *Shun* many things, *Do* many things that their B*odily Health* may not be impaired. But now, from your own Conduct about The *Health* of a *Body,* Learn what your Conduct must be that a SOUL may *Prosper and be in Health.* If you *Spiritualize* your Care about your *Bodily Health,* you will see how careful you ought to be that your *Spiritual Health* may be provided for.[56]

For many in the American religious colony, disease was sin, an imbalance in the soul that voiced itself through the body. The body stricken with smallpox made public the secrets of the soul. Because the religious doctrines were so strongly ingrained among many of the believers, religious arguments had been very persuasive during the debate. Those destined to die from smallpox would die. Were the Inoculators assuming a position of the Supreme Arbiter by promising relief from the scourge through their technique? For those operating within this ideology, medical practice could have only involved somewhat limited efforts; otherwise, a surrender to one's fate or one's reward was expected. The abundance of prayer in *Angel of Bethesda* competes with more practical physical treatments. Yet, the notion of Puritan thought needs to remain complicated. If religion and prayer were all that were needed to cure one's ills, Mather would not have written a lengthy book documenting every known cure and treatment with the largest chapter on the inoculation against smallpox; nor would he have risked his own life and those of his family on the controversial project. We see in this chapter how these beliefs provided many savvy rhetorical strategies through which both proponents and opponents of inoculation could argue.

During the smallpox controversy, a number of the elements had begun to re-formulate power over the Boston colonials. Discourses, institutions, laws and regulations, architectural forms, administrative measures, and various philosophical and juridical propositions are all part of power relations as they had begun to disorganize and reorganize in this time period.[57] It is necessary to closely examine some of the arguments that feature the rhetoric of the church, its dogma, its laws and regulations, as well as the "Law of Physick" in that context. How had those against inoculation, mostly physicians and citizens, used these doctrines to challenge the church's own previous control over the parishioner's body.

The parishioners of Boston were very well informed about their own traditional, religious doctrines, so the framing of the discourse fit neatly into their well-developed schema. Thus arguments from the standpoint of religious dogma and its attendant rhetorics were used successfully by physicians, the "common people," including some of those in Mather's own congregation, as well as by the editors of two of the three newspapers in Boston against the ministers. Of course *The New-England Courant* was the most effective medium for the Anti-Inoculators.[58] This reversal in rhetoric with the ministers' arguments based on current and developing medical science and the doctors and their adherents' arguments based on religious rhetoric began almost immediately after Boylston began the first inoculations June 26, 1721 on his son and two of his own enslaved Africans. Both religion and Physick (medicine) had been seen as and framed verbally as "law," whether doctrinal law or law of Physick, and in colonial, theocratic Boston, the law and Christianity had often been fused together.[59]

Charges of "Illegality" and the Laws of Physick

A line of argument in the frequent attacks on Boylston questioned his use of inoculation on the basis of his using a technique outside of the "Law of Physick." Because variolation was new and broached a new paradigm, it was regarded as outside the Law of Physick and consequently "illegal and unlawful." "Law" and "legality" became key tropes and framing devices in the war of pamphlets and newspaper articles, and one necessary pole for power according to Foucault.[60] And in his lectures, he laid out the following:

> In England it is the bourgeoisie against the absolute monarchy of the Stuarts, and *religious dissidents* from the start of the seventeenth century. In short, the opposition always makes a legal objection to *raison d'Etat* and consequently uses juridical reflection, legal rules, and legal authority against it. In a word, let's just say that in the seventeenth and eighteenth centuries public law is oppositional, although it is true that some theorists favorable towards royal power took up the problem and tried to integrate questions of law, legal questioning, within *raison d' Etat* … .[61]

The Puritans, the original colonists, were of course religious dissidents. When the colonials used arguments against the Royalty (in their case, the British governor over Massachusetts and Rhode Island colonies), they had used the law to back up their claims. The Anti-Inoculators, especially the Franklins and those that favored their newspaper (many Bostonians) were being urged to use legal arguments against both the royalty and the old theocracy of the Puritan Mathers. Cotton Mather also was resistant to certain Governors over the colony, but he had also curried favor with some in seats of power at home, and also with those abroad, such as those in the Royal Society.

John Williams, the apothecary and tobacconist, had been one of the most frequent and passionate writers and contributors to the debate on the side of the Anti-Inoculators. He was also known as "Mundungus," an obsolete slang term, for cheap and rank tobacco or "stinky tobacco."[62] This member of the opposition was well known to be almost illiterate, and when he did write, did so in strangely formal syllogisms and scribbles; apparently his spelling, although spelling wasn't standardized then, was almost impossible to decipher.

Thus, someone must have had to heavily edit and revise any letter he sent in or tract he had printed at James Franklin's printing house; therefore, the editors would most likely have been James and/or the young Ben Franklin, or perhaps a more literate Anti-Inoculator. Cotton Mather said of Williams in an unpublished letter to his friend, Dr. James Jurin, that Mundungus could not even "spell the word *English*, ... and could not read his own Manuscript, but pray'd the printer to find out Ye meaning, and make English of it."[63] Because Mundungus's reputation as an illiterate had been clearly established, one might wonder if the tobacconist/apothecary had been used so frequently as one of the Anti-vaxxers' mouthpieces to persuade the "common" people, those who were not part of the elite class of ministers and physicians. His texts would have been (and whether intended or not, *were*) an effective strategy to insure that this issue had not looked like a gentlemen's debate among the *literati*. It can also be hypothesized, given the firebombings and resistance to inoculation that represented a more emotional and incendiary type of verbiage, that this targeting of the audience via spokespersons such as the tobacconist had been successful rhetoric to incite reactionary and more violent measures among a certain portion of his audience.

There are other reasons Mundungus was so persuasive. He had played the role of the buffoon yet represented populist wisdom that confronted the sedate and powerful ministerial alliance. This writer/Anti-Inoculator succeeded in launching for this already complicated debate, a comic frame. Burke referred to such a technique or rhetorical strategy as the "comic corrective." He described the comic corrective as a method that is "neither wholly euphemistic, nor wholly debunking—hence it provides the charitable attitude towards people that is required for purposes of persuasion and co-operation, but at the same time maintains a shrewdness concerning the simplicities of 'cashing in.'"[64] In such a serious debate it also provided some welcome space to introduce the flaws and criticisms of the Mather family and the ministry in general, while at the same time seeming somewhat good-humored. While in the individual sense, Burke saw the "comic corrective" as enabling transcendence for a single person, in the group sense, it is a way to challenge the ruling group and cultural norms ideologically by highlighting their failures at the same time keeping basic order intact, at least intact most of the time. Mundungus offered commonplaces or *topoi* aka shared understandings to a very large audience of Bostonians. Poking fun at the "power elite" caused a further undermining of the family dynasty, Mather theocratic leadership, in which cracks had already begun to appear. Into this complex mix, Mundungus also cleverly interjects questions of legality, of utmost importance to the colonists under British rule.

Like those of many of the other Anti-Inoculators, Mundungus's claims in his letter of December 4, 1721 were centered on the illegality of inoculation: against the Queen, against the laws of nature and Physick, and against God. Although George I was on the English throne at the time, the colonists most often referred to Queen Anne's laws, those laws passed during her reign.

Most germane in this situation was the law that prohibited a physician or "quack" from spreading a contagion or disease. She was well known for a number of laws such as the assurance of a continuation of Protestant not Catholic rulers of England, called the Act of Settlement, and the first copyright laws for books and the protection of authors. The copyright law had been meant to encourage learning. In the first part of Williams's (i.e. Mundungus's) letter, he set out to prove Mather's project was against the law of natural Physick. This was an easy argument to make because the new method against smallpox was indeed innovative and a departure. Mather was proposing that it should become part of the practice of medicine, which challenged and frightened Bostonians. Mundungus's claim had been an easy one to prove since inoculation or variolation was outside the accepted law of Physick, thus it could not be part of the very long-settled dogmas that any new discovery in medicine would have to confront.[65]

Williams's first argument was brief: "If inoculating the Small Pox be not contained in the Rules of Natural Physick, then it is not lawful. But, Inoculating the Small Pox is not contained in the Rules of Natural Physick. Therefore, it is unlawful."[66] Like much of his style, which produces arguments through syllogistic reasoning, Williams brings his proof that the rules of "Natural Physick are Two ... Sympathy and Antipathy" and that nothing outside either of these is not a part of the "Physick."[67] Here he is invoking Galenic medicine in citing "sympathy and antipathy," since this medical model was one that used "contraries and analogues." As pointed out earlier though, the fluid from a live pox could be used in such a way to ward off a harder case of smallpox. The concept of using a small amount of a similar substance to treat a patient with a particular illness should have been somewhat familiar under the paradigm of Physick. In addition to Mather's later compendium, this form of "sympathy" was mentioned, for example, in Nicolas Culpeper's *English Physitian,* printed in 1652 in London and available in the colonies. However, Culpeper's listings did not of course include vaccinations against smallpox.

Once Mundungus made the claim that inoculation falls outside the purview of medicine accepted at that time, he then brought a "proof text," a Biblical verse that supported his claim:

> Now Inoculating the Small Pox is not in Sympathy with, not Antipathy with a Wound or Disease already received, but making a wound in order to communicate a disease, which is an Abuse unto that text, Math. 9. 12: 'They that are whole need not a Physician, but they that are sick,' and a horrid violation of the Intent that our Lord said it for.[68]

He had chosen to ignore the idea that using drops from a pustule of smallpox could be a treatment that could fall under the category of "sympathy."

While the style of sprinkling proof texts throughout one's argument is not unique to Williams, because he was not a minister, his using this genre in an argument by a non-cleric against the clergy was an interesting rhetorical strategy to have chosen. It was also not unusual at this time to use *Biblical* quotations as proof texts, but these were used most often by the educated, including preachers, scholars, and readers.[69] This copying of the ministerial discourse in every stylistic detail, as well as the content, could also be seen as a mocking of the powerful ministers, especially those who had been on the pinnacle of theocratic power. More recently, the clergy had been in some contention with the Selectmen, the Bostonian city council, all of whom were still situated under the Governor sent by the Crown. Williams was also mocking or imitating the educated, of which he was not a member, by using evidence for his claims and not using the common parlance of conversational or informal writing. Especially given Williams's ethos as a buffoon and a jokester, this Anti-inoculator's imitation of a ministerial style could widely be seen as poking fun. However, in comparing Williams's prose to Mather's sermons, while logical connections between claims and most Biblical verses quoted by Mather and others had been apparent, sometimes Mundungus's connections had not been as clear or logical. In addition to Williams's writing skills being dubious, his use of some of his Biblical evidence for the claims he made had not been well chosen. Even if his writings had been heavily edited, most likely by Ben Franklin, as Kittredge suggested, his particularly compromised claims had not always been corrected.[70] Perhaps, too, in this debate it had not mattered. To frame the argument in religious and legal terms perhaps had been effective enough for his audience without such attention to detail. Most of Williams's many arguments retained the syllogistic and proof-text format.

Williams had also been aware that he was held by the educated in poor regard, because he had appealed to his audience to believe that he was a good man. He had invoked the Biblical narrative of David and Goliath to gain acceptance for his rhetoric; he was the powerless and small David going up against the theocratic or ministerial Goliath. Using appeals to pathos and ethos, the apothecary had pleaded in his own behalf for his value as a spokesperson:

> Say not that he is a Mechanick, and an illiterate Man, for there is good Mettal sometimes under mean Soil; ... I know the Wall which I attempt to scale is very high; that it is defended by Men ... of a great Stature [Goliath-like] and I but a Stripling, and have not that Armour which is good for Defence: Yet the work is the Lord's, on whom I depend for Assistance.[71]

While Mundungus's first letter argued that inoculation was outside the Law of Physick, his second letter challenged the technique as being outside the Queen's Law. However, in addition to the medical and royal/governmental legality of inoculation, Williams also invoked in his letters and tracts a sense of inoculation being "unlawful" in religious law. This argument went beyond the stylistic use of biblical verses as proof texts. There were, in the eyes of many Colonists, fundamental ideological challenges to religious doctrine by the inoculation project. Those are not just found in Mundungus's text here, but in numerous tracts, folios, pamphlets, and newspapers. The sometimes violent reactions on the part of the Bostonians were informed by and heightened within the religious doctrines and practices at the time. After the witchcraft trials and the realization by Massachusetts clergy and Colonists that their actions had gone so far astray, the citizens of the colony held some reasonable expectations that they would not indulge in the same mass hysteria that promulgated the earlier incidents some 30 years earlier. However, many of the same doctrinal tenets held true some 30 years later and surfaced again during the smallpox epidemic, particularly in light of Cotton Mather's central involvement in the persecution of witches. Many of the opponents articulated views that re-invoked these strongly held religious beliefs within Calvinism that functioned as law in the minds of Bostonians.

Religious Arguments against Inoculation: More Williams's, Grainger's, and Douglass's Tracts

In the main part of his texts, Williams enumerated his religious arguments against inoculation rather than just his arguments based on Physick. He often numbered his various claims, as scholars did. To further document this particular Calvinistic religious claim, he again constructed a syllogism, in which the premises and conclusion were set up to prove that only human actions that reflected God's will could be appropriate actions.

Williams maintained that "There is no rule in the Word of God to found Inoculation upon."[72] He quoted a passage that maintained that the rights of the stranger, fatherless, and widow cannot be perverted, and that these were "helpless ones" dependent on the goodness of others. His next claim was that the inoculation project took away such rights. Williams showed how he and the other Anti-Inoculators were not only protecting the rights of others but also seeking to act in the common good. His conclusion then was that inoculation was an unrighteous action because it perverted the judgment of the defenseless (i.e. strangers, orphans and widows) and led these groups astray from God's plan for them.

Another argument Williams brought forward was a clearer and stronger syllogism: "Arg. 4. If Inoculation be a doing Violence unto the Law of Nature, and the Pattern that God hath set us, then it is unholy. But, Inoculation *is* a doing Violence unto the Law of Nature, and the Pattern Which God hath set us, (which we are to imitate.) Therefore, Inoculation is unholy …" (emphasis added).[73] He continued, "Now, that Inoculation is unrighteous and unholy, I shall demonstrate thus: Every Man has a natural Right to" exist.[74] Here he used two more pages to lay out an argument based on the commandment to do unto others as you would have them do unto you. He built a long trajectory informed by Biblical passages showing that one must not bring hazard to one's neighbors. Then he connected the commandment to inoculation, because he claimed that by a neighbor contracting a lighter version of the disease through the inoculation procedure, he endangered all his neighbors by bringing a case of the smallpox back into his home in close proximity to others. Thus, he used this argument as one of the fundamental *religious* reasons against vaccination, supporting his argument with logical and ethical Biblical appeals. In reality, Mather and Boylston made sure to quarantine those with light cases after inoculation. However, to protect those individuals, this caution might not have been advertised widely in the town.

Williams continued his argument by means of questions to the audience: The first question he posed: was not the smallpox perhaps a strange work of God and would not inoculation be a "fighting with the Most High"?[75] He positioned the inoculators as vying with God for power, much as the Pharaohs' magicians did, who had been summarily dispatched by God. The second question: "Was not smallpox perhaps a punishment sent by God?"[76]

> Whether the Small Pox be not a Punishment from a righteous God, upon a People for their Sins? And hath it not a crying voice to them saying, *Cease to do evil, and learn to do good?* And whether the labouring to avert the Stroke in the way of Inoculation, doth answer this crying Voice; or whether it be not to provoke him more and more?[77]

This question figured prominently as a justification again for the argument that to attempt to prevent smallpox was interfering with God's power and will.

The third question was much like his first claim, was the smallpox inoculation not against the will of God as the giver and taker away of health and life? Thus this claim/question based again on predestination is repetitive, perhaps purposefully to enforce the fear such a question engendered among religious people for whom this concern strongly resonated. According to Mundungus, the God of the Colonists was a punitive and wrathful God who took vengeance when His parishioners flaunted His will.

His next question was a more charged one and one more difficult to back up: could not the increased mortality rates from smallpox in the town of Boston be blamed on the inoculations?[78] By increased mortality he meant among the citizenry who had been inoculated, had a light case, and then spread it to others. He offered no evidence: numbers, anecdotes, names, etc. Williams answered his own question in the affirmative and listed the following reasons: He set up a cause-effect argument in one of his "Reasons" with evidence again presented using a formal, logical structure of numbered premises.[79] He contended that in the summer months the deaths from smallpox were few, and the variolations were few. In the fall weather and more temperate climate, the number of deaths from smallpox increased at the same time as the number of inoculations grew.[80] His set-up of a cause-effect argument and false equivalence that claimed the increased cases were caused by immunization had ignored the fact that both trends were coincidental or co-relational and not causal; however, setting up it up the way he did could also be very persuasive for his audience. Only six had died of the almost 300 inoculated, and only a couple from smallpox. This number was much, much lower than those that contracted smallpox without having been vaccinated.

As in the example above, some of Williams's claims veered away from religious doctrine, but they concentrated on reinforcing the natural fears of his audience. His second "Reason" in support of his claims was again medical: that the wound made by variolation was worse (and the pustules formed as a result were worse) than those occurring in smallpox in "putrefaction," smell, and length of healing.[81] Boylston's documentation of the cases he followed claimed the opposite: that in fact the pustules were usually less severe, fewer, and lasted a shorter time than those from "natural" infection. Although the cases were local, the results would have been difficult to track for anyone outside the immediate family, as the patients quarantined in their homes or the homes of others who had been inoculated. Because they were not visible to the townspeople, such misinformation could be easily spread and the Anti-Inoculators had been able to claim failure on the part of variolations.[82]

In his next "Reason" in this section of his tract, the Anti-Inoculator challenged Mather and Boylston to produce or publicize the results of their inoculations. The Inoculators sent the numbers of inoculated to London, especially to *The Royal Society*. Because Mather and Boylston were both being threatened with harm, and Mather's home had been attacked, they were loath to share the information. It was possible that they had feared for those who received the inoculations, lest they, too, be attacked. The names of those inoculated were not revealed until Boylston met with physicians in London and his data was published, many months after the vaccinations had ended.

Mundungus's fourth claim was a falsification of the usual outcome of variolation, which he said was

> … drawn from the fatal event that Inoculation hath had on those that have took the Small Pox of them: Where are they? How few are there of those living, that we have reason to think took the Infection of them? Now to save Life, by giving Death for it, it is but a *swapping,* and very dear, though the purchaser may think he hath a good *bargain* (emphasis added).[83]

Williams again falsely reported fatalities among the inoculated. In a fearful populace where death from smallpox was happening to many in the epidemic of 1721–1722, such a false claim had also been persuasive.

With the segue that Williams made in the fourth reason, he turned back to more religious claims in the last two reasons (5 and 6) and conclusion. In his tract, Reason 5 for rejecting inoculation was that it was being practiced amid God-fearing people, and God said he would punish his people for their iniquities. This claim was a strong one, given the colonists' beliefs that regarded disease, drought, and other phenomena as punishments from their god because of their own actions, unhealthy thoughts, or lack of piety. The element of religious dogma for the colonies was continually and effectively reinforced and strengthened by Mundungus's and other Anti-inoculators' arguments through their religious rhetoric.

Reason 6 had drawn on still more Biblical support, in this case from the Old Testament. "Because God is a jealous God; *Deuteronomy 32: 22: They have provoked me to Anger with their Vanities; I will move them to Jealousy*. That is, as we walk contrary to God, so God walks contrary to us."[84] Williams framed his deity as a kind of "tit-for-tat" being, a positioning drawn more closely, as was the Biblical passage, from the view of Jehovah pictured in the Old Testament. His conclusion continued in this vein, calling again on Deuteronomy, the passage in the 28th chapter that was used most frequently by the Anti-Inoculators perhaps because it seemed most germane when writing about smallpox: "*The Lord doth smite them with a Fever, with an Inflamation, and with Spots which cannot be healed; and* as to very many *the Physicians be of no value.*"[85] Now the author had returned to the idea of predestination and that it was the deity that gave illness and death, healing and life, and that humans should not interfere in the mysterious workings of their god, who sends punishments on the parishioners who have sinned and deserve illness. Williams also had advanced the argument that members of the congregation could, if they had survived such a disease, perhaps learn to be better Christians. Suffering in general was accepted by this religious audience as being part of the learning process, so again to interfere would take away the opportunity for Christians to improve their devotion and faith. This close reading of Williams's text in particular, because of its highlighting of religious claims and positioning the inoculation project as contrary to God's law, is very representative of the religious claims the Anti-inoculators were making, and Mundungus/Williams was one of their most frequently published spokespersons. Either the physicians had used Williams to help make these particular claims or his own fervor had happened to have served all of their purposes.

As mentioned above, Williams's use of arguments, questions, and reasons adhered more closely to the use of proof texts in the sermonic discourse of ministers and also the syllogistic scholastic argument structure of the time. These tracts written by a non-academic and almost "illiterate" tradesman in an academic argument style portrayed a clever, rhetorical strategy, not that his use of secular and religious reasons was always consistent. His reasons posed as answers to his questions were not always answers but rhetorical strategies that sometimes did not clearly follow from the argument he had outlined, and there was no dearth of circular arguments. There were also certainly well-framed reasons in the cultural context for rejecting vaccination overall, which would have been the overarching purpose of Williams's publications. Although Mundungus was thought of with less respect and considered to be a colorful character by the *literati* and later critics, his rhetoric was much appreciated by a particular audience at the time and can still be considered representative of the religious rhetoric against the project in its frequent invocations of religious doctrine and religious law, particularly through Biblical citations or proof texts.

He was not the only Anti-Inoculator making these arguments, however. It's also important to note that juxtaposing fears of contagion with *fear* of God's wrath was most obvious in this particular tract, but was also found in others. Samuel Grainger, another Anti-inoculator, also took up the Anti-Inoculators' cause. Grainger was a headmaster of long-standing and was a highly literate Bostonian. He, like Williams, also took up religious arguments against the project. His "The Imposition of Inoculation as a Duty Religiously Considered in a Leter[sic] to a Gentleman in the Country Inclin'd to Admit It … Boston in N.E." was a long tract given exclusively to religious arguments and claims. In it, he echoed many of Williams's premises, "Reasons," or evidence and attacked the inoculation project as being against God's law. Grainger chose one of the same commandments Mundungus highlighted above:

> IT IS LAWFUL TO SAVE LIFE, and a *Duty* incumbent upon us, but the Means us'd for the preservation of mine, must no ways offend or endanger My Neighbours' safety, for it is written, *Thou shalt love thy Neighbour as thy Self.* You have seen (doubtless) what has been offered to the Publick in Defence of *Inoculation* as a lawful Practice, & to enforce it as a Duty.[86]

Grainger was responding here to Mather's resistance to a claim that inoculation was a "duty" that appeared previously in a tract by the Inoculators. This response had perhaps less emotional valence at this point, as it was not juxtaposing fear of their deity's wrath, but debating point-by-point in a more *logos*-centered claim. However, this claim was repeated many times in the various texts of the physicians and other Anti-Inoculators; it was debated back and forth in numerous documents and not just by these two authors, Mundungus and Grainger, against the Inoculators/Ministers.

Because the God of the Puritans was the wrathful one of the Old Testament (although providing "grace" if the sinners repented), other sections of Grainger's tract did call upon some more fearful connections/tenets within the theology for his points. For example, in the following, in which he asked his readers the following question: "When the Almighty sends his Judgments among us to punish and humble us for our Sins, Especially a wasting and Pestilential Distemper, what are the *Means* which may be *lawfully* us'd for our Preservation FROM his desolating Judgments"?[87] Grainger then asked the rhetorical question: "Whether the new method of

Inoculation is a *lawful means* and as such is capable of Relieving us from our *present Calamity.*"[88] The headmaster set this premise up as a "straw man" and quickly followed it with the answer that: inoculation would only be lawful if it is "*Warranted by God's Word.*"[89] Using a formal logical structure, Grainger argued that only God's mercy can relieve or save the people from what he characterized as a "*National Judgment.*"[90] One has only to invoke the common American memory of Jonathan Edwards's "Sinners in the Hands of an Angry God," preached 20 years later in 1741, to understand the fearfulness with which many parishioners in the American colonies regarded their deity.

The jeremiad was pivotal in Grainger's tract and one found frequently in texts of the Anti-Inoculators:

> Examine that [mercy] carefully, I beseech you Sir, and produce if you can, *any other appointed Means* for preventing or removing a *National Judgment*, and then that of a *National Repentance and Reformation.* And I hope you'll allow the best means of deliverance from National Calamities, are those of *Gods Appointment,* not our own.[91]

Like Mundungus, Grainger was positing the wrath of a vengeful God as a major argument against inoculation. The fear of God was quite literal; if one believed that one's sinful thoughts and actions would bring down disease on a whole colony of people and also believed that interference in God's will for punishment could engender even more retribution, then how could such an invasive medical technique be supported or arguments against inoculation be refuted if man tried to take away God's process? The deity sends disease; parishioners increase prayers; then they repent. Only afterwards does the deity offer mercy and the opportunity to be saved.

Such a carefully worked-out dogma and process of thinking on the part of colonists illustrates how power worked and the body was sublimated. While the arguments and claims presented by Williams and Grainger had not been very subtle, the actual personal internalization of the process and the way it works was subtle. The above is one such snapshot of the distributions, mechanisms, reciprocal controls, and adjustments used to garner biopower on the part of church.[92] Given the exigence of the smallpox epidemic and the smallpox inoculation in response, other factors must have indeed appeared to defend against a perceived threat to shore up a reigning religious paradigm and to ward off the incursion of a possible new scientific or medical intervention. Both Anti-inoculators and their rhetorics used the discursive elements in their arsenal in addition to Biblical texts, such as liturgies, histories, theologies, etc. to persuade an audience well-steeped in religious tradition.

It seemed that every minister in Boston had lined up behind the Mathers in support of the inoculation project. However, the degreed doctor against inoculation, Douglass, in addition to some religious arguments in his own texts against the inoculation, also questioned the *number* of Boston's ministers who were involved in supporting inoculation. In the introduction to his tract, "The Abuses and Scandals of Some Late Pamphlets in Favour of Inoculation of the Small Pox ...," Douglass questioned the authority and credibility of the committed ministers by challenging their numbers: "If a Stranger to the Affair were to read their Writings, he could not think other ways than that all the Ministers of Boston are Inoculators, all at Variance with the Practitioners in Physick; in short, that they all are guilty of those Things alledg'd against a few."[93] Douglass supported his point by asserting that "There are in Boston Sixteen Settled Ministers; and of them, Six only are transiently said to have by Subscription insured the Inoculation."[94] Even of those, Douglass insisted only two or three have written in support of the plan—including Increase and Cotton Mather; he didn't take into account Benjamin Colman and William Cooper, both at Brattleboro Church.

He wrote that other ministers were more appropriately "meek" (this "meekness" did not include Increase and Cotton Mather in his view).[95] Once the "appropriate" pastors had found that their congregations were in an uproar, and that ministerial support of inoculation had caused "contentions" among them, the appropriately "meek" ones chose not to further inflame "animosities," according to Douglass.[96] Instead they admitted that because as "Parsons" they were outside of their professional knowledge, if they had opinions on medical matters, they might have indeed been "fallible" in their belief that inoculation was a valid procedure for saving lives.[97] As pointed out above, in the earliest times in the theocratic Colonies, ministerial duties and those of the physician often overlapped; the presence of more medical practitioners in Boston as well as the arrival of Douglass could perhaps be expected to cause a rupture in the tradition of ministers caring for both the bodies and souls of their parishioners.[98]

In addition to religious issues, questions of credibility and expertise in a field arose especially in Douglass's arguments and claims. After first writing against Boylston, he personally attacked Cotton Mather. This new tactic was an expansion of the campaign against inoculation; Douglass was no longer just attacking one in his own profession. Scientific and religious paradigms were being challenged; they were no longer seen as compatible as they had been in earlier times in the Colonies but were beginning to confront each other but not without considerable ironies. The Anti-inoculators more often presented religious arguments, while Cotton Mather and the other Inoculators had been presenting a scientific medical technique and empirical knowledge gained through African lived experience, Royal Society papers, and first-person testimonials. Douglass's arguments were often less centered on scripture than those of his fellow Anti-Inoculators and medical practitioners who served as mouthpieces against inoculation, but he did chastise C. Mather in print for his conduct as a minister and his loyalty to his religion and parishioners. "To compare the difficulties they [Inoculators] meet with, [which they complain about in published letters, etc.] in their Promotion of Spreading of infection, to those our Saviour met with in the propagation of the Gospel, is this not an *Abuse of the Scriptures?*"[99] In addition, Douglass, the leader of the professional opposition, had also written that the doctor, Zabdiel Boylston, was mischievously "propagating the infection in the most Publick Trading Place of the town."[100] He then used a religious call to the ministers to determine "how trusting more the extra groundless Machinations of Men than to our Preserver in the ordinary course of Nature, may be consistent with that Devotion and Subjection we owe to the all-wise Providence of GOD Almighty." He also suggested that legally inoculation could be interpreted as "Propagating of Infection and Criminal."[101] While Williams, Douglass, and some other Anti-Inoculators had earlier given a polite nod to the sincerity of Increase Mather and occasionally to Cotton and other of the Inoculators, Douglass soon forgot his earlier regard for the minister and took on Cotton with a vengeance. It could have been understandable had the degreed doctor's anger against Boylston been fueled by the breaking of ranks by a fellow physician, but it was also clear that he had greatly resented the ministerial interference in his field.

An Inoculator's Refutations: William Cooper's Tracts

One of the ministers that Douglass did not count in his tally of opponents, William Cooper (minister and defender of the Inoculators), in *A Letter to a Friend in the Country: [Re] a Solution of the Scruples and Objections of Conscientious or Religious Nature, Commonly Made Against the New Way of Receiving the Small-pox,* which was his answer to the many tracts against inoculation, outlined and refuted the Anti-Inoculators' religious objections.[102] Some of Cooper's claims directly answered the doctrinal claims of Mundungus above. The ministers needed such refutations to use against religious arguments in order to fight like with like, although Mather's and other inoculators' reliance on African testimonials, the Royal Society's publications, and the microscope stands out in their arguments in support of inoculation. Just like many of the other texts, Cooper's letter was published and circulated widely.

In the first part of Cooper's tract, he acknowledged that like the Reverend Increase Mather, he agreed that those who were conscientious in their real concerns about the good people of Boston deserved to be honored and commended, including the Anti-Inoculators. This move was considered a politeness feature, one also seen in Douglass's tract above and a norm of gentlemanly prose. He had then attacked the false arguments (scruples) of Douglass and the other Anti-Inoculators, characterizing them as "preposterous."[103] Cooper stated his purpose: "... that which you want Satisfaction about is, the *Scruples* and Objections of a *Conscientious* or Religious Nature, which are commonly offer'd by People against this Method [inoculation]. These, I shall endeavour to answer and resolve, as I am able, in a few words; and if they afford you any Light or Satisfaction respecting the same, you may communicate them to whom you please."[104]

As a minister, Cooper had the authority to address those concerns regarding the religious nature of claims being made by the Anti-Inoculators. In addition, because Cotton Mather had been charged with being a "meddler," Cooper set out to draw a very clear linkage to the previous claims and charges: "... and if it should be tho't worth while to make them public, I think none can censure me for starting out my Line, or *medling* with what is none of my Business, since the thing I am now upon relates to *Religion and Conscience*" (emphasis added).[105] Here Cooper, as minister, is affirming that he is perfectly within his area by writing about religion and not medical practice.

Cooper's first refutation took on the claim made by one of the Anti-inoculators that one should not make oneself ill: "That it is not lawful for me to make my self sick when I am well."[106] The Colonists were urged to stay within the laws their deity delivered to them in order to live and flourish, especially in a new country of many dangers. The minister's counter to this claim concerned the Law of Physick as well as religion, that if one made oneself sick (i.e. was inoculated) to ward off a worse case of a serious disease, then that would be "... fitting and Reasonable, and therefore lawful."[107] He gave as evidence other examples of health care practices in the Colonies: "This is every day practic'd among People without any Scruple, in Vomits and Purges, and other things in Medical Use. Now if I may lawfully make my self Sick, by putting something in at my *Mouth*, why not by putting something in at my *Arm*."[108] He also made the case in refuting the argument that he would be "presumptuous" to be inoculated when his neighbors around him were all being "visited" with the "Distemper [smallpox]" naturally and to expect God to save him with "Extraordinary Preservation."[109] He argued that the "Law of Self-Preservation" was also God's law, and that it was through God's blessing that a disease had a remedy.[110] Here one sees the lens revelatory of the early colonists' thought process: in theological debates, issues are weighed through the framing of logical argument and carefully constructed discourse of reasoned prose. This genre was part of the culture and reflected education and class. Most colonists responded to the religious nature of the claims and accepted the dogma because of its regular oral transmission via the ministers' pulpits. The upper classes found this style of discourse easiest to reproduce, and the ministers were more educated than the wider public in that era.

Cooper, as he wrote his refutation, seemed to take these arguments in order of importance or at least frequency, addressing the question frequently posed by the opponents, "Will you not wait God's time?" This religious argument had also been frequently, that to "rush" God, in effect, was to question his judgment and attempt to intervene in the sending of a plague or disease for the punishment of his people. The minister answered this charge in this way: that God's time for sending a remedy was during a time of "imminent and immediate" danger to the people, thus it was indeed "God's time" to subject oneself to inoculation.[111] When also confronted in this part of the refutation with an accusation of a lack of trust in God, Cooper responded: "I suppose every body will allow that Use of Means is not inconsistent with Trust in GOD; and why there can't be trust of GOD in the Use of *this* means as well as other, I can not imagine."[112] This claim uses both logical and ethical appeals and draws a very fine point of distinction for an audience that one had hoped could appreciate the skill with which it had been turned back on itself.

Cooper also alluded to something Mundungus had brought up in his tract above that the dependence on man for healing rather than God was also a dangerous enterprise. Cooper addressed this argument directly: "What then, can't we make use of Men and Means in a time of danger without going from God?"[113] He also wrote that those who are inoculated, and he had been an eyewitness, spent much time in prayer prior to inoculation and after, invoking God's help. He then built a logical scaffold for readers to follow:

> But still some say, this Practice looks to them like *taking God's Work out of His hand.* — Indeed this Distemper can arrest none without a Commission from God. But yet it is not inflicted by God's *immediate hand;* we receive it in a *natural way,* and by means of *Second Causes*; and *this we do in the way of Inoculation,* as well as of common infection. If we have Small Pox in either of these ways, it is still the Work of God. For all Second Causes act under Him the first Cause.[114]

Cooper had carefully parsed the opponents' claims, meeting them point by point and had created a parallel structure that saw the colonists' deity as the "first cause" of all that happens to the parishioners and the inoculation as the "second cause." Making these two "means" of contracting smallpox equal aimed at changing the view of inoculation as outside the laws of God and Physick, and outside of their obedience as subjects.

Cooper addressed this fear even more concretely in his next part of the argument, because the opponents and others thought that if smallpox was a judgment from God sent to punish and humble them for their sins, an evasion of the disease could be interpreted as an affront to the deity. Cooper here used the rhetorical strategy of acceding to the opinion of the majority and creating a commonplace for them: "I fully agree to it, that it is a sore Judgment of God upon us for our Sins, which we have much deserved; …."[115] Then he argued again: "But is it Unlawful to use means for our Prevention against a desolating Judgment? *Especially*, if at the very time that God sends His judgment, He shews us a way to escape the *Extremity* and Destruction at least, if not the Touch of it."[116] Here he's using logic, but not in the very simple syllogisms of Mundungus, but reasoning in an enthymematic format which means that the audience must draw its own conclusions that if God sent both the destruction and means of escape, then clearly the deity intended that his populace use his gift.

Next Cooper extended this point by highlighting gratitude as a response, "If a gracious God shews us so much *Mercy* as this under the Judgment, does it become us to *put it away from our Selves,* or rather should we not accept it with *Adoring Thankfulness?*"[117] There was strong, doctrinal support that along with fearing the wrath of God, the Colonists must also show gratitude to their deity. Lastly, the minister used a simple analogy to further support his main point. He wrote that "If this Town was to suffer an *Inundation,* that would be a more terrible Judgment than this, ...; yet would any refuse to make use of a *Boat,* or a *Plank that might providentially come in his Way,* thinking that to do it would be criminal Evading the Judgment? *I trow not* ... ."[118]

This analogy should have been an effective one, as it was simple and clear.

At the same time these religious people had suffered under the many fears that beset them in a difficult and less "civilized" place, one of the arguments against inoculation was that the method of inoculation "tends to take off the fears of this Distemper from the Minds of the People; and who knows of what Spiritual advantage these fears might be to them?"[119] This argument was also mentioned in the Williams's tract above and was in many of the texts attacking the inoculation project. Fear was regarded as a useful emotion in the religion of the Colonists. If a parishioner was not afraid of getting smallpox, then what difficulty would present itself as an opportunity for faith and deliverance? The power of the church and Crown experienced ongoing rumbles and ruptures; in the case of the smallpox inoculation and this particular epidemic, power was both challenged and reinscribed in various ways. Often a series of what appear to be minor processes make up a new political anatomy especially during a crisis like an epidemic.[120] The fear was thought to impel one to be more religiously motivated in reading the Biblical texts and awaiting deliverance. Cooper's answer to this was to ask if God's Mercy might not also lead the people into sinless behavior after inoculation.[121]

One of the fears in play in the debate continued to be predestination and Mundungus's argument above had maintained that it was against the will of God to inoculate as He alone was the giver and taker away of health and life. Cooper addressed this objection by countering that this argument might as well be brought against the "use of *all Physick, nay even of Food,* against the Practice."[122] His argument repeated his earlier premises used in setting up the first- and second-cause arguments above, so that pattern was one he relied on for thornier questions. Again he used the strategy of first agreeing with the premise, a major tenet of the religion he shared and, as minister, led and taught: "God has predetermined and fixed the Period of everyone's life ...; so that if this time be come, Inoculation will not save the person's life."[123] He suggested that in addition to the deity having "fix'd the Period of every one's Life, he also has done it with a *Regard to Second Causes*, or that course of Nature which He has established; *the End and Means are determined together.*"[124] Then the argument featured a very skillful challenge to the claim that inoculation changed the outcome of one's life. Cooper asked in this part of his response how parishioners knew that the inoculation was not preordained to extend the life of the person to his or her appointed time?[125] He cited as his evidence that conventional means had caused or could not stop death, but they had not been objected to. He listed two cases: one person he knew died of a "Vomit" or emetic treatment, while another bled to death after the simple extraction of a tooth.[126]

Later in the passage he admitted that he, too, had once been of "another mind" toward the project, gaining greater *ethos* or credibility through this confession, but then gave his eyewitness account of those inoculated:

> And for my own part, as much as I am now for Inoculation, I am not at all shy to say, that a Person may miscarry under it; for GOD *is Sovereign,* and will keep us in a Dependence upon Him in the use of all Means … . if one in an hundred should die in this way, while there is a *Demonstration,* … that it is *ten times* as safe as the common way of infection, This I humbly conceive, would be sufficient to justify my going into it.[127]

The minister is saying that if a person's time has arrived coincident with the variolation procedure, that congregant can still die, but those odds, since there were about two in a hundred in this particular vaccination, were superior by far than the much higher death rate if one contracted smallpox naturally. This fact alone, he claimed, would have persuaded him to undergo vaccination (and possibly already had). Eyewitnesses' accounts as support exhibit tremendous strength, and those combined here with the admission that Cooper himself had once been of "another mind" should have also given this part of his refutation great persuasive ability and should have enhanced his own ethos.

In addressing the claim above, he had also brought up another question that could be on a colonist's mind (because dying was a time of religious reflection): what if he might die after the inoculation? Would he not have a particularly "dark" hour knowing that he had brought such an affliction onto himself?[128] He candidly admitted that this question most occupied him in the debate, but that he had reasoned that even if a person died from the inoculation, he would have the satisfaction of knowing that he had used "the most *likely* means … to save his life in a time of common peril."[129] While this claim seemed weaker, because it was framed in effect as doing "due diligence" as a believer, it, too, should have fallen on some sympathetic colonial ears.

Charges of "Illegality" against the Crown

Both the Inoculators and Anti-Inoculators had frequent and different authors and genres of writings going forward to the public and answering each other's claims. In the many letters, tracts, and newspaper articles, inoculation as an "unlawful" practice was raised frequently in another sense, too. In addition to the medical sense of "legal" (a practice lying within the bounds of traditional medicine or "Physick") and the religious sense of "legal" (acting according to God's laws), there were other applications of the law as understood at the time on the part of the people of Boston and the city's officials.

Because Boston was still part of a New World colony and under the protection and law of a Governor from England, the Crown's representative, colonists had been fearful of going outside of English *law* as well as medical and religious "law." Several letters of the Anti-Inoculators, including those written by Williams, addressed going against English law. His first letter was written in response to Increase Mather's tract: *Several Reasons Proving that Inoculating or Transplanting the Small pox, Is a Lawful Practice, and That It Has Been Blessed by God for the Saving of Many a life*[130] and *Sentiments on the Small Pox Inoculated* by an anonymous author, but thought to be written by Cotton.[131] Williams's responses to both of the tracts above were published in October or November of 1721 and advertised in James Franklin's *Courant* at least four times between November of 1721 and January of 1722, indicating the intense response of the Franklins' newspaper, the *New-England Courant.*

In the tract, "Several Arguments, Proving, that Inoculating the Small Pox Is Not Contained in the Laws of Physick," Williams suggested that Mather's invocation of the idea that some of the royalty in England had let the inoculation method be used on their children against the smallpox was not a strong argument for using the method in Boston.[132] This was the Lady Montagu and her Turkish connection to inoculation occurring around the same time as the Boston controversy. Williams again used a Biblical support for his counter claim: "The matter was not disputed by the Pharisees, whether their Children did cast out Devils by *Beelzebub;* the reflection that our Lord cast upon them was, that they did it *unlawfully.*"[133] In other words, Mundungus points out that the Pharisees in Israel had been in support of a certain action of the people, but their deity had castigated the people because the action had been illegal, whether supported by the religious leaders or not. He goes on to argue in this tract: "*The King and the Prince have accepted of it as Means to save the Lives of the Subject:* But yet I remember, they have not proved what you have undertaken to do ... ."[134] The tobacconist's point is that even if church leaders had approved such an action, that is no proof that inoculation was legal. His other use of such terms, *prince* and *king*, was of course slurs on the Mathers. Cotton Mather had been referred to as the Prince in other attacks, and Increase, his father, the King. There was enough anti-monarchy and anti-theocracy in Boston even at this time to make this substitution rhetorically very effective. Williams had delighted in poking fun at both ministers.

Even more to the point of arguing against the authority of the colony and the crown, after Cooper's meeting Mundungus's objections above with religious arguments in response, Williams responded with another tract, this time a 20-page one, in which he answers Cooper: "An Answer to a Late Pamphlet, Intitled, 'A Letter to a Friend in the Country, attempting a Solution to the Scruples and Objections of a Conscientious or Religious Nature, Commonly Made Against a New Way of Receiving the Small Pox.' By a Minister of Boston. Together with a Short History of the Late Divisions Among Us in Affairs of State, and Some Account of the First Cause of Them ...." In this tract, Williams introduced an edict by Queen Anne, as reported by Dr. Robert Richards in the College of Physicians in England. In the Second Act Queen Anne had signed, according to Richards, she had ordered that "if any Doctor, Quack or any other person, shall do anything to spread a mortal or contagious disease, 'they shall suffer death.'"[135] Williams threatened that if someone had done such a thing (inoculated with smallpox in this case) and had been taken to court, he would have found a bill against him (a law enforced in a royal colony) and be put to death in Boston. This quote had been featured very prominently in the book; when Williams wrote the tract, he dedicated it to the Selectmen, but included this threat in the dedication itself. He had also written as part of this dedication, "Now by this Time I hope it appears, that if any Person will be so hardy, as to go on in a Practice against Reason and Law, the Grand Jury will not be at a Loss to find a Bill against them."[136]

With this appeal to English Law, Williams upped the ante in his and his compatriots' war of words against the inoculation project in an attempt to push the Selectmen to put a legal stop to the technique. Framing the inoculation in terms not only of the Law of Physick and God's Law, but of the Queen's Law, was an important device used by the opponents of the procedure to incite fear among the colonists. The colony existed in an often difficult situation vis-à-vis the colonizer. Frequently there were rigorous debates and objections raised to being colonized, long before the revolution itself took place. English laws were still well known by the colonists, Queen Anne's particularly, even after her death. Although she had earlier made laws against dissenters (including Puritans), she had also insured the Protestant rather than Catholic reign, and when there was need for some pressure along political lines, such reference back to monarchical law could be relied upon to instill fear and compliance.

Foucault claimed that a "whole set of regulations," which constituted a register, had been developed by philosophers and physicians who used "empirical and calculated methods relating to the army, the school and the hospital, for controlling or correcting the operations of the body."[137] If one changes philosophers to theologians or theocrats, one sees that the church of the colonials also used their regulations to control the "docile bodies" of the parishioners, especially in earlier times. In Boston the "discipline" of medicine had been divided among a few physicians, surgeons, midwives, herbalists, and apothecaries yet overseen for the most part by the ministers in the absence, except for the Selectmen, of local government or control. Such a formula for domination had reigned for some time in this colony, not so much a disciplinary function of medicine but more of a complete domination by the theocracy and, although there were some exceptions, by the Crown. When Williams made the threat using Queen Anne's edict, he had been calling on the Crown's representative and the Selectmen to exercise their power against the Mathers, a challenge to the previous power elite of the Puritans.

This threat showed that relatively early in the debate the discourse was already a mixture of appeals, on one hand the use of *logos* (emphasis on law, legality, reasoning, and syllogistic reasoning) and *ethos* (who has the authority to speak; who has credibility; who is the good person speaking well). *Pathos*, the emotional appeal in discourse, occurred via the situation itself with fear of contagion, fear of being punished for breaking laws, and fear of the deity's wrath. Although Mundungus's letter was published in July 1721, it was continually circulated (and advertised as noted above) in succeeding months. The fire-bombings and threats, which in reality threatened Mather's, Boylston's, and their families' lives, occurred in November that same year. However, this emphasis on law also served to challenge the authority of the Inoculators, particularly the Mathers, characterized above by Williams as "Pharisees" and royalty: "the King and the Prince." Thus, by invoking the Crown and Queen Anne as authorities, Williams played on the colonial audience's fear of and vulnerability to the English monarchy, another source of control over the bodies, both individual and the body politic.

One (the last shown here) objection that Cooper refuted was "frequently in the Mouths of People—that [inoculation] is originally from the Devil."[138] This claim, too, was a frequent charge of the Anti-Inoculators.[139] There was much more to this particular invocation than meets the eye, however. This fear of the Devil being involved in inoculation was not just the peoples' religious fear of the Devil as a real and cogent influence in their lives, but in addition had invoked Cotton Mather's involvement some 30 years earlier as a young man and activist in the witchcraft trials. Such framing was not accidental, but knowingly invoked even more serious challenges to the variolation project. This topic will be explored in more depth in the next chapter.

Examining the legal and religious arguments leads to real insight into the magisterial and spiritual views of early American predecessors; hearing them debate the pros and cons of inoculation reveals the motivating forces on both sides, as well as how and why the reactions were so charged regarding this new method of disease prevention. The religio/legal arguments had been among the weightiest for and against smallpox variolation. Both sides knew that to use such arguments would enhance the chance of their arguments being accepted, so such framing was well chosen. Among the various reasons given for or against inoculation, in the various texts, the religious and legal ones were the most numerous. These types of claims most directly articulated by the Anti-Inoculators, the majority of whom were physicians or apothecaries and not religious leaders, had been ironic but not unsuccessful. The ministers, the Mathers and others, had used first-person testimonials, Royal Society natural philosophy (scientific letters), and their own scientific investigations, but those arguments often had fallen on deaf ears. However, as strong as religio/legal discourse could be in its persuasive ability, issues of religion and law were not the only reasons for resistance to inoculation, as will be seen in the following chapters.

Notes

1 *A Catalogue of the City: Councils of Boston, 1822–1908, Roxbury, 1846–1867, Charlestown, 1847–1873 and of the Selectmen of Boston, 1634–1822: also of Various Other Town and Municipal Officers*. Accessed 25 November 2012. https://archives.cityofboston.gov/repositories/2/digital_objects/230

2 Zabdiel Boylston, *An Historical Account of the Smallpox Inoculated in New England Upon All Sorts of Persons, Whites, Blacks, and of All Ages and Constitutions: With Some Account of the Nature of the Infection in the Natural and Inoculated Way, and Their Different Effects on Human Bodies: with Some Short Directions to the Unexperienced in this Method of Practice/ Humbly Dedicated to Her Royal Highness the Princess of Wales* (London: Printed for S. Chandler, at the Cross-Keys in the Poultry, 1726); (Boston in N.E.: Re-printed at S. Gerrish in Cornhill, and T. Hancock at the Bible and Three Crowns in Ann Street, 1730), "Appendix," 51–52.

3 *A Catalogue of the City*, 230.

4 Boylston, 51–52.

5 George Lyman Kittredge, "Introduction." *Several Reasons Proving That Inoculating or Transplanting the Small Pox, Is a Lawful Practice, and That It Has Been Blessed by God for the Saving of Many a Life*. By Increase Mather. *Sentiments on the Small Pox Inoculated*. By Cotton Mather (Cleveland, OH: 1921), 10.

6 Selectmen. *New-England Courant* (Boston: Franklin Press, August 15, 1721).

7 Kittredge, 10.

8 Keith Krawczynski, *Daily Life in the Colonial City* (Santa Barbara, CA: ABC-CLIO, 2013), 467.

9 Krawczynski, *Daily*, 467.

10 Academic Partnerships, "Literacy" (Accessed June 7, 2022). https://academicpartnerships.education/brief-history-of-literacy.aspx

11 Krawczynski, *Daily Life*, 467–468.

12 M. Best, A. Katamba, and D. Neuhauser, "Making the Right Decision: Benjamin Franklin's Son Dies of Smallpox in 1736," in *Quality and Safety in Health Care* (December 2007) 16.6, 478.

13 Arneil, Barbara, *John Locke and America: The Defense of English Colonialism* (Oxford: Clarendon Press, 1996), 49.

14 Thomas Kuhn, *The Structure of Scientific Revolutions* (Chicago: University of Chicago Press, 1962).

15 John Chynoweth Burnham, *What Is Medical History?* (Cambridge, UK: Polity, 2005). According to John Chynoweth Burnham, a "stroker" is "the seventeenth-century Irish "stroker" who treated and healed the ill by touching them.

16 Kittredge, 69.

17 Michel Foucault, "The Politics of Health in the Eighteenth Century," in *Foucault Studies*, No. 18, pp. 113–127, October 2014.

18 Michel Foucault, *Discipline and Punish* (New York: Pantheon, 1977), 184.
19 Kuhn, 84.
20 Kuhn, 84.
21 Kuhn, 85.
22 S. E. D. Shortt, "Physicians, Science, and Status: Issues in the Professionalization of Anglo-American Medicine in the Nineteenth Century," in *Medical History* 27 (1983), 53.
23 Shortt, "Physicians, Science, and Status," 53.
24 *Boston News-Letter*, July 24–July 31, 1721.
25 Cotton Mather, *An Account of the Method and Success of Inoculating the Small-Pox, in Boston, in New England* (London: 1722), 12.
26 C. Mather, *An Account of the Method*, 12.
27 Often shortened from *New England Courant* to *Courant* in references.
28 "The Boston News-letter," *Eighteenth-Century American Newspapers in the Library of Congress,* 344 (Boston: Bartholomew Green. August 28, 1721).
29 "The Boston Gazette," *Eighteenth-Century American Newspapers in the Library of Congress,* 280 (Boston: Philip Musgrave. September 4, 1721).
30 This was a common practice of the time, to use a penname and thus remain somewhat anonymous, even as Ben Franklin had written under the pseudonym "Silence Dogood."
31 Kittredge, 12.
32 Kittredge, 3.
33 Boylston, *An Historical Account*, 2.
34 Best, M., D. Neuhauser, L. Slavin, "'Cotton Mather, you dog, dam you! I'll inoculate you with this; with a pox to you': Smallpox Inoculation, Boston, 1721," in *Quality and Safety in Health Care.* (2004). 13.1: 82–83.
35 "Letter." *News-Letter,* 7/24/1721.
36 Kittredge, 13.
37 Gordon W. Jones, "Introduction," to *Angel of Bethesda* by Cotton Mather. (Barre, MA: American Antiquarian Society and Barre Publishers, 1972), xii.
38 I. John Hesselink, "Calvin's Theology." *The Cambridge Companion to Calvin*, ed. Donald K. McKim (Cambridge: Cambridge University Press, 2004), 74.
39 T.H.L. Parker, *John Calvin* (Oxford: Lion Hudson Plc., 1975), 30.
40 Herbert W. Armstrong, *Who's Who in Christian History,* ed. J. D. Douglas with Philip W. Comfort and Donald Mitchell (Wheaton, IL: Tyndale House Publishers, Inc. 1992), 132.
41 Armstrong, *Who's Who,* 132–133.
42 Wilhelm Niesel, *The Theology of Calvin* (Grand Rapids, MI: Baker Book House, 1980), 13–14.
43 Samuel Storms, *Reformation Theology* (Accessed June 2014), https://www.samstorms.com/all-articles/post/whats-your-theology, n.p.
44 Storms, *Reformation Theology.*
45 Parker, *John Calvin,* 97.
46 Niesel, *The Theology of Calvin,* 78–79.
47 Parker, *John Calvin,* 47.
48 Patricia Roberts-Miller, *Voices in the Wilderness: The Paradox of the Puritan Public Sphere* (Tuscaloosa, AL: University of Alabama Press, 1999), 23–24.
49 Roberts-Miller, *Voices in the Wilderness,* 24.
50 Armstrong, *Who's Who,* 131.
51 P. Stearns and George Pasti, Jr., "Remarks Upon the Introduction of Inoculation for Smallpox in England," in *Bulletin of the History of Medicine xxiv* (1950), 106–08.

52 Samuel Storms, *Reformation Theology*, n.p.
53 Barbara Arneil, *John Locke*, 49.
54 Foucault, "The Politics of Health," 114.
55 Richard H. Shryock, *Medicine and Society in America: 1660–1860* (Cornell, NY: Cornell University Press, 1960), 9.
56 C. Mather, *Angel*, 13.
57 Foucault, *Power/Knowledge: Selected Interviews and Other Writings 1972–1977*, ed. Colin Gordon (New York: Pantheon, 1981), 194.
58 M. Best, A. Katamba, and D. Neuhauser, "Making the Right Decision," 478.
59 Arneil, *John Locke*, 49.
60 Michel Foucault, *The History of Sexuality*, trans. Robert Hurley (New York: Random House, 1978), 139.
61 Michel Foucault, "10 January 1979," in *The Birth of Biopolitics*, ed. Michel Senellart (New York: Palgrave Macmillan, 2004), 9.
62 The *OED* also mentions an even earlier meaning from a Spanish term meaning tripe or waste parts of animal entrails. However, the apothecary here was also a tobacconist.
63 C. Mather, "Unpublished Letter to Dr. James Jurin" (Worcester, MA: American Antiquarian Society Archives, 5/4/1723), 14.
64 Kenneth Burke, *Attitudes Toward History* (Oakland, CA: University of California Press, 1984), 166.
65 Kittredge, "Introduction," 27.
66 John Williams (Mundungus), *Several Arguments, Proving, that Inoculating the Small Pox Is Not Contained in the Laws of Physick* (Boston, J. Franklin, 1721), 1.
67 Williams, *Several Arguments*, 1.
68 Williams, *Several Arguments*, 1.
69 John W. Welch, "Biblical Law in America: Historical Perspectives and Potentials for Reform," in *Brigham Young University Law Review*, 3 (2002), 614.
70 Kittredge, "Introduction," 27.
71 Williams, "Dedication," *Several Arguments*, 1.
72 Williams, *Several Arguments*, 2.
73 Williams, *Several Arguments*, 2, my emphasis.
74 Williams, *Several Arguments*, 2.
75 Williams, *Several Arguments*, 4.
76 Williams, *Several Arguments*, 5.
77 Williams, *Several Arguments*, 5.
78 Williams, *Several Arguments*, 5.
79 Williams, *Several Arguments*, 5.
80 Williams, *Several Arguments*, 5.
81 Williams, *Several Arguments*, 5–6.
82 Zabdiel Boylston, *An Historical Account*, 286.
83 Williams, *Several Arguments*, 6.
84 Williams, *Several Arguments*, 6.
85 Williams, *Several Arguments*, 7.
86 Samuel Grainger, *The Imposition of Inoculation as a Duty Religiously Considered in a Letter to a Gentleman in the Country* (Boston, MA: Nicholas Boone, 1721), 2.
87 Grainger, *The Imposition of Inoculation*, 4.
88 Grainger, *The Imposition of Inoculation*, 4.
89 Grainger, *The Imposition of Inoculation*, 4.
90 Grainger, *The Imposition of Inoculation*, 4.
91 Grainger, *The Imposition of Inoculation*, 4.

92 Michel Foucault, "Body/Power" in *Power/Knowledge,* ed. Colin Gordon (New York: Pantheon, 1981), 62.
93 William Douglass, *The Abuses and Scandals of Some Late Pamphlets in Favour of Inoculation of the Small Pox* (Boston: J. Franklin, 1722), 1.
94 Douglass, *The Abuses,* 1.
95 Douglass, *The Abuses,* 1.
96 Douglass, *The Abuses,* 1.
97 Douglass, *The Abuses,* 1.
98 Michel Foucault, *The Archaeology of Knowledge* (New York: Routledge, 1972), 4.
99 Douglass, *The Abuses,* 3.
100 John B. Blake, "The Inoculation Controversy in Boston: 1721–1722," in *The New England Quarterly,* 25, no. 4 (December 1952), 493.
101 Douglass, *News-Letter* (July 24, 1721).
102 William Cooper, *A Letter to a Friend in the Country* (Boston: S. Gerrish, 1721).
103 Kittredge, "Introduction," 33.
104 Cooper, *A Letter,* 3.
105 Cooper, *A Letter*, 3.
106 Cooper, *A Letter*, 3.
107 Cooper, *A Letter*, 3.
108 Cooper, *A Letter*, 3.
109 Cooper, *A Letter*, 5.
110 Cooper, *A Letter*, 5.
111 Cooper, *A Letter*, 5.
112 Cooper, *A Letter*, 5.
113 Cooper, *A Letter*, 5.
114 Cooper, *A Letter*, 6.
115 Cooper, *A Letter*, 7.
116 Cooper, *A Letter*, 7.
117 Cooper, *A Letter*, 7.
118 Cooper, *A Letter*, 7.
119 Cooper, *A Letter*, 7–8.
120 Foucault, *Discipline*, 138.
121 Cooper, *A Letter,* 8.
122 Cooper, *A Letter,* 8.
123 Cooper, *A Letter,* 8.
124 Cooper, *A Letter,* 8.
125 Cooper, *A Letter,* 8.
126 Cooper, *A Letter,* 8.
127 Cooper, *A Letter,* 10.
128 Cooper, *A Letter,* 11.
129 Cooper, *A Letter,* 11.
130 Increase Mather, *Several Reasons Proving that Inoculating or Transplanting the Small pox, Is a Lawful Practice, and That It Has Been Blessed by God for the Saving of Many a life* (Boston: Original Folio Single Sheet, 1721), (Cleveland, OH: 1921).
131 Cotton Mather, *Sentiments on the Small Pox Inoculated* (Boston: 1721), (Cleveland, OH: 1921).
132 Hervé Bazin, *Vaccination: A History from Lady Montague to Genetic Engineering* (Esher, UK: John Eurotext Ltd., 2011), 25.
133 Williams, *Several Arguments*, 7.
134 Williams, *Several Arguments*, 7.

135 John Williams, *An Answer to a Late Pamphlet Intitled, A Letter to a Friend in the Country* (Boston: J. Franklin, 1722), 2.
136 Williams, *An Answer*, 2.
137 Foucault, *Discipline*, 136.
138 Cooper, *A Letter*, 11.
139 Williams, *Several Arguments*, 6.

Bibliography

Academic Partnerships. "Literacy." Accessed June 7, 2022. https://academicpartnerships.uta.edu/articles/education/brief-history-of-literacy.aspx

Armstrong, Herbert W. *Who's Who in Christian History*, ed. J. D. Douglas with, Philip W. Comfort and Donald Mitchell. Wheaton, IL: Tyndale House Publishers, Inc., 1992.

Arneil, Barbara. *John Locke and America: The Defense of English Colonialism*. Oxford: Clarendon Press, 1996.

Bazin, Hervé. *Vaccination: A History from Lady Montague to Genetic Engineering*. Esher, UK: John Eurotext Ltd., 2011.

Best, M., D. Neuhauser, and L. Slavin. "'Cotton Mather, you dog, dam you! I'll inoculate you with this; with a pox to you': Smallpox Inoculation, Boston, 1721" In *Quality and Safety in Health Care*, 13, no. 1 (2004).

Best, M., A. Katamba, and D. Neuhauser, "Making the Right Decision: Benjamin Franklin's Son Dies of Smallpox in 1736" In *Quality and Safety in Health Care* 16, no. 6 (December 2007).

Blake, John B., "The Inoculation Controversy in Boston: 1721–1722" In *The New England Quarterly*, 25, no. 4 (December 1952).

The Boston Gazette. *Eighteenth-Century American Newspapers in the Library of Congress*. 280. Boston: Philip Musgrave, September 4, 1721.

The Boston News-Letter. *Eighteenth-Century American Newspapers in the Library of Congress*. 344. Boston: Bartholomew Greene, July 24–July 31, 1721; August 28, 1721.

Boylston, Zabdiel. *An Historical Account of the Smallpox Inoculated in New England Upon All Sorts of Persons, Whites, Blacks, and of All Ages and Constitutions: With Some Account of the Nature of the Infection in the Natural and Inoculated Way, and Their Different Effects on Human Bodies: with Some Short Directions to the Unexperienced in this Method of Practice/Humbly Dedicated to Her Royal Highness the Princess of Wales*, S. Chandler, at the Cross-Keys in the Poultry, 1726; Boston in N.E.: Re-printed at S. Gerrish in Cornhill, and T. Hancock at the Bible and Three Crowns in Ann Street, 1730.

Burke, Kenneth. *Attitudes Toward History*. Oakland, CA: University of California Press, 1984.

Burnham, John Chynoweth. *What Is Medical History?* Cambridge, UK: Polity, 2005.

A Catalogue of the City: Councils of Boston, 1822–1908, Roxbury, 1846–1867, Charlestown, 1847–1873 and of the Selectmen of Boston, 1634–1822: also of Various Other Town and Municipal Officers. Accessed 25 November 2012. https://archives.cityofboston.gov/repositories/2/digital_objects/

Cooper, William. *A Letter to a Friend in the Country*. Boston, MA: S. Gerrish, 1721.

Douglass, William. *The Abuses and Scandals of Some Late Pamphlets in Favour of Inoculation of the Small Pox*. Boston: J. Franklin, 1722.

Foucault, Michel. *The Archaeology* of Knowledge. New York: Routledge, 1972.

Foucault, Michel. "Body/Power" In *Power/Knowledge*, ed. Colin Gordon. New York: Pantheon, 1981.

Foucault, Michel. *Discipline and Punish*. New York: Pantheon, 1977.

Foucault, Michel. *The History of Sexuality*, trans. Robert Hurley. New York: Random House, 1978.

Foucault, Michel. "10 January 1979" In *The Birth of Biopolitics*, ed. Michel Senellart. New York: Palgrave Macmillan, 2004.

Foucault, Michel. "The Politics of Health in the Eighteenth Century" In *Foucault Studies*, no. 18 (October 2014).

Foucault, Michel. *Power/Knowledge: Selected Interviews and Other Writings 1972–1977*, ed. Colin Gordon. New York: Pantheon, 1981.

Grainger, Samuel. *The Imposition of Inoculation as a Duty Religiously Considered in a Letter to a Gentleman in the Country*. Boston, MA: Nicholas Boone, 1721.

Hesselink, I. John. "Calvin's Theology" In *The Cambridge Companion to Calvin*, ed. Donald K. McKim (Cambridge: Cambridge University Press, 2004).

Jones, Gordon W. "Introduction" to *Angel of Bethesda* by Cotton Mather. Barre, MA: American Antiquarian Society and Barre Publishers, 1972.

Kittredge, George L. "Introduction" to *Several Reasons Proving That Inoculating or Transplanting the Small Pox, Is a Lawful Practice, and That It Has Been Blessed by God for the Saving of Many a Life.* By Increase Mather. *Sentiments on the Small Pox Inoculated.* By Cotton Mather. Cleveland, OH, 1921.

Krawczynski, Keith. *Daily Life in the Colonial City*. Santa Barbara, CA: ABC-CLIO, 2013.

Kuhn, Thomas. *The Structure of Scientific Revolutions*. Chicago: University of Chicago Press, 1962.

Mather, Cotton. *An Account of the Method and Success of Inoculating the Small-Pox, in Boston, in New England*. London, 1722.

Mather, Cotton. "Unpublished Letter to Dr. James Jurin" Worcester, MA: American Antiquarian Society Archives. (May 4, 1723).

Mather, Increase. *Several Reasons Proving that Inoculating or Transplanting the Small pox, Is a Lawful Practice, and That It Has Been Blessed by God for the Saving of Many a life*. Boston: Original Folio Single Sheet, 1721.

Niesel, Wilhelm. *The Theology of Calvin*. Grand Rapids, MI: Baker Book House, 1980.

Parker, T. H. L. *John Calvin*. Oxford: Lion Hudson Plc., 1975.

Roberts-Miller, Patricia. *Voices in the Wilderness: The Paradox of the Puritan Public Sphere*. Tuscaloosa, AL: University of Alabama Press, 1999.

Shortt, S. E. D. "Physicians, Science, and Status: Issues in the Professionalization of Anglo-American Medicine in the Nineteenth Century" In *Medical History* 27 (1983).

Shryock, Richard H. *Medicine and Society in America: 1660–1860*. Cornell, NY: Cornell University Press, 1960.

Stearns, P. and George Pasti, Jr., "Remarks Upon the Introduction of Inoculation for Smallpox in England" In *Bulletin of the History of Medicine XXVI* (1950).

Storms, Samuel. *Reformation Theology*. Accessed June 2014. https://www.samstorms.com/all-articles/post/whats-your-theology

Welch, John W. "Biblical Law in America: Historical Perspectives and Potentials for Reform" In *Brigham Young University Law Review*, 3 (2002).

Williams, John (Mundungus). *An Answer to a Late Pamphlet Intitled, A Letter to a Friend in the Country*. Boston: J. Franklin, 1722.

Williams, John (Mundungus). *Several Arguments, Proving, that Inoculating the Small Pox Is Not Contained in the Laws of Physick*. Boston, MA: J. Franklin, 1721.

3 Echoes of the Witchcraft Trials: The Power of the "Invisible"

Witchcraft Trials and the Microscope

As important as religious arguments were in the debate about the pros and cons of the smallpox inoculation, Mather's reputation and the "Devil" also played large roles. The Anti-Inoculators who played on Mather's past role in the witchcraft trials of the 1690s had been sure that they could invoke some terrible memories for those living in Massachusetts some 30 years earlier. The specter of the horrific events would be strategically resurrected to be used against Cotton Mather's latest project. In addition to the questions of judgment and character, an explication of the language used to describe Mather's microscopy is also important. The trope of "invisibility" served to paint the variolation project with a brush dipped in the spectral evidence of the witchcraft trials in Massachusetts.

The history of Mather's role in publicizing the witchcraft trials almost thirty years earlier in Salem challenged the purpose, wisdom, and validity of the minister's efforts in the inoculation project, thus also affecting his *ethos* in the debate. Toward the end of and after the witchcraft trials, many Massachusetts colonists and clergy realized that their actions had gone far astray. There was some reasonable expectation that the colonists would never again indulge in the same mass hysteria that promulgated the earlier incidents. Yet, in the texts written during the years of the inoculation project, Mather's prior history and reputation were invoked in the memories of those of his generation, now the leaders and most active citizens of Boston and its environs. While in earlier chapters, the Mathers' authority and privilege were emphasized, that's only a part of the complicated picture. Cotton Mather's reputation had been damaged as a young man during the earlier debacle. Some of the language he had used to defend the smallpox project and gain adherents years later was reminiscent of his texts from the witchcraft trial era and reminded Anti-Inoculators of the earlier hysteria even though the minister was now in his 50s. Such reminders raised further alarms in an already frightened populace during an epidemic, and a number of his opponents connected Mather's role in the witchcraft trials directly with the inoculation project.

DOI: 10.4324/9781003312369-4

Because of the emotional valence of the past happenings, to hear similar language in the new project triggered strong, negative, emotional reactions in many of Boston's citizens. A certain term had framed the discourse about the project in a way that made it difficult for the vaccination project to find acceptance. In this case, a "terministic screen" served to include both projects, finding "witches" or evidence of Satanic influence and "germs (little animals"), both *invisible* to the naked eye, while excluding differences between the two. Terministic screens refer to words that act in inclusive and exclusive ways to construct meaning, anchoring a rhetorical understanding of language and its lack of neutrality.[1]

In *Order of Discourse* Foucault illustrated how these underpinnings (or the grammar) of discourse (based on conditions of possibility) enabled social power to work. The theorist found that the regularization of social practices of "appropriation, control and policing" merged with certain principles articulated within the discourse, much in the way social construction works.[2] However, social construction does not articulate its tenets as "policing;" that was Foucault's contribution, particularly in line with his earlier more negative view of the functioning of power. This power should not be thought of as "substantializing" but as "relational."[3] Power itself establishes "certain relationships between heterogeneous elements" and the functioning of those power relations and the conditions within which these connections could take place. Foucault saw the practice then contextualized within a "terrain of operations."[4] In only a certain moment in history, would such human practices be possible and also be only finitely modifiable, rather than infinitely modifiable. In other words, there would be only so many paths that these practices could take given the constraints set up surrounding the possible actions of certain actors within a particular context.

In the Mather project, social relations are highlighted in the discursive practices of the earlier local incident (the witchcraft trials) and the later local episode (variolation). These rhetorics "are implicitly situated as local episodes within a more general history of the political" and made up only part of the resistance to the project.[5] Resistance to power, in some cases, enables a disinheriting of an old "norm" of earlier social practices, in this case the social hysteria of the late 1680s and early 1690s in the Massachusetts colony, which most of the populace had later rejected. The very strong resistance to Cotton Mather's "ideas" and to revisiting what the Bostonians interpreted as a new hysteria was colored by the previous rejection and a reluctance to return to an earlier norm of believing in the "invisible," as spectral evidence had loomed so large during the witchcraft tragedy. Foucault emphasized our need to study the resistance as well as the strength of the particular set of power-relations extant during any period. The project within the hysteria about variolation, where "the field of strategies is the field of conflicts," is so situated as to provide a rich area of study of resistance and the play of certain discursive strategies, including appeals to *pathos*.[6]

The Scene of the Earlier Witchcraft Debacle

Given the purpose of this text centered on the smallpox vaccination debate itself, only a cursory exploration of the history of Salem's witchcraft debacle is possible. However, to further contextualize the earlier disaster, some background is necessary in order to understand Cotton Mather's role in the medical intervention and how his involvement as a young man might have caused further skepticism and a loss of *ethos* for him later in life. It must be remembered that in England alone, for example, around one thousand people suspected of being witches were hanged from about the 1550s to the end of the 1600s. All of them had been suspected of *bargaining* or having some association with the devil. In the English colonies, especially in New England, witchcraft fears figured prominently as part of 17th-century religious practices.[7] Colonists and most of Europe believed in witches and in their minds connected such activity with the belief in a personal Devil that worked on a daily basis in their lives. Colonists also believed that the Devil had bewitched and worked through the witches to cause harm. After the horror of the innocent victims' imprisonment, tortures, and murders, most colonists recoiled from their involvement. Many citizens then simply rationalized that the devil had worked in the "witch finders" and prosecutors to hang harmless people.[8] However, given that another dramatic action arose years later in the same region with some of the same active perpetrators, it was not surprising to find that such terms as *devil, invisible,* and *witchcraft* functioned as persuasive rhetorical strategies when used by the Anti-Inoculators. Both the Mathers (Increase and Cotton) had written and participated in the past incident, although in very different ways. Cotton Mather's prodigious writings and actions had supported the persecutions of so-called witches.

In Mundungus's writings regarding the "legality" of inoculation, he had made a religious argument against the practice that in his view invoked "bargaining" with the devil. Williams challenged the Inoculators saying that maybe inoculations were fatal. "Now to save Life, by giving Death for it, it is but a *swapping,* and very dear, though the purchaser may think he hath a good *bargain.*"[9] Williams invoked fears of death in those inoculated (although none of the ones inoculated at the time had died) by replacing inoculation with "Death," a metonymy. In addition, at this time in the Colonies and particularly after the witchcraft incidents of the 1690s, "bargaining" or "swapping" were terms that invoked deals made with the devil; the idea of selling one's soul to escape death or gaining other rewards had been still very real at this time and particularly for this audience. Using these terms was an effective strategy if one's purpose was to evoke fear and painful memories of other, deleterious "bargains" in the past, as had been accused of the so-called witches. This claim could rekindle a terrible memory in those who had suffered through the witchcraft turmoil.

Many historians and cultural studies scholars have written excellently and at length about the late 1600s' phenomenon and unearthed numerous contributing factors to the tragedy. Some of these factors include, according to Paul Boyer and Stephen Nissenbaum, history of the occult, adolescent psychology, Puritan repression, and cyclic mass hysteria in Western society.[10] Other historians, such as Frances Hill, Peter Hoffer, Carol F. Karlsen, Douglas Linder, Bernard Rosenthal, and others have interpreted the crisis as a class, gender, and/or power struggle through their close readings of court records, tax receipts, census documents, genealogies, and other cultural artefacts. Some of the authors above also found that inheritance laws and their enforcement (or lack of) made women especially vulnerable,[11] and also found discrimination toward Native Americans, Catholics, and the Irish.[12]

When the witchcraft hysteria began, C. Mather had written that adolescent girls had been "led away with little sorceries."[13] Those seemed to include some innocent fortune-telling, including the young girls' seeking to know whom they might marry.[14] Soon followed unusual behaviors among many adolescent and pre-adolescent girls and then grown women and men. At first, when presented with the so-called evidence of witchcraft, including the confession of Tituba and other unfortunate answers and behaviors from other girls and women, Increase Mather himself intervened and had implored that the communities would not use "spectral evidence" to convict "witches."[15] His role was thought by later historians to be a somewhat more positive one than that of his son.

The only conviction Increase Mather ever supported was that of George Burroughs because it had not been founded on spectral evidence (but on other types of physical tests); he himself attended that trial, but it was the only one he attended, and he was not a judge.[16] In addition, Increase Mather not only questioned the lack of empirical evidence (he did value such evidence as confessions), but he also wrote in his *Cases* that the credibility of witnesses had to be taken into account. Thus he largely ignored, as not credible, testimonies of children, although he had not completely renounced the testimonies of the three girls of Salem Village (immortalized in *The Crucible*).[17] He had insisted on evidence to be presented and then had subjected each case to a careful review "with the logical thoroughness and seriousness of the Puritan sermon form."[18] Almost all cases, he had determined, did not stand up under such scrutiny.

At the same time, Boyer and Nissenbaum are careful not to paint Increase "Mather as a lone and heroic figure battling for a return to reason in a society gone mad with witch hysteria."[19] In their view Increase's approach had been much more logical, in that it examined situations rationally, legally, and ethically in an attempt to establish a new paradigm to stabilize a society infected with murders of its own citizens.

> Undeniably too, there were instances of gross injustice—injustice by the standards of the day as well as of our own. But when all this has been conceded, what emerges from the records is the sense of a society, confronted with a tenacious outbreak of a particularly baffling crime at a time of severe political and legal disruption, nevertheless striving, in an equitable way, to administer justice and to restore order.[20]

Thus, in a time when the persecutions, prosecutions, and subsequent murders of innocent women, and men who had been branded as witches were taking place, the judicial system and particularly Increase Mather had been trying to put some brakes on the runaway train.[21] The persecution and hysteria, however, had not been easy to stop.

Increase Mather had been instrumental on a somewhat more positive side of this debacle, while *Cotton* Mather, on the other hand, garnered much blame for being associated *with* the abhorrent practice. Of interest is that on the subject of witchcraft, the son's activities were so different from those of his father, although both father and son believed in the possibility and even probability of witches, as did so many others in America and Europe. Cotton had embraced the persecutions fully, and while present-day scholars can be indebted to him for his prodigious writings, his accounts during the time most likely led to more mischief than amelioration. His detailed and long descriptions of those bewitched or involved in witchcraft were widely read and discussed throughout Puritan New England.

Because the belief in witches was so widespread in Puritan communities, it insured that parishioners were susceptible to manipulation while hiding other agendas. Even small happenings that had transpired in the 1680s and 1690s in colonial Massachusetts without a mention of witchcraft were no longer ignored. Instead there were many attempts to connect disparate happenings, for example a woman's piercing glance when angry at a neighbor, followed two days later by the neighbor's cow's death; this connection would have been reason enough to charge the angry woman with witchcraft. Often these types of connections were successful in further increasing the vulnerability of the villagers of Salem, as each incident fed on the previous one. The framing of each event was all important, and if each incident was framed as evidence of satanic activity, the cumulative effect grew. Like social media, villagers were eager to have a story, invent their own narrative, so that they could add their testimonial to the greater whole. Thus they were using the lens of witchcraft, even as Mather used his microscopic observances as a lens to see a possible cause of illness, to see feuds, slights, losses, etc., as evidence of devilish behaviors affecting their lives.

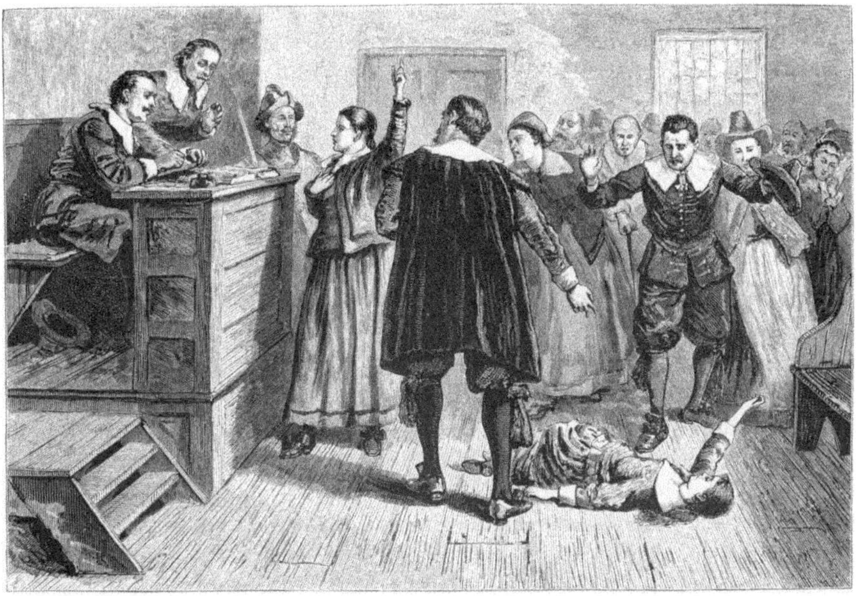

Figure 3.1 Witchcraft Trial of Mary Walcott, Public Domain.

Memorable Providences and Wonders of the Invisible World

Mather's first witchcraft text, *Memorable Providences, Relating to Witchcrafts and Possessions* was a bestseller in 1689, detailing, among others, an episode of supposed witchcraft a year earlier involving the Irish washerwoman, Ann Glover.[22] Mather had introduced into his text the widowed woman, the most usual subject of accusation during the Salem witchcraft trials, although it's not clear she had much property. However, her holdings could have been tied up in the courts. Much research has been done to show that often widowed women who owned the properties of their deceased husbands had been targeted with accusations of witchcraft to wrench their property from them in the avaricious land grab taking place in the colonies at the time; however, the situation is more complicated according to Karlsen, who tracked the economic situation of many of the victims. For example, she found that the wider inheritance laws were most important in the formulation of accusations and not just those for widows.[23] Economic considerations, then, do appear to have been at work in the New England witchcraft cases. But the issue was not simply poverty—or wealth—of the accused witches or their families. It was the special position of most accused witches vis-à-vis their society's rules for transferring wealth from one generation to another.[24] Although there were rules of inheritance in place, ones that could award widows with real property, there were also several ways that magistrates could manipulate the situation to make it impossible for women to get their inheritance. This was especially true when widows had only daughters (no sons) and " … the women who stood to benefit economically also assumed a position of unusual vulnerability."[25] At the same time, it should be noted that the first accusation of witchcraft by the two young girls in Salem had been made against the Parris's enslaved woman, who had no means and no inheritance.

Those in power at the time and seeking to maintain their power were the Puritan and Congregationalist ministers, the Mathers, and others. They were male and the power elite. Yet Mather did not frame the arguments he made regarding witchcraft in any way that acknowledged the power situation, although by its very nature those persecuting the victims had ultimate power. Instead he wrote very dramatic descriptions that he, in his twenties, found persuasive and popular to an audience and were framed in ways to perhaps provide a channel of resistance to the very straight jackets of Puritan behavior that he preached on Sundays in two 90-minute sermons. Yet these *pathetic* appeals to an audience that was vulnerable to old superstitions, which the young Mather (he was in his twenties in the 1680s and early 1690s) also believed, had been effective. He also wrote about and supported the continuance of power within his own class and profession, although at a later age. He had been perhaps also an unwilling or unconscious player/actor within the apparatus that had long ago been set up and had survived via frequent reinforcement of biased social norms by such writers of compelling arguments as he had been.

In fact, Cotton Mather had become one of the main instruments of operation within the event. The courts, the townspeople, the accusers, the victims, the ministers, all had operated or been operated upon through discourses and institutions in the effort to reinforce religion and "control" or "police" behaviors of the docile bodies of the citizens.

Also in his first text on witchcraft, *Memorable Providences …*, Mather had articulated his commitment to the reality of witches and witchcraft, reinforcing his *ethos* at that time:

> I was my self an Eye-witness to a large part of what I tell; and I hope my neighbours have long thought, That I have otherwise learned Christ, than to ly unto the World. Yea, there is, I believe, scarce any one particular, in this with which any man that shall go to impose. The things of most Concernment in it, were before many Critical Observers; and the Whole happened in the Metropolis of the English America, unto a religious and industrious [people] … I shall count that man Ignorant who shall suspect, but I shall count him down-right Impudent if he Assert the Non-Existence of things which we have had such palpable Convictions of.[26]

Mather had articulated his commitment to the reality of witches and witchcraft, imagining that he was reinforcing his *ethos*.

In some cases, Mather had not only forwarded reports from his personal observations of the first girls of Salem Village, Betty Parris, and Abigail Williams, to the magistrates but also examined the suspected perpetrator, Tituba, the Parris family's enslaved woman, testing her and evaluating her himself, then sending out his observations again. In this way, he had become one of the main instruments of operation within the event. Perhaps as a young man, he was also seeking to prove his own place in the social order, although conceivably it had already been cemented by his family, education, and profession.

Clearly we can see the functioning (acts) of the courts, the townspeople, the accusers, the victims, the ministers, all operating through both discourses and institutions. We see the functioning of the laws, both of the church and the government, religious tenets and philosophies, and Puritan regulations regarding behaviors, especially of women, but of men, too, particularly those who could not "control" or "police" their own women. Part of the apparatus was discrimination because that is learned behavior, biases, and prejudicial practices communicated to and passed on to community members.

Early in *Wonders of the Invisible World* (1693), Mather's second text on witchcraft, there are many sermonic passages about the devil and "his" effect on the colony. It's clear that preaching against the devil had been very much a part of the ministerial duties. The practices of Satan had then been more easily interpreted in the actions and behaviors of the accused witches. Given the hardships of the earliest colonists in this part of the Americas and the belief system within the religion, there was much paranoia about the devil at work in New England and the need to please their God in order not to empower the devil. As Mather gives a brief history of his own colony, he writes:

> There is a *little room* for hope, that the *great wrath* of the Devil, will not prove the present ruine of our poor *New-England* in particular. I believe, there never was a poor Plantation, more pursued by the *wrath* of the *Devil*, than our poor *New-England*; and that which makes our condition very much the more deplorable is, that the *wrath* of the *great God* Himself, at the same time also presses hard upon us. It was a rousing *alarm* to the Devil, when a great Company of English *Protestants* and *Puritans*, came to erect Evangelical Churches, in a corner of the World, where he had reign'd without any controul for many Ages; and it is a vexing *Eye-sore* to the Devil, that our Lord Christ should be known, and own'd, and preached in this *howling Wilderness*. Wherefor he has left no *Stone unturned*, that so he might undermine his Plantation, and force us out of our Country.[27]

In addition to sermonizing and elaborating on the work of the devil, Cotton Mather had access to all the trial records of the happenings in his colony. *Wonders* was written after the witchcraft trials in New England, and Mather not only documented those cases, but added witchcraft trials and horrors from Europe, Scotland, and England. He incorporated other sources and experiences into his book. As Mather had articulated his commitment to the reality of witches and witchcraft, he must have imagined that he was reinforcing his *ethos*. Had witchcraft needed a publicist, Mather could not have been more skilled at popularizing and keeping the issue in front of the people of Massachusetts.

Because Cotton Mather had clearly gone to some pains to establish himself as an expert in the area of witchcraft during the events of the late 1600s, an association of him with the horrendous happenings of the time would have been very natural among the people of Boston. In addition, his associates had also been very much involved in the ordeal. According to Douglas Linder, "three of the five judges appointed to the Court of Oyer and Terminer that would hear the Salem witchcraft trials were friends of Mather and members of his church," presumably William Stoughton, Major John Richards, and Samuel Sewall. Unlike his father, Increase, C. Mather had advised the three judges, and in particular, John Richards to give consideration to spectral evidence, giving it, in fact, such weight as "it will bear," thus contradicting his more prudent minister/father.[28]

As the trials began and continued through 1692, Cotton Mather delivered a sermon on August 4 of that year, warning that the Last Judgment was near and that he and other community leaders were leading a battle against the Devil and his minions.[29] On August 19, Cotton had, like his father, attended the execution of ex-minister, George Burroughs. However, on Gallows Hill, Burroughs had recited the entire Lord's Prayer, a recitation that had been thought impossible for witches. A number of spectators asked for the execution to be stopped, but C. Mather had intervened and insisted that Burroughs, convicted by a jury, be killed.[30] Mather's book, *Wonders of the Invisible World,* was based on the official records of the Salem trials, which were given to the minister/writer by the judges who hoped Mather would write at length extolling their (the judges') virtues.[31] In this text, the author, C. Mather, had written "an account of seven of the trials at Salem, compar[ing] the doings of the witches in New England with those in other parts of the world, and add[ing] an elaborate dissertation on witchcraft in general."[32]

William Stoughton, the chief judge and a wealthy politician, in a letter after receiving the Mather manuscript, *Wonders,* urged that it be printed, and he expressed "Obligation and Thankfulness" for Mather's "so great Pains."[33] After confessed witches had begun to recant previous testimony, C. Mather might have started to doubt himself. He began to change his own position on the use of spectral evidence to match his father's stance and attempted to no avail to minimize his considerable personal role in the trials. Later in life, certainly by the time of the inoculation project, some thirty years later, he had turned away from the supernatural and perhaps even questioned his own earlier observations.[34] It might be worth noting that the unguarded enthusiasm which C. Mather had for the witchhunt might have been more typical of a 25-year-old and, as a 57-year-old with much more life experience during the variolation project, perhaps the world had looked quite different to him. In fact, it looked somewhat different to him after just four years, although he was his usual contradictory self.

Although in C. Mather's first text, *Memorable Providences, Relating to Witchcraft and Possessions,* detailing the witchcraft activities and declaring the validity of his own observations and personally urging the execution of the Widow Glover and Burroughs, by 1693 in *Wonders,* he was singing another tune: "For my own part, I was not Present at any of Them [the trials]; nor ever Had I any personal prejudice at the persons thus brought upon the Stage; much less at the Surviving Relations of those persons, with and for whom I would be as Hearty a mourner as any man Living in the World: … ."[35] It was possible of course that he had not been at any of the trials, although other sources maintain otherwise, but would had advised judges, attended at least the one execution cited above, as well as been on hand for examining Widow Glover before her execution. Because he had received many of the court documents, Mather further averred that he could "do no other than shortly Relate the Chief Matters of fact, which occurr'd in the Trials of some that were Executed … . I have only singled out Four or Five [trials], which may serve to Illustrate the way of dealing, wherein Witchcrafts use to be concerned; and I Report matters *not as an Advocate but as an Historian*"(emphasis added).[36] This language and the establishment of *ethos* here was markedly different from the previous text on witchcraft. He had backed off of wanting to be an authority, leader, and advocate of the persecutions and prosecutions, at this point in the text claiming just the authority of reporter, historian, or chronicler, exhibiting the *ethos* of a more disinterested party, some uninterested observer. His rhetorical strategy and the declaration of his purpose *seemed* to have changed very abruptly.

What is confusing, though, is that although Mather says he had no advocacy role, he also seemingly contradicted himself in his continued fervor in this same text as shown in some of the previous quotations and in: "I have indeed set my self to Countermine the whole Plot of the Devil against New-England, in every Branch of it, as far as one of my Darkness can comprehend such a Work of Darkness."[37] Silverman had earlier pointed out the contradictory nature of Mather's addresses throughout his life, a kind of waffling or wanting-to-have-it-both-ways style of writing and speaking, which incited Mather's peers to refer to him as the "ambidexter." In some of his writings, Silverman identified the minister's tendencies as causing historians to accept contradictory views of his opinions.[38] In this case, Cotton may have wanted to make clear to an audience that he was vigorous in leading a righteous life as a minister, as one could ill afford to be perceived as being "soft" on the Devil. At times his tone displayed peevishness, and he displayed both anger and pique at his treatment by others. His audience could also have needed the reassurance in such a charged time. "A certain degree of reaction ... appeared to be taking place, and the magistrates who had conducted the proceedings had begun to be alarmed, and to have some doubts of the wisdom of their proceedings. Cotton Mather was called upon by the governor to employ his pen in justifying what had been done; ... "[39]

Mather had a different purpose in mind as he had written these two lengthy works on witchcraft. In addition, in Mather's positioning himself as protector, righteous minister, and historian so carefully, he in this text made it clear to his readers that he had still another audience, not just the local one:

> I may add, that I have herein also aimed at the Information and Satisfaction of Good men in another Countrey, a Thousand Leagues off, where I have, it may be, More, or however, more Considerable Friends, than in My Own; And I do what I can to have that Countrey, now as well as alwayes, in the best Terms with My Own.[40]

Mather is referring here to England and the Royal Society. It was very important to Mather to be highly regarded by Society members, which brought him no small ridicule by Bostonians during the smallpox inoculation debate.[41] During Mather's own visitations with Angels, which Silverman described at some length, one of them had promised Mather a broad reach, "Explaining Ezekiel's prediction of the '*greatness, in the Length of his Branches,*' as referring to the books Mather would publish not only in America, but also in Europe, the angel in effect promised him a transatlantic penis."[42] Note that he also had not found favor with his own friends, claiming that he had more friends abroad. "More, or however, more Considerable Friends," insulted his colleagues in Boston and the environs, who might have suddenly viewed themselves as not thought of as "considerable" or of as high a status as Mather's friends abroad. While his claim might have been quite honest, it could be seen as being somewhat peevish, too. This statement hints to us that Cotton Mather had gotten some criticism for his involvement in the witchcraft debacle.

Mather continued his lengthy statement of purpose and explanation of his own positioning:

> But while I am doing these things, I have been driven a little to do something likewise for My self; I mean, by taking off the false Reports and hard Censures about my Opinion in these matters, the Parters Portion, which my pursuit of Peace has procured me among the Keen. My hitherto Unvaried Thoughts are here Published; and, I believe, they

> will be owned by most of the Ministers of God in these Colonies; nor can amends be well made me, for the wrong done me, by other sorts of Representations.[43]

In this passage his tone increased in peevishness, and he displayed both anger and pique at treatment by others, showing that at the ages between 25 and 29, he had indeed become a controversial figure, an identification that stayed with him throughout his life, although he had supporters, too. The past seemed to have also had an impact on his ability to reach people with the new medical intervention he most wanted to deliver to them. He ended the passage on the note of some hopelessness, saying that he had realized that he himself could not be successful in changing the views of others toward him through his own efforts, even in his new work on witchcraft.[44]

The first trial he had written about in *Wonders* was that of George Burroughs, who had been accused by nine people of feats of strength and extraordinary lifting. There had apparently been enough testimonies gathered against Burroughs for those feats plus other unspecified charges that he had "qualified" for being labeled as a witch.[45] Those "victims" who had felt bewitched by him, had testified that they had been tortured every day by "*Invisible* Hands," presumably belonging to the "specters" of Burroughs.[46] Mather had written that these ideas could not possibly have been made up or invented, and victims believed he (Burroughs) was attempting to kill them.[47]

Although Mather's disclaimer at the beginning of *Wonders* had suggested he was not an observer or participant and was simply a "historian in his detailed accounts of the trials, he had narrated the trial not in full as an exchange of questions and views, but as a litany of details against the accused." For example, those tormented had claimed to have teeth marks showing in their skin after being beset by Burroughs's specters and Mather insisted in his text that those marks "could be distinguished from those of some other men's."[48] Burroughs had claimed at the end of his trial as part of his defense that there was no such thing as a witch and for the authority on such a claim, he had quoted a text that he had pulled from his pocket, which Mather recognized as having been written by Thomas Ady, an author and English Catholic very skeptical about the existence of witches. Ady's work had boldly taken to task the Catholic Church and its persecution of "witches;" he had been one of the few brave enough to make such claims in 1656.[49]

In neither edition were Burroughs's exact words at the trial found, but a number of ministers and lay people had been familiar with the arguments advanced there; Mather had felt Ady's arguments against witches had generated enough skepticism to possibly threaten the exoneration both he and the judges had hoped to receive through the publication of his *Wonders of the Invisible World*.[50] Thus Cotton had chosen to mention Ady in

Wonders ... in reference to the paper Burroughs pulled out of his pocket. The accused

> Only gave in a paper to the Jury; wherein, altho' he had many times before granted, not only that there are Witches, ... yet he now goes to evince it, That there neither are, nor ever were Witches, that having made a compact with Divel, can send a Divel to Torment other people at a distance. This paper was Transcribed out of Ady; which the Court presently knew, as soon as they heard it.[51]

Earlier as a minister who eschewed such long prayers, sermons, and the norms of the Puritan ministry, and then as an accused man who did not believe in witches and had a source to back him up, Burroughs showed strong resistance to the theocratic authorities.

Although Mather had obtained the trial records, the judges had at first been reluctant to release them to him. As mentioned above, some authors believed the judges wanted to be exonerated by Mather's text, and yet there seemed to have been second thoughts about the whole enterprise by the judges. So Mather's purpose more and more appears as an attempt to regain his own authority and credibility. As a result, Mather reported on a relatively small number of cases out of the hundreds arrested. Reading some of the original documents of the trials, one could quickly understand that there were very many more people brought to trial than ultimately executed.[52] But all the cases C. Mather did report were in such detail, there was a sense of the author's possible fascination with witchcraft. Often conclusions he made did not fit with his stated role as a mere "historian." Perhaps instead, then, his purpose of gaining *ethos* as an honorable and impartial historian fell short of the mark. Mather's fascination as evidenced in the text itself further reinforced the earlier view of him as an impassioned advocate, unable to resist being drawn in again to the witchcraft drama. As noted on the chapter on religion, however, whenever there was a concurrence with religious beliefs and local practices, there seemed to have been more willingness to accept non-logical proofs. In the case of the witchcraft trials, much of the acceptance settled on the invocation of the Devil. The trials and persecutions finally ended, and in 1692, Martha Corey was the last innocent woman to be hanged.

Mather's "Curiosities"

In *Wonders of the Invisible World,* Mather wrote a section that he called "Curiosities;" these musings are of great interest, and, in fact, "curiosities" 300 years later helps in understanding some conflation by his opponents of Mather's extensive writings on witchcraft with his interest in some new process of inoculation or variolation. In "*Curiosities*" (he lists four), in a rare style shift, Mather asked a number of rhetorical questions based on charges the accusers had made. His questions concerned the actions those accused of consorting with the devil were supposed to have executed:

> "What is their striking down with a fierce Look? What is their making of the Afflicted Rise, with a touch of their Hand? What is their Transportation thro' the Air? What is their Travelling in Spirit, while their Body is cast into a Trance? ... What is their Entering their Names in a Book? What is their coming together from all parts, at the Sound of a Trumpet? ... *What is their Covering of themselves and their Instruments with Invisibility*?"[53]

Mather's "Second Curiositie" was again this **invisibility**, on which he dwelt at length. *Invisibility* had become a trope throughout the period of witchcraft fascination and was deeply embedded in the colonists' experience; how could a person whose life is centered around religion and the "invisibility" of the spirit and of a god's intervening in one's life not believe in another form of spirit? In fact, the "spectral evidence" that C. Mather had supported and that I. Mather had not, was the combination of invisible visitations, violent actions by invisible actors, etc. The witches (and devil) themselves had been characterized by this same invisibility as the actions of those possessed have illustrated. Mather had written:

> In all the Witchcraft which now Grievously Vexes us, I know not whether any thing be more Unaccountable, than the Trick which the Witches have, to render themselves and their Tools *Invisible*. Witchcraft seems to be the Skill of Applying the Plastic Spirit of the World unto some unlawful purposes, by means of a Confederacy with Evil Spirits. Yet one would wonder how the Evil Spirits themselves can do some things: especially at *Invisibilizing* of the Grossest Bodies. I can tell the Name of an Ancient Author, who pretends to show the way, how a man may come to walk about *Invisible,* and I can tell the Name of another Ancient Author, who pretends to Explode that way.[54] ... The notion of procuring *Invisibility*, by any Natural Expedient yet known, is, I Believe, a meer Plinyism;[55] ... (emphasis added).[56]

In this section, Mather contributed many examples in which "Spectres," also invisible, had teased, tormented, and annoyed victims. He had cited these stories as proofs and to make visible the invisibility.[57]

Although Mather had claimed to have written *Wonders of the Invisible World* as an objective "historian," he had not been able to refrain from writing about the spectral/invisible "evidence" in compellingly rich detail in spite of his father's warning. He had also not been able to restrain himself from writing his "Curiosities," which amounted to further justification for the executions. His texts on witchcraft, although written as a younger man, still marked him in the minds of the colonists, although certainly not the only one nor the most blameworthy, perhaps, but certainly as one intimately involved in the crisis and writing to justify the abhorrent actions of the judges who later sought absolution. All the incidents during the time of the witchcraft trials would later be repudiated by most of the colonists.

A period of self-examination began in the colony following the release of those surviving colonists who had been accused of being witches (of the 100–200 in all who had been accused and imprisoned). By December 1696, one of the judges, Samuel Sewall, issued a public apology for his role in the witchcraft trials, although it took a number of years for the changes in attitude to occur.[58] In addition, Sewall wrote a proclamation for a day of fasting, repentance, and even reparation by the government for their individual and collective sins during the witchcraft trials. Each year after 1697, the judge continued to set aside a day for his own prayer and fasting, during which he asked for forgiveness for his sins of participation in the Salem trials. A number of jurors also came forward to confess that they had been "sadly deluded and mistaken" in their judgments.[59] Others had not been as honest or generous and had either blamed others or just refused to accept blame or apologize.[60]

The Trope of Invisibility and the Inoculation Project

Mather had framed his discourse on witchcraft in both texts using the terms *invisible, invisibility,* and even *invisibilizing* over and over again. In his second witchcraft text, *Wonders* … , he documented the many cases of spectral evidence in the list here: "and the houses of the good people there are filled with the doleful shrieks of their children and servants, tormented by *invisible* hands, with tortures altogether preternatural"[61] "I will venture to say thus much, That we are safe, when we make just as much use of all Advice from the *invisible* World, as God sends it for;"[62] "The people thus afflicted, are miserably scratched and bitten, so that the Marks are most visible to all the World, but the causes utterly *invisible*; and the same *Invisible* Furies do most visibly stick Pins into the bodies;"[63] "They appear'd in *Spectre* then to Torture those that were before their Fellow-Sufferers;"[64] "The *Witches* which by their covenant with the Devil, are become Owners of *Spectres*, are oftentimes by their own *Spectres* required and compelled to give their consent, for the molestation of some, which they had no mind otherwise to fall upon;"[65] "In the Prosecution of these Witchcrafts, among a thousand other unaccountable things, the *Spectres* have an odd faculty of cloathing the most substantial and corporeal Instruments of Torture, with Invisibility, while the wounds thereby given have been the most palpable things in the World;"[66] "Sufferers assaulted with Instruments of Iron, wholly *unseen* to the standers by;"[67] "She one Day caught an *Invisible Mouse*, and throwing it into the Fire, it Flash'd like to Gun-Powder. None besides the Child saw the *Mouse*, but every one saw the *Flash*."[68] These are just a few examples from the second text. Becoming the reporter and documentarian of such events that were later strongly repudiated by the citizens of Salem and Boston had eventual repercussions for the minister, who had been so industrious a chronicler in his early twenties and throughout his life.

While many renounced their involvement in the witchcraft trials, others did not and one cannot assume that superstition and beliefs in the supernatural were no longer any part of the culture of Boston and other areas of Massachusetts (and other colonies) in 1722. In fact, in the Franklins' paper: *The Courant,* the following account appeared in the March 26–April 2, 1722 issue: "This last Winter there was a Women dy'd at Narraganset of the smallpox, and since she was buried, there has appeared upon her Grave chiefly, and in various other Places, a bright Light, as the Appearance of Fire. This Appearance commonly begins about 9 to 10 of Clock at Night, and sometimes as soon as it is dark."[69] The description of the phenomenon suggested that

> It appears variously as to Time, Place, Shape and Magnitude, but commonly on or about the Grave, and sometimes about ... the barn and adjacent Trees; sometimes in several Parts, but commonly one entire Body ... When it is at the Highth, they can see Sparks fly from the Appearance like Sparks of Fire, and the Likeness of a Person in the midst wrapt in a Sheer with its Arms folded."[70]

This specter was certainly indicated that some readers would be interested in and continue to believe in the supernatural. In addition, this apparition had been described as having magical powers: "This Appearance moves with incredible Swiftness, Sometimes the Distance of half a Mile from one Place to another in the Twinkling of an Eye. It commonly appears every Night, and continues till Break of Day. A Woman in That Neighbourhood says she has seen it every Night for these Six Weeks past."[71] Belief in the supernatural appeared to be alive and well in Massachusetts.

Mather's connection with witchcraft and his earlier zeal for the outings, trials, and executions of witches continued to be part of the common knowledge of his past. When Mather then had begun to talk about the inoculation project, that earlier history haunted his attempts to introduce a measure of protection against a horrendous disease because of how he wrote about his microscopic observations of phenomena not visible to the naked eye. Mather's earlier writings and the trope of *invisibility* functioned unconsciously and then rhetorically as one of the several factors marshaling bias against his intervention in the smallpox epidemic in Boston. The minister had multiple sources for the procedure itself, but when he wrote about his use of the microscope and the observations he recorded, he used similar terms of invisibility to describe what he saw, as what he was seeing was always *invisible* without a microscopic lens. This discourse and the invisibility trope used in the inoculation controversy had become conflated with his support of what had been an erroneous belief in witchcraft and the putting to death of nineteen innocent victims.

Mather had written in the chapter on smallpox in *Angel of Bethesda*, "It begins now to be Vehemently Suspected That the Small-Pox may be more of an Animalculated Business, than we have been generally aware of. The Millions of—which the Microscopes discover in the Pustules, have Confirmed the Suspicion."[72] The blank illustrated that Mather had no term for what he was seeing in his microscope. These bacteria that the Puritan minister might have seen would not have been the smallpox virus because microscopic lenses at the time were too coarse to see it, but nevertheless what he observed were some type of *animalculae* (little animals in Latin) that he characterized as *invisible* to the naked eye. When Mather wrote and spoke about his findings with his parishioners, other ministers, and citizens of Boston, he had explained what he had seen when looking through his microscope in those terms. Those that read or had heard the terms at best thought his descriptions implausible and ludicrous, but at worst they heard such references to invisible tiny animals as more sinister.

A number of Anti-Inoculators, both named and anonymous in various texts, connected his fascination with the previous wonders of the invisible world (e.g. devilish activities, apparitions, "Spectres," and invisible attacks and tortures) to his present fascination with the new wonders of an invisible world inside a smallpox pustule. Silva evoked Breen's more theological reading of the connection of the invisibility of the germs that Mather thinks he sees via the microscope. He saw the analog of the invisible physical world with the invisible spiritual world of the Puritans (159). While this is somewhat obvious, the invisibility arguments of the inoculation controversy also strongly reflect the witchcraft connection of Cotton Mather, which had not been previously explored.[73]

After Cotton Mather had begun to fight back in letters and various tracts against those attacking the inoculation project in print and literally attacking his home with a firebomb, the *Courant* featured this "conversation" between clergy (*Cler.*) and laypeople (*Laym.*) in a January 1722 issue:

Cler: I would have the Blame center on the Guilty; and then I am sure it will not all fall on the Clergy.

Laym: I pray Sir, Who have been Instruments of Mischief and Trouble both in Church and State, from the Witchcraft to Inoculation? who is it that takes the Liberty to Villify a whole Town, in Words too black to be repeated? Who is that in common Conversation, makes no Bones of calling the Town a MOB? and whose Disciple is he who has lately done the same?

Cler: But you must not Condemn all because some are Imprudent.[74]

When the Layman asked "who have been Instruments of Mischief and Trouble," the author was referring to the Mathers, particularly Cotton. The minister had recently released texts that called the citizens of Boston a "mob" for attacking his home in November 1721, as well as threatening Boylston. Boylston and the other Inoculators had also written in defense of Cotton's scientific explorations and condemned the violence used against them.

Like the Franklins, Douglass, John Williams (Mundungus), and other Anti-Inoculators made the connection between the witchcraft history and the inoculation project in their "An Answer to a Late Pamphlet," although it was published with only John Williams as the author. He wrote that it was the devil who devised the inoculation to destroy the bodies of Christians and capture their souls.[75] In one such connection Mundungus had written:

> I do seriously believe its [inoculation is] a Delusion of the Devil; and there was never the like Delusion in New-England, since the Time of the Witchcraft at Salem, when so many innocent Persons lost their Lives, and afterwards some of them that were instrumental in taking their Lives away, made a Recantation.[76]

Williams et al claimed to believe that the devil had duped the prosecutors and deluded those who were intent on executing the "witches," just as the Devil was now deluding the Mathers, Boylston, and the other Inoculators. Mundungus had already been a very effective spokesperson for the Anti-Inoculators, and his rhetoric here would have been persuasive particularly with those Bostonians outside the intelligentsia, while Douglass weighed in to influence the more educated audience.

The Scottish doctor confirmed the idea of Mather's involvement in the two misbegotten projects: the execution of innocent people accused of witchcraft and the killing of innocent victims by variolation. In addition, Douglass, in one of his missives, had included in the list of Mather's dangerous misdeeds a third one in reference to the Quakers:

> All *Countrys*, or Bodys Politick, (our own Mother Country not excepted) have been subject to *Infatuations*: These in this Country seem always to have proceeded from some of those who call themselves *Sons* of *Levi*. The *Persecution of the Quakers* about the year 1658, the *hanging of those suspected of Witchcraft*, about the year 1691, Etc. and *Inoculation*, or *Self-procuring* the *Small-Pox*, in the year of 1721.[77]

Kittredge maintained that James Franklin wrote the introduction to this letter; the letter definitely had come from Franklin's press.[78] Silva suggested that when Douglass connected the three events directly: persecutions of Quakers, witchcraft trials, and inoculation, he performed a "rhetorical revision." In fact, it is a logical fallacy, in that it does not charge the three events as being dangers to the colony because of an over-zealous religion, but instead pinpoints the ministers as the grave affliction.[79] The doctor also falsely compares three quite different events as equal, which is also a fallacy of inconsistency. Cotton, born in 1663, could not have been included in the banishment of Quakers. The attacks against the theocracy and the ministers in general would have been concurrent with the purpose of James Franklin, though. In the *Courant,* on May 21, 1722, was a notice from the Selectmen that smallpox had ended its hold on Boston, and "Douglass gloated that Mather's infatuation left just as his infatuation with witchcraft left 30 years ago," again tying two events (witchcraft and the inoculation project) together in print. Douglass characterized those inoculated as "victims":

> Last January *Inoculation* made a sort of *Exit,* like the Infatuation Thirty Years ago, after several had fallen Victims to the Notions by *Dr. M----r* and other Learned Clerks concerning Witchcraft. But finding Inoculation in this Town, like Serpents in Summer, beginning to crawl abroad again the last Week, it was in time, and effectually crushed in the Bud, by the *Justices, Select-Men* and the *unanimous Vote* of a general Town-Meeting.[80]

Using this fallacy of inconsistency, Douglass and Williams could cause the audience to believe that those two events were identical, rather than parsing the similarities and differences of the two very different events. This strategy had been quite effective, and one could see how the colonists who remembered the former horror could have recoiled at a life-saving process they hadn't had much possibility, perhaps, of understanding.

Other ideas of Mather's had been challenged, as well, to undercut his credibility. Various rhetorical strategies had been used thus far to challenge Mather's ideas had questioned his role in the witchcraft debacle, his wisdom in the inoculation project, and his claim that he was a fellow in the Royal Society. Now, in addition, another letter he had written was exposed to ridicule by Douglass. Mather had written a letter to Dr. Woodward on November 18, 1712, (and a note says to see the *Philosophical Transactions*, Volume 29), "the wild Pidgeons, when they leave New-England at certain Seasons, repair to some undiscover'd Satellite, accompanying the Earth at a near distance."[81] This argument against Mather's character by the Anti-Inoculators was a strong one, in that it called into question Mather's more imaginative ideas, such as witchcraft, spectral evidence, and satellites, and positioned doubt in the readers' minds that perhaps the inoculation project was of the same genus or kind. The Anti-Inoculators had also mentioned in this letter the squaring of the circle, which had been likened before to the Black Arts, and was thought by mathematicians to be unsolvable. Mather had also claimed to have solved the puzzle of squaring the circle in a letter he sent to the Royal Society.[82] The authors drove their point home with the statement: "A man guilty of such *Absurdities,* is no good Voucher for an Experiment [smallpox variolation] of such Consequence."[83] These attacks on Mather's credibility were indeed a challenge for the Inoculators, and the minister's own writings had clearly cast doubts about his advocacy of the smallpox vaccination, as well as ministerial authority and power relations in the colony. Cotton Mather had indeed written about numerous strange ideas to the Royal Society in particular. Those types of letters were not made up by the Anti-Inoculators.

Certainly the power used against people in the witchcraft trials and executions can be seen as the most negative social construction that enforced adherence to social practices as the worst kind of ... "control and policing."[84] The policing had not only been perpetrated by the magistrates, but also by ministers, by the community members, and most insidiously by small children like the Goodwins, most likely guided by older children or even adults. Children had been taught to pinpoint neighbors as witches; men with political power wielded their authority to keep inheritance laws from working against their own material interests; discrimination was undergirded in the persecutions of women who did not always act within the strict confines of Puritan regulations and sometimes did nothing wrong other than survive their husbands or give birth only to daughters rather than sons.

Although some of the accused tried to mount some resistance against the charges, arrests, etc., of so-called "witches," such resistance would have ended up costing them their own lives. It was only at the end of the hundreds of arrests and nineteen executions that the persecutions stopped, and the people in Salem and Boston and its environs recoiled in horror. Mather's attempt in *Wonders* to exonerate himself was unsuccessful, although among the judges, especially the Chief Justice of the Court of Oyer and Terminer, William Stoughton escaped humiliation apparently unscathed and went on to the highest political office of the times. Most interestingly, the trope of invisibility that figured so predominately in the debate pro and con "spectral evidence," a debate that separated father (Increase Mather) and son (Cotton Mather), had surfaced again some thirty years later.

The trope of invisibility that Mather had used in the 1720s to describe his microscopic findings in a smallpox pustule teeming with "tiny animals" had put his character once again into grave doubt. This accidental echo reminded community members who were part of the Salem and Boston witchcraft scenes of the horror that had transpired three decades ago. It would take powerful persuasion to make his audience want to repeat their past errors. He was, after all, referring to an object, the microscope, that was not something commonly used by Bostonians, even though the advent of the microscope predated the smallpox inoculation project by seventy years. At most in that era, it would have been part of a polite, wealthier society parlor game, to observe some natural plant or other objects under a microscope and exclaim about the intricacies, rather than yield important data regarding a dreaded disease.

The Role of the Microscope and Early Germ Theory

While the origins of Mather's belief in inoculation as a viable panacea included accounts by Onesimus and other West Africans as well as the writings of Europeans about the use of inoculation in Turkey and other parts of the "Levant," this third origin of Mather's knowledge came from his observations via the microscope.

> Historically, Mather's reference to microorganisms marks a turning point in Colonial American medicine and places his text on the 'cusp' of this discursive change; however, early germ theory had a very long cusp. Certainly, Mather's discussions in print were ground-breaking in the American colonies because of his discussion of germ theory in the compendium, including in his description of the inoculation project itself.[85]

The discovery of the animalculae in that vitreous smallpox matter was one of two chapters when Mather had discussed microscopy and early germ theory in his compendium, Chapter 7: "Conjecturalies, or Some Touches Upon a New Theory of Many Diseases" and Chapter 20: "Variolae Trimphatae. The Small-Pox Encountered." He was not alone but was part of a group of other researchers (although none he cited were in the Colonies) known as animalculists. At this point, the early researchers had not yet been able to distinguish between viruses, bacteria, corpuscles, or "worms." For example, Nicholas Hartsoeker (1656–1725) had written in his studies of semen in various animals that he was "the first to see the spermatic animalcula but thought it indelicate to announce his discovery to the world."[86] Among the majority, though, prevailing knowledge held that bad air was to blame for many illnesses, a.k.a. the miasma theory in addition to humoral imbalances. The inclusion of such attention to a fledgling germ theory in Mather's medical compendium could have been the first textual evidence of the transformation of medicine in *America* from a craft still based on miasmas, humors, Galen, and Hippocrates to a science.

In *The Invisible World: Early Modern Philosophy and the Invention of the Microscope,* Catherine Wilson argued against the conventional wisdom and scholarship that holds that early germ theory began with Pasteur, or with the mid-18th century Italians whose work preceded his.[87] She also suggested that the view that Pasteur's and later Koch's work were *not* based on earlier formulations and ideas of microorganisms causing disease was "incorrect."[88] Wilson advocated for reexamining that view and questioned, "Why the historical evolution of the theory of animate contagion should have been overlooked or denied is something of a historiographical mystery."[89] Through her research, she found that "a theory of animate contagion can thus be said to have emerged between 1650 and 1720," which puts Mather at the end of the first development phase although possibly quite early or the first in the Americas.[90] While Wilson found a number of proofs and much evidence for her claim, a few of which are mentioned here, there were others in Mather's compendium. Mather, like Wilson, cited Athanasius Kircher, Antoni van Leeuwenhoek, Nicholas Andry, Nicholas Hartsoeker, Benjamin Marten, and August Hauptmann. All of the above are mentioned in his chapter in *Angel* called "Conjecturales."

Jutta Schickore noted that some historians had suggested use of the microscope was on the decline in the 18th century; she also argued that such a "portrayal of eighteenth-century microscopy is in need of revision."[91] In addition, Schickore mentioned other historians, although she doesn't say which ones, had begun to challenge such a view. A substantial amount of scientific facts and ideas had been established in the era as a result of vigorous discussions.[92] Most interesting for my purposes in this text was her claim that aligns with mine that "recent studies on the social and cultural contexts of eighteenth-century science imply that contrary to Ruestow's diagnosis, social and institutional structures did exist."[93] Use of the microscope has become known of late as "polite science," and Alice N. Walters said it flourished both in the "formal public sphere of the lecture" and the "comparatively informal domestic space of the home."[94] Such sites of microscopy had been part of both "polite science" and "polite society," and among the upper-class citizens who could afford microscopes. Texts written concomitantly to appeal to such audiences did not mean that such instruments and explorations did not also have epistemological and methodological agendas.[95]

One example of such usage was Mather's "*Conjecturalies.* Or, Some Touches upon, A *New Theory* of *Diseases.*"[96] In discussing the *causes* of diseases, he analyzes the Bostonian physicians' rhetoric, who were against inoculation, as the following: "[T]heir Talk is very *Conjectural,* very *Uncertain,* very *Ambiguous;* and often times a meer *Jargon;* and in it, they are full of *Contradiction* to One another."[97] Mather was familiar with and frequently cited others who had written on microscopy and early germ theory, in support of his own explorations, such as Benjamin Marten. Marten's text, *A New Theory of Consumption,* had been published in London in 1720. Charles J. Singer claimed that Marten/Martin was "a neglected predecessor of Pasteur."[98] Marten had written: "How can we better account for the regular Types [of diseases] … than by concluding they are severally caus'd by innumerable *Animalcula* … that variously offend us according as their Species are different … ."[99] Anne Davis suggests that Marten's 1720 text was "amazing," having been written 26 years after Leeuwenhoek's "opening a new world of microscopical vistas" and that it was anticipating germ theory.[100] Gordon Jones believed Mather owned a copy of Marten's text. Richard Shryock had maintained about Mather that no other American had discussed germ theory until John Crawford in 1811; Marten was English, but Shryock had neglected to mention Mather's work possibly because his history on American medicine came out in 1960, and

Mather's compendium was not available to the public until 1972.[101] Mather had bitterly complained that no one would publish it in 1724 when it was completed.

In "Conjecturalies" in the compendium, Mather described what had been discovered via microscopes and invisible to the naked eye in the following: "Every Part of Matter is *Peopled.* Every *Green Leaf* swarms with *Inhabitants.* The Surfaces of Animals are covered with other *Animals.*"[102] In addition, Mather speculated about cells, which had been written about previously by Europeans.

> Yea, the most Solid *Bodies,* even *Marble* itself, have innumerable Cells, which are crouded with imperceptible Inmates. As there are Infinite Numbers of these, which the *Microscopes* bring to our View, so there may be inconceivable Myriads yet Smaller than these, which no glasses have yet reach'd unto.[103]

About the "animals" or germs themselves, Mather had written that "The *Animals* that themselves are much *more* than Thousands of times *Less* than the finest Grain of Sand … may insinuate by the *Air,* and with our Ailments, yea thro' the Pores of our skin; and soon get into the Juices of our Bodies.[104] For an audience unaware of such discoveries and those texts, Mather's descriptions could sound alarming. But were the Bostonian physicians all unaware of such writings and did they have microscopes themselves? Douglass read The Royal Society's *Transactions;* that is known for sure, as it was the source of Timoni's and Pilarino's testimonials that he has passed on to Cotton before the inoculation controversy.

Cotton had cited others who have suggested that these tiny animals caused disease and said that the animalculae "may have a *greater Share in producing many of our Diseases than is commonly imagined.*"[105] In Mather's prose, he usually had italicized one or two of the most important words that he wanted to stress in a sentence. In the above phrase, because he seldom italicized all of the words in a clause, this point would have been major for him, and he had made his point very visible. Others that he had read through the Royal Society *Transactions* and cited regarding his argument were August Hauptmann (1607–1674), a German doctor who had studied parasites and thought diseases were caused by microscopic worms. Mather had also written about Athanasius Kircher (1602–1680), a German microscopist who had believed that the plague was the result of minute organisms infesting human bodies.[106] The scientist had written about observing an insect that laid microscopic eggs and that when those had been inhaled by a dog, the animal had developed plague-like symptoms and died.[107] Kircher had had access to microscopes as early as 1634 and published illustrations from them by 1646.[108] Mather had asserted that both Kircher and Hauptmann had claimed that "*Malignant Fevers* never proceed from any other Cause than Little Animals" and also that Blancard

(Blankaard) had corroborated that the "*Microscope* discovers the *Blood* in *Fevers* to be full of *Animals.*"[109] Hauptmann is credited with the "elevation of the animalculist theory to prominence."[110] Kircher and Hauptmann also worked together to corroborate each other's work and to combat their critics.[111] Kircher, especially, seemed to have come under considerable ridicule, although he was not excluded from the community experimenters and had even been consulted by them.[112] Microscopists had also speculated about the air is carrying insects and microscopic animalculae. Seeming to treat such an episteme as a commonplace, Mather had suggested that in addition to air being able to transmit disease, that it might be carried from different countries and climates via "Bodies or Cloathes or Goods of Travellers."[113]

While it is obvious that Mather had been well-read, one can surmise that with the completion of the medical compendium and his initiation of and extensive involvement in the smallpox inoculation project and medicine, that early science had been a prime interest of many years before he died in 1728. In addition to the authors he had mentioned above in his work on microscopy, Cotton also had cited: Michael Ettmuller (1644–1683), Martin Lister (1638–1712), Theodore de Mayerne (Mayem, 1573–1655), and Giovanni Alfonso Borelli (Borellus) (1608–1679).[114] Hartsoeker and Andry had agreed together that there were two kinds of "worms," spermatic ones and flesh-eating ones, but the spermatic variety was not exactly made up of worms. However, the sick who had the flesh-eating type in their bodies had "an infinite variety of invisible *Insects,* who grow and devour everything that comes in their way."[115] Mather added the following quotation from Borelli to his own work after commenting on the "*Animals*" on wound dressings observed by the Italian iatromechanicist: "*Thus we are held of many Diseases which come from Invisible Animals, or such as can only be perceived by Microscopes.*"[116]

To add to the plausibility of his claims, Mather had credited Dr. Nicholas Andry with noting that smallpox pustules were full of animalculae, as was blood and urine in "*Venereal Distemper;*" the entire body was full of them.[117] Although Andry is better known to many now as the father of Orthopedics, Paolo Palladino notes Andry's role in genetics and also discusses Foucault's use of his illustration in *Discipline.*[118] Andry had also written on worm-like creatures and spermatozoa and was considered an animalculist, as was Mather.[119] Jones's note in *Angel* suggested that Andry's 1700 text was "widely known in the colonies and undoubtedly on Mather's shelves."[120] Julie Grissom argues that "Andry's practical helminthology text, … in translation, *An account of the Breeding of Worms in Human Bodies* (1701), is illustrative of the importance of worms in eighteenth-century medical theory as the potential source of a remarkable number of diseases."[121] She also notes "Andry's numerous references to the experiences of other physicians, through the inclusion of their illustrations, case histories, and letters."[122] Mather also had the idea that easterly winds carried "animalculae" from Tartar to Europe. "When the *Plague* raged in *London*, that these places that had Scents probably Kill'd or Chas'd away these *Animals*, were kept from the Infection."[123]

Oddly, Mather at first appeared to have discredited all his earlier source work in the chapter when he followed up the "Scents" quotation with "This conjecture about the *Origin of Diseases*, may be as good as many as have been Confidently Obtruded and more generally Received."[124] It's not quite clear why he had maximized winds and scents or seemed to overstate this point in the book, especially given that the theory about disease and his work with microscope were one of the three legs supporting his inoculation project. Possibly he had meant more to express exasperation about the reception of early germ theory or discoveries of "animalculae" because of the rejection of smallpox variolation in Boston rather than doubting his own beliefs. He may also have been ironic given the rejection of the citizenry of his ideas regarding microscopy and the invisible animalculae or even simply had resorted back to his ambidextrous self. Even though the compendium had been finished several years after the controversy, he had clearly continued to be convinced of the instrument's and the theory's validity in spite of the negative reception of early germ theory and to his own discoveries of "animalculae." The rejection of smallpox variolation in Boston and the ridiculing of his rhetoric on invisible animals not only had not dissuaded him but perhaps had even encouraged him to cite such exhaustive examples of other experimenters of microscopy in the compendium. In short, his review of the literature was exhaustive and impressive.

He characteristically (most chapters have such examples) had followed up his interesting "conjectures" with religious exhortations. For example, Mather had asked the rhetorical question following his origin of disease work: "But what *Remarks* are to be made upon it; what *Sentiments of PIETY* to be produced?"[125] In the early modern period generally, epidemics could still be looked at as acts of providence calling sinners to repent and reform.[126] Mather then had continued with "How much does our *Life* ly at the Mercy of our God! How much do we walk thro' *unseen Armies of* Numberless Living Things, ready to Seize and Prey upon us! ... What *Unknown Armies* has the Holy One, wherewith to Chastise and Even destroy, the Children of Men? Millions of Billions of Trillions of Invisible *Velites!*"[127] Mather used another military metaphor here, in addition to "Armies." *Velites* were a type of light infantry Roman warrior, who had fought on foot in light armor and used spears. They were known for quickness, agility, and mobility.[128] His hyperbolic and exhortative phrasing was typical of his writing style as well. This ending to the chapter had employed pathos and metaphors in contrast to the majority of his discussion on microscopy, which was much more weighted toward the logical and ethical appeals. Mather employed such language to show his familiarity with and connection to the major figures who investigated "animalculae" and other phenomena via early microscopes.

From the above section, it's clear that like Latour and Woolgar's work in *Laboratory Life,* Mather had been part of a discourse community through the multitudinous letters of the Royal Society and his own library if not *in situ* as in the laboratories of more recent times. The *Transactions* were, in addition to major European universities and the Mather family's own extensive libraries, the structure for the collaborative process involved in "the construction of scientific facts." It's also clear that "[T]he information provided by scientists [or natural philosophers] will have a significant effect in shaping investigators' reports and that the information provided depends, in turn, on the nature of the relationship between scientist and investigator."[129] The heavy citation practices in this particular chapter of *Angel* highlighted his interest and scholarship and offered still another valuable insight into Mather's belief in and enthusiasm for an inoculation project.

New Places to Look and New Ways to Observe

Juxtaposed in *Angel of Bethesda* were both the old medical terms and the beginnings of the new biomedical (scientific) terminology. Both Michel Foucault and Kenneth Burke referred to a "new way of seeing," and both examined the interactions of language and perceptions within the culture and within particular areas of culture.[130] Burke argued that "Not only does the nature of our terms affect the nature of our observations, in the sense that the terms direct the attention to one field rather than to another … [but] many of the 'observations' are but implications of the particular terminology in … which the observations are made."[131] Foucault also acknowledged the importance of the microscope: "On the side of origins or motives, we place the new privileges accorded to observation: the powers attributed to it since Bacon and the technical improvements introduced in it by the invention of the microscope."[132] Like Burke, Foucault also recognized that there were exclusions within the microscopic gaze or certain restrictions. He thought perhaps it might "be claimed that the use of the microscope compensates for these restrictions; although sensory experience was being restricted in the direction of its more doubtful frontiers, it was nevertheless being extended towards the new objects of a technically controlled form of observation."[133] For natural philosophers such as Mather, though, his discourse regarding his discoveries through microscopic lenses did not gain him greater power, but perhaps contributed to a further ebbing of it, at least when it came to the inoculation project. Wilson noted Bachelard's comments that the microscope could have functioned as more of an impediment in the 1600s and 1700s because it drew more attention to the beauties of nature than to theory formation when it had been used as part of polite science. The theorist felt that that phenomenon might have distracted from the importance of the discoveries themselves and could have been an example of "bad timing."[134] It seems that much of science was regarded as "Curiosities," and the theorist confirmed that the microscope was also an instrument for entertainment, thus the use of it in polite society. Those who had been able to afford such an instrument enjoyed looking at a flower petal or some other object and had exclaimed perhaps over its great beauty or strange shapes when magnified. One can see that Mather's claims regarding the microscope, if more known as entertainment and a parlor game, would have still been discredited or cause suspicion in the midst of a smallpox epidemic.

The new observations that informed medical discourse, including Mather's in the 1700s, were a result of two developments, not just one, coinciding almost simultaneously: microscopy and autopsy. "Hooke's *Micrographia* described the microscope as a prosthetic device, as a tool to regain the lost unity with nature. In contrast, for 18th-century microscopists, the microscope appeared as an extension of vision into entirely new regions. It provided the observer with a new sense that gave access to the wonders of the microworld.[135] Microscopy was not the only new way seeing had been configured in the discourse community of natural philosophy; the increased use of autopsy in Europe and in America presented another new way of seeing disease. Mather had permitted his son, Joseph, to be autopsied and reported it in his diary. This child was born in 1693 to Mather and his first wife, and the baby died after three days. Such was his fascination with science that he had observed his own son's autopsy.[136] Dissection had been done frequently in Europe since the 16th century, but had been practiced less often in Colonial America. Making the interior of the patient visible to the physicians' eyes would eventually change the previous concepts of anatomy, physiology, and their terminology. Mather had been at the forefront of this alteration in colonial America.

Smallpox *itself* was a very visible and obvious disease process that also carried its own visual, written, and spoken rhetoric in colonial Boston. Colonials believed such a disease was sent to punish people as a group, since so many would be affected and suffer, but also to punish individually for a person's sinful activities or sins of omission. Sins of omission could include a lack of prayerful attitude or penitence, a very invisible and silent inner process made visible by the ugly pustules of the disease. This framing and overall mindset of the people had spoken louder than the discovery of "animalculae" as tangible evidence of a cause for such a loathsome disease. The framing of the importance of his evidence in this chapter did not mean that Mather himself had recognized the importance of his own discovery without continuing to hold his religious worldviews. Just as the previous example of his religious exhortations showed, the minister himself continued to hold multiple conceptual frames within his mind at the same time, those of both science and religion, which was not unusual for those in the midst of a societal rupture or a paradigmatic change for the colonials.

Although Mather relied heavily on the writings from the Royal Society, microscopy and autopsy were important because in his own observations the invisible became visible. For example, in the 16th century, Vesalius (1514–1546) had through post-mortem autopsy corrected some of Galenic medicine and had begun to decipher the mysterious symptoms and signs of tuberculosis.[137] Such findings would lead to a break-up of the paradigm in which the gaze shifted from external observable to the internal observable for a few, forcing profound redefinitions in medicine. The importance of this systemization and direct observance was that it brought into play new vocabulary and, concomitantly, profound alterations in the relationship between patient and doctor, between the patient and her own body, and between "medicine" and "society." What used to be observable to each patient and to the community in which she lived, to her minister, and to her God (in Puritan America), was destined to become observable only to those who were privileged to see through special lenses: those found at the end of a microscope or in the autopsy theater. With microscopy it was possible to observe what was going on below the surface in the disease process. This ability eventually enabled scientists to set up direct relations between certain microbes and certain diseases, breaking down the old humoral system, which classified symptoms as diseases according to the ancient system based on the four elements and the concomitant fluids. The discourse had to change to reflect these alterations in relationships as well. That same privileged visibility occurs today, in that practitioners and researchers have access to materials and understandings of internal disease processes, which even in our media-rich environment the ordinary citizen does not necessarily have. In Mather's time, though, the experience of microscopy was so rare in the colonies, that even his communications would not be enough, as relatively few citizens in Boston had familiarity with or reference points for microscopic observations. It was, in short, difficult to relate to the idea of looking through a small apparatus with lenses to see something not visible to the naked eye. Thus even an advanced concept within the life sciences and medicine could be framed at that time by Anti-Inoculators as something similar to another strange and deadly concept the minister had held in the past as just another figment of Mather's imagination.

Historically, Mather's reference to microorganisms marked a turning point in Colonial American medicine and placed his text and his research at the beginning of this discursive change, particularly vis-à-vis the mention of germ theory found in his 1724 medical compendium. Mather's reaction at the time, to write his exhaustive and thorough work covering all "medical" treatments, had been a scholarly one. The death rate in the colonies, the disease itself, and the frustration of having a rejected means of preventing this scourge, could well have been the exigencies that had impelled Mather to finish his compendium. Some believe in difficult colonial lives, religious fervor might have reflected an effort to simply give harsh reality some meaning. Mather's action of recording his observations must also be contextualized within the time period, as there was a "contempt" for the human body, which was

> related to a general attitude to death; and, in such an attitude, one can detect not only the values proper to Christianity, but a demographical, in a sense biological, situation: the ravages of disease and hunger, the periodic massacres of the epidemics, the formidable child mortality rate, the precariousness of the bio-economic balances—all this made death familiar and gave rise to rituals intended to integrate it, to make it acceptable and to give a meaning to its permanent aggression.[138]

These attitudes and "rituals" vis-à-vis death and disease would continue to militate against new discoveries in medicine for the following decades until a qualitative change could be effected.

The timing of this text was also of note. Mather continued writing and finished his compendium after the "failed" project, in 1724, perhaps as a gift to what must have seemed to him a very shortsighted and resistant community. Mather's contributions, the inoculation project, and the discussion of "animalculae" could have had a more important impact on the then-current medical treatment in his community. However, no one would publish the tome unlike his usual success in publication of his many works. The hostile reaction during the inoculation project imposed a rejection of Mather's credibility on medical topics, especially those based on poor evidence in the eyes of his audience. Jones reminds us that the hostility came from the physicians *and* the populace, not from other clergy.[139] However, it could be assumed that some of the physicians and other intelligentsia in Boston would have had some knowledge of microscopy because the *Philosophical Transactions of the Royal Society* and texts written on such topics would have been available to those audiences. However, the invisibility trope, religious objections, observations through unfamiliar instruments, and even common sense might not have been the only factors. The primary texts of the debate, the ones we have access to, reveal still other negative possibilities to add to the mix. While Mather had found a distant audience and a conversation among those working with microscopy and sharing their work in the Royal Society's *Transactions,* his rhetoric and the invisibility trope were not able to persuade his local audience in Boston and those he hoped to save from smallpox. C. Mather's ethos had suffered from the blow by the Anti-Inoculists, and the trope of invisibility had also contributed; his prodigious writings and enthusiastic embrace of those things he could not explain to his local audience had constructed yet another obstacle along the path and postponed a discovery of a preventative that if used more widely would have indeed saved even more lives. Although even had Mather's compendium been finished, published, and distributed, it is doubtful that his wide reading of others about microscopy and germ theory in *Angel* would have been persuasive, as a large gap and division had begun to open up between those very educated (the small minority who attended Harvard or had been educated in Europe) and those who made up the rest of Boston's citizenry. In fact, great resentment on the part of others regarding the elite or literati and their years of control under the Puritan ministers played a large role in the debate as will be seen in the original texts of their arguments in Chapter Four. The irony was that the Anti-Inoculator Dr. William Douglass considered himself to be the only truly educated physician because he had gone to a university in Europe. However, he was aided and abetted by strong voices against the elite and Harvard-educated by Mundungus, the Franklins, and others in his fight against the vaccination project.

Notes

1 See Kenneth Burke's *Language as Symbolic Action.*

2 Michel Foucault, "Afterword," *Power/Knowledge: Selected Interviews and Other Writings, 1972–1977.* Colin Gordon, ed. (New York: Pantheon, 1981), 245.

3 Foucault, "Afterword," *Power/Knowledge*, 245.

4 Foucault, "Afterword," *Power/Knowledge*, 245.

5 Foucault, "Afterword," *Power/Knowledge*, 256.

6 Foucault, "Afterword," *Power/Knowledge*, 255.

7 John Corrigan and Lynn S. Neal, eds. *Religious Intolerance in America* (Chapel Hill: University of North Carolina Press, 2010), 34.

8 Kittredge, "Introduction," 36.

9 Williams, *Several Arguments*, 6.

10 Paul Boyer and Stephen Nissenbaum, *Salem Possessed: The Social Origins of Witchcraft* (Cambridge: Harvard University Press, 1982), xi.

11 Carol F. Karlsen, *The Devil in the Shape of a Woman* (New York: W. W. Norton, 1987), 82–83.

12 Goody Glover Historic Gravesite. https://www.google.com/search?q=goody+glover+historic+plaque+image&safe=active&rlz=1C1CHBF_enUS797US797&tbm=isch&source=iu&ictx=1&fir=QWyKR8HpCGgDqM%253A%252C0CTfd6B65lpIcM%252C_&vet=1&usg=AI4_kRJr1eWGWh8_pbRh8F_YH1XWzwb6g&sa=X&ved=2ahUKEwiF95iH7efjAhXsT98KHXTjC98Q9QEwAXoECAkQCQ#imgrc=QWyKR8HpCGgDqM:

13 Cotton Mather. *The Life of His Excellency, Sir William Phips* (Boston: 1697), 130–131.

14 Boyer and Nissenbaum, *Salem Possessed*, 15.

15 Increase Mather, *Cases of Conscience Concerning Evil Spirits Impersonating Men, Witchcrafts, Infallible Proofs of Guilt* (Boston: 1693).

16 Increase Mather, *Cases of Conscience,* 59, 65–66.

17 Increase Mather, *Cases,* 41–45.

18 Boyer and Nissenbaum, *Salem Possessed*, 18.

19 Boyer and Nissenbaum, *Salem Possessed*, 19.

20 Boyer and Nissenbaum, *Salem Possessed*, 19.

21 Boyer and Nissenbaum, *Salem Possessed*, 19.

22 Douglas Linder, *Famous American Trials.* "Salem Witchcraft Trials." Accessed June 2009. https://www.famous-trials.com/salem.

23 Karlsen, *The Devil*, 80.

24 Karlsen, *The Devil*, 80.

25 Karlsen, *The Devil*, 83–84.

26 Cotton Mather, *Memorable Providences, Relating to Witchcraft and Possessions …* (Boston: R. P., 1689), "Section XXXIII."

27 Cotton Mather, *Memorable Providences,* "Conjecture 3."
28 Douglas Linder, *Famous American Trials.* "Salem Witchcraft Trials: 1692." Accessed December 2012, https://famous-trials.com/salem
29 Douglas Linder, *Famous American.*
30 Douglas Linder, *Famous American.*
31 Douglas Linder, *Famous American.*
32 Anonymous, "Introduction," in Cotton Mather's *Wonders of the Invisible World, from Narratives of the Witchcraft Cases* (Boston, 1693). The Project Gutenberg EBooks # 28513, viii.
33 William Stoughton, "Letter from William Stoughton," in *Wonders of the Invisible World, from Narratives of the Witchcraft Cases* (Boston, 1693). The Project Gutenberg EBook # 28513, 6.
34 Douglas Linder, *Famous American.*
35 Cotton Mather, *Wonders of the Invisible World, from Narratives of the Witchcraft Cases* (Boston, 1693). The Project Gutenberg EBook # 28513, 110.
36 C. Mather, *Wonders of the Invisible*, 110.
37 C. Mather, *Wonders of the Invisible*, 112.
38 Kenneth Silverman, *The Life and Times of Cotton Mather* (New York, NY: Welcome Rain Pub., 2001), 144.
39 Anonymous, "Introduction," viii.
40 C. Mather, *Wonders of the Invisible*, 5.
41 For more about the importance of the Royal Society to Mather and Douglass's responses regarding this issue, see Chapter Four.
42 Kenneth Silverman, *The Life and Times*, 129.
43 C. Mather, *Wonders of the Invisible,* 5.
44 C. Mather, *Wonders of the Invisible*, 5.
45 C. Mather, *Wonders of the Invisible*, 126.
46 C. Mather, *Wonders of the Invisible*, 128.
47 Burroughs was the previous minister of the church Reverent Parris, father of the children who started accusations in Salem, had taken over.
48 Cotton Mather, *Wonders of the Invisible,* 122.
49 George Lincoln Burr, ed. *Narratives of the Witchcraft Cases, 1648-1706* (New York: Scribner's Sons, 1914), 221.
50 Burr, ed. *Narratives*, 221.
51 C. Mather, *Wonders of the Invisible*, 129.
52 Anonymous, *Records of Salem Witchcraft*, Vols. I and II (New York: Sagwan Press, 2018).
53 C. Mather, *Wonders of the Invisible,* 161.
54 *Mather* here was referring to two authors in addition to Pliny, Ralph Cudworth (*Intellectual System*) and through him "Cambridge Platonism" and Cudworth's work on demonology as well as the Danish theologian Nicholas Hemming (Niels Hemmingsen) in his *Admonitio de Superstitionibus Magicis vitandis* (Copenhagen, 1575), fol. C2 verso.
55 A plinyism is a statement of doubtful truth or accuracy, as in some of the statements in Pliny's *Natural History.*
56 C. Mather, *Wonders of the Invisible*, 162.
57 C. Mather, *Wonders of the Invisible*, 162.
58 Linder, "Sewall."
59 Linder, "Sewall."
60 Benjamin Ray and The University of Virginia. *Salem Witchcraft Trials Documentary Archive and Transcription Project.* Accessed Jan. 2022. https://salem.lib.virginia.edu/home.html.
61 C. Mather, *Wonders of the Invisible*, 15.

62 C. Mather, *Wonders of the Invisible*, 28.
63 C. Mather, *Wonders of the Invisible*, 81.
64 C. Mather, *Wonders of the Invisible*, 82.
65 C. Mather, *Wonders of the Invisible*, 82.
66 C. Mather, *Wonders of the Invisible*, 82
67 C. Mather, *Wonders of the Invisible*, 82.
68 C. Mather, *Wonders of the Invisible*, 115.
69 *The New-England Courant* Overleaf (Boston: J. Franklin, March 26, 1722).
70 *Courant* Overleaf, Mar. 26, 1722.
71 *Courant* Overleaf, Mar. 26, 1722.
72 C. Mather, *Angel of Bethesda*. Barre, MA: American Antiquarian Society and Barre Publishing, *94*.
73 Cristobal Silva, *Miraculous Plagues: An Epidemiology of Early New England,* Oxford, UK: Oxford University Press, 2011, 159; Louise Breen, *Cotton Mather*, the 'Angelic Ministry' and Inoculation." *Journal of History of Medicine and Allied Sciences*. 46 (July 1991): 159.
74 *Courant*, Jan. 1722.
75 Kittredge, "Introduction," 35.
76 John Williams, "An Answer," 4.
77 Douglass, *Inoculation Considered.*
78 Kittredge, "Introduction," 39.
79 Silva, *Miraculous Plagues,* 146.
80 Douglass, *Abuses and Scandals*, 6.
81 Douglass, *Abuses and Scandals*, 6.
82 Douglass, *Abuses and Scandals*, 6.
83 Douglass, *Abuses and Scandals*, 7.
84 Michel Foucault, *Power/Knowledge*, 245.
85 Barbara Heifferon, "The New Smallpox: An Epidemic of Words?" in *Rhetoric Review* 25, no. 1 (2006), 86.
86 Catherine Wilson, *The Invisible World: Early Modern Philosophy and the Invention of the Microscope* (Princeton, NJ: Princeton University Press, 133.
87 Wilson, *Invisible World,* 140.
88 Wilson, *Invisible World,* 140.
89 Wilson, *Invisible World,* 140.
90 Wilson, *Invisible World,* 174.
91 Jutta Schickore, *The Microscope and the Eye* (Chicago: University of Chicago Press, 2007), 17.
92 Schickore, *Microscope and the Eye,* 17.
93 Schickore, *Microscope and the Eye, 17.*
94 Alice N. Walters, "Conversation Pieces: Science and Politeness in 18th Century England" in *History of Science,* 35 (1997), 122.
95 Schickore, *Microscope and the Eye,* 18.
96 C. Mather, *Angel of Bethesda,* 43.
97 C. Mather, *Angel of Bethesda,* 43.
98 Charles J. Singer, "Benjamin Marten, A Neglected Predecessor of Louis Pasteur" in *Janus,* 16 (1911), 81.
99 Benjamin Marten, *A New Theory of Consumption* (London, 1720), 65.
100 Anne L. Davis, "A Historical Perspective on Tuberculosis and Its Control of Tuberculosis" in *Tuberculosis: A Comprehensive International Approach,* ed. Lee B. Reichman and Earl S. Hershfield (2005), 7.
101 G. Jones, "Preface," in *Angel of Bethesda* by Cotton Mather. Barre, MA: American Antiquarian Society and Barre Publishing, ix.
102 C. Mather, *Angel of Bethesda,* 43.

103 C. Mather, *Angel*, 43.
104 C. Mather, *Angel*, 43.
105 C. Mather, *Angel*, 44.
106 C. Mather, *Angel*, 44.
107 Athanasius Kircher, *Scrutinum Physico-Medicum* (Rome, 1658), 229.
108 Wilson, *Invisible World*, 76.
109 C. Mather, *Angel*, 44; Steven Blankaard, *The Physical Dictionary* (London: J. D., 1702), 136.
110 Wilson, *Invisible World*, 155.
111 Wilson, *Invisible World*, 155.
112 Wilson, *Invisible World*, 223.
113 C. Mather, *Angel*, 45.
114 C. Mather, *Angel*, 45.
115 Nicolas Hartsoeker. *Principes de Physique* (Paris: J. Annison, 1696), 216–217.
116 C. Mather, *Angel*, 45.
117 C. Mather, *Angel*, 45.
118 Paul Paladino, *Plants, Patients, and the Historian* (Manchester, UK: Manchester University Press, 2002), 11–12.
119 Punnett, R.C. "Ovists and Animalculists." *The American Naturalist* 62. (November-December 1928): 481–507. Remi Kohler, "Nicolas Andry de Bois-Regard: The Inventor of the Word 'Orthopaedics' and the Father of Parasitology" in *Journal of Child Orthopedics,* 4, no. 4 (2010), 349.
120 G. Jones, "Introduction" in *Angel of Bethesda* by Cotton Mather. Barre, MA: American Antiquarian Society and Barre Publishing, 36.
121 Julie Hayden Grisson, *Parasitic Worms in Early Modern Science and Medicine 1650-1810* (PhD. Dissertation, University of Oklahoma, 2014), 10–11.
122 Grisson, *Parasitic*, 10–11.
123 C. Mather, *Angel,* 46–47.
124 C. Mather, *Angel*, 47.
125 C. Mather, *Angel*, 47.
126 Sara Stidstone Gronim, "Imagining Inoculation: Smallpox, the Body, and Social Relations of Healing in the Eighteenth Century" in *Bulletin of History of Medicine,* 80, no.2 (2006), 260.
127 C. Mather, *Angel*, 47.
128 Linda Alchin, "Velites." *Roman Coliseum Tour,* 2014. http://jakesyl.insomnia247.nl/www.tribunesandtriumphs.org/gladiators/velites.htm.
129 Bruno Latour and Steven Woolgar, *Laboratory Life: The Construction of Scientific Facts* (Princeton, NJ: Princeton University Press, 1986, 20.
130 Kenneth Burke, *Language as Symbolic Action* (Berkeley, CA: University of California Press, 1966); Michel Foucault, *The Order of Things* (New York: Knopf, 2012).
131 Burke, *Language as Symbolic*, 46.
132 Foucault, *The Order of Things Order of Things: An Archaeology of the Human Sciences.* (New York: Vintage, 1994), 133.
133 Foucault, *Order of Things,* 133.
134 Wilson, *Invisible World,* 251; quoting Bachelard, Gaston (*La Formation de L'Esprit Scientifique,* 8th ed. Paris: J. Vrin, 1972), 161.
135 Schickore, *Microscope and the Eye,* 4.
136 G. Jones, xxxv.
137 Lee B. Reichman and Earl S. Hershfield, *Tuberculosis: A Comprehensive International Approach.* 2nd ed. (Basel: Marcel Dekker, 2000), 6.
138 Foucault, *Discipline,* 54.
139 G. Jones, xxxiv.

Bibliography

Alchin, Linda. "Velites." *Roman Coliseum Tour*, 2014. Accessed June 22, 2014. http://jakesyl.insomnia247.nl/www.tribunesandtriumphs.org/gladiators/velites.htm

Anonymous, "Introduction" to Cotton Mather's *Wonders of the Invisible World, from Narratives of the Witchcraft Cases*. Boston, 1693. The Project Gutenberg EBooks # 28513, viii.

Anonymous. *Records of Salem Witchcraft*, Vols. I and II. New York: Sagwan Press, 2018.

Bachelard, Gaston. *La Formation de L'Esprit Scientifique*. 8th ed. Paris: J. Vrin, 1972.

Blankaard, Steven. *The Physical Dictionary*. London: J. D., 1702.

Boyer, Paul and Stephen Nissenbaum, *Salem Possessed: The Social Origins of Witchcraft*. Cambridge: Harvard University Press, 1982.

Breen, Louise. "Cotton Mather, the 'Angelic Ministry' and Inoculation" In *Journal of History of Medicine and Allied Sciences* 46 (July 1991).

Burke, Kenneth. *Language as Symbolic Action: Essays on Life, Literature, and Method*. Berkeley: University of California Press, 1966.

Burr, George Lincoln, ed. *Narratives of the Witchcraft Cases, 1648–1706*. New York: Scribner's Sons, 1914.

Corrigan, John and Lynn S. Neal, eds. *Religious Intolerance in America*. Chapel Hill: University of North Carolina Press, 2010.

Cudworth, Ralph. The True Intellectual System of the Universe. London, 1678.

Davis, Anne L. "A Historical Perspective on Tuberculosis and Its Control of Tuberculosis" In *Tuberculosis: A Comprehensive International Approach*, eds. Lee B. Reichman and Earl S. Hershfield (2005).

Douglass, William. *The Abuses and Scandals of Some Late Pamphlets in Favour of Inoculation of the Small Pox*. Boston: J. Franklin, 1722.

Douglass, William. *Inoculation of the Small Pox as Practised in Boston, Considered in a Letter to A[lexander] S[tuart], M. D. F. R. S., in London*. 1722.

Foucault, Michel. "Afterword" In *Power/Knowledge: Selected Interviews and Other Writings, 1972–1977*, ed. Colin Gordon. New York: Pantheon, 1981.

Foucault, Michel. *The Order of Things: An Archaeology of the Human Sciences*. New York: Vintage, 1994.

Foucault, Michel. *Power/Knowledge: Selected Interviews and Other Writings, 1972–1977*, ed. Colin Gordon. New York: Pantheon, 1981.

Grisson, Julie Hayden. "Parasitic Worms in Early Modern Science and Medicine 1650–1810" PhD diss. University of Oklahoma, 2014.

Gronim, Sara Stidstone. "Imagining Inoculation: Smallpox, the Body, and Social Relations of Healing in the Eighteenth Century" In *Bulletin of History of Medicine*, 80, no. 2 (2006).

Hartsoeker, Nicolas. *Principes de Physique*. Paris: J. Annison, 1696.

Heifferon, Barbara. "The New Smallpox: An Epidemic of Words?" In *Rhetoric Review* 25, no. 1 (2006).

Hemmingsen, Niels. *Admonitio de Superstitionibus Magicis Vitandis*. Copenhagen, 1575.

Jones, Gordon G. "Preface" In *Angel of Bethesda* by Cotton Mather. Barre, MA: American Antiquarian Society and Barre Publishing, 1972.

Karlsen, Carol F. *The Devil in the Shape of a Woman*. New York: W. W. Norton, 1987.

Kircher, Athanasius. *Scrutinum Physico-Medicum*. Rome, 1658.

Kittredge, George L. "Introduction" to Increase Mather's and Anonymous's [Cotton Mather's] *Several Reasons for Transplanting the Small Pox, Is a Lawful Practice, and That It Has Been Blessed by God for the Saving of Many a Life. Etc.* and Cotton Mather's *Sentiments Written on the Small Pox Inoculated*. Cleveland, OH, 1921.

Kohler, Remi. "Nicolas Andry de Bois-Regard: The Inventor of the Word 'Orthopaedics' and the Father of Parasitology" In *Journal of Child Orthopedics* 4, no. 4 (2010).

Latour, Bruno and Steven Woolgar, *Laboratory Life: The Construction of Scientific Facts*. Princeton, NJ: Princeton University Press, 1986.

Linder, Douglas. *Famous American Trials*. "Salem Witchcraft Trials." Accessed June 2009, December 2012. https://www.famous-trials.com/salem.

Marten, Benjamin. *A New Theory of Consumption*. London, 1720.

Mather, Cotton. *Angel of Bethesda*. Barre, MA: American Antiquarian Society and Barre Publishing, 1972.

Mather, Cotton. *The Life of His Excellency, Sir William Phips*. Boston, 1697.

Mather, Cotton. *Memorable Providences, Relating to Witchcraft and Possessions*. Boston: R. P., 1689.

Mather, Cotton. *Wonders of the Invisible World, from Narratives of the Witchcraft Cases* by Cotton Mather. Boston, 1693. The Project Gutenberg EBook # 28513.

Mather, Increase. *Cases of Conscience Concerning Evil Spirits Impersonating Men, Witchcrafts, Infallible Proofs of Guilt*. Boston, 1693.

The New-England Courant [Courant], Boston, January 1722; Overleaf, Mar. 26, 1722.

Paladino, Paul. *Plants, Patients, and the Historian*. Manchester, UK: Manchester University Press, 2002.

Pliny. *Natural History*. New York: Penguin, 1991. Reprint.

Punnett, R. C. "Ovists and Animalculists" In *The American Naturalist* 62, (November-December 1928).

Ray, Benjamin and The University of Virginia. *Salem Witchcraft Trials Documentary Archive and Transcription Project*. Accessed January 2022. https://salem.lib.virginia.edu/home.html

Reichman, Lee B. and Earl S. Hershfield, *Tuberculosis: A Comprehensive International Approach*. 2nd ed., Basel: Marcel Dekker, 2000.

Schickore, Jutta. *The Microscope and the Eye*. Chicago: University of Chicago Press, 2007.

Silva, Cristobal. *Miraculous Plagues: An Epidemiology of Early New England*. Oxford, UK: Oxford University Press, 2011.

Silverman, Kenneth. *The Life and Times of Cotton Mather*. New York, NY: Welcome Rain Publishers, 2001.

Singer, Charles J. "Benjamin Marten, A Neglected Predecessor of Louis Pasteur" In *Janus*, 16 (1911).

Stoughton, William. "Letter from William Stoughton" In *Wonders of the Invisible World, from Narratives of the Witchcraft Cases* by Cotton Mather. Boston, 1693. The Project Gutenberg EBook # 28513.

Walters, Alice N. "Conversation Pieces: Science and Politeness in 18th Century England" In *History of Science* 35, 1997.

Wilson, Catherine. *The Invisible World: Early Modern Philosophy and the Invention of the Microscope*. Princeton, NJ: Princeton University Press, 1995.

4 Class and Education in The "Academicus Dialogues," other Commentary, and Silence Dogood

Introduction

In addition to Mather's reputation from the past, especially the witchcraft trials and the trope of invisibility, and religious objections, there were other social forces that played roles in the controversy: intellectualism, anti-intellectualism, the class system, and early stirrings of revolution. The Mathers had long been regarded at least by some as the Bostonian intellectuals and the "elites." Increase Mather had been President of Harvard, acting President in 1685–1686; rector from 1686–1692; and again President from 1692–1701. Cotton Mather's paternal grandfather, Richard Mather, had been a Harvard Overseer. Increase had entered Harvard as a student at 12 and Cotton at 11. The year Increase had been asked to assume the Presidency of Harvard, he in many ways had acted as a less-than-engaged Rector and commuted from his home as he hated Cambridge and preferred to live in what was then Boston proper.[1] Anti-intellectualism was personified and well represented by the figure of "Mundungus" or John Williams, the semi-illiterate fellow who had become curiously literate in his written attacks on the Inoculators. An apothecary and tobacconist by trade, Williams was well known for his rowdy and outlandish behavior and believed to have been responsible for the tar or glue on what he mistakenly thought was Boylston's horse's saddle as it was "parked" next door to his tobacco establishment.[2]

Mundungus's use of religious language, unlike that of some of the other Anti-Inoculators, seemed to be posing serious arguments referencing doctrinal points, perhaps to make fun of the Mathers and other Bostonian ministers rallying behind them. Especially given his outrageous behavior and well-deserved reputation, putting such religious language in this self-ordained buffoon's mouth parodied the academically-trained Boston clergy. Because he had not been regarded as in the same class as the educated men of the town (specifically, the doctors who made up the other Anti-Inoculators and the ministers who made up the Inoculators), Mundungus's letters to James and Ben Franklin's paper had been especially effective in rallying the "common folk" and further enraging them against the Mathers

DOI: 10.4324/9781003312369-5

and other "Inoculators." In addition, the dialogue featured below between Academicus (thought to be Isaac Greenwood and possibly Cotton) and Sawny (thought to be Williams and Douglass) provided an extended debate that played out class difference at least on one level, and that fostered resistance to the theocracy and the power structure at another level. The text clearly highlighted the resentment toward the "Academics," Mathers, and other Inoculators, who as ministers usually had also been Harvard-educated. Although William Douglass is a "character" in the dialogue or debate, it's thought that Greenwood and Williams wrote and exchanged the two dialogues, each written by one of them, but both most likely had had extensive assistance. Some believe Mather with Greenwood penned some or most of the first dialogue, while most believed Douglass or one of the Franklins had penned some of Williams's answer to Greenwood.[3] The dialogues are often ethopoetic in that they had assumed each other's roles and had written from those stances to more vividly portray certain points. The Academicus Dialogues (March 1722) and letters to Alexander Stuart (February 1722) and other attempts by young Harvard scholars to defend their elder alums and mentors point to the schism that had developed between the classes and/or between those formally educated and those who were not. Also, disruptions had taken place among student social and political groups from the 1710s to the 1720s.[4] The friction impacted the inoculation project. In addition, the rhetoric of these texts exposed cracks in a soon-to-be-former theocratic rule that had begun to show signs of movement and change in the power relations of this colony. The genre of the dialogues is particularly interesting in light of the other serious tracts, newspaper entries, and pamphlets in which both science and religion were discussed in very solemn tones. To fully analyze the inoculation debate, one would be remiss in not taking up this parody.

The evidence for the suspicion that Mather had penned much of the first dialogue was because of a diary entry of Mather's: that he had penned an "excellent Contrivance" at this particular juncture. For him to publish the dialogue under his own name would have been much less effective. By 1722 Mather had become very much aware of the increasingly problematic nature of his own credibility and authority. Douglass had suggested that Mather had written the dialogue in the *Courant*: "It can be no other than the Performance of some Ill-Bred School-Boy (a Chip off the old Block) with the Assistance of the Author perhaps of an *Essay to shake of* [off] *a Viper,* because several of the Ingredients are to be found nowhere but in his Museum or Shop."[5] The "Ill-Bred School-Boy" could have been a thinly veiled allusion to Cotton or Samuel Mather, as well as the "Chip off the old Block;" the "old Block" could have been Increase or Cotton Mather. Samuel Mather, Cotton's only ministerial son, had been a stout defender of his father in numerous controversies. Douglass's colorful language suggested that the style of the dialogue was very much similar in style to Cotton

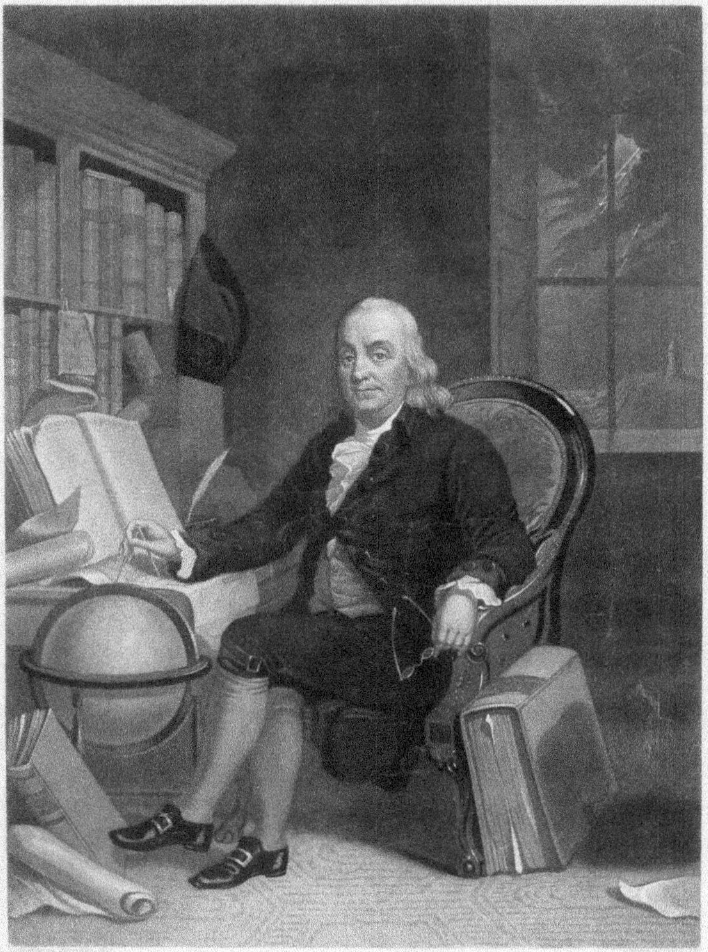

Figure 4.1 Benjamin Franklin, "Courtesy, American Antiquarian Society".

Mather's. Yet most research points to Isaac Greenwood, a student at Harvard; Douglass would have been guessing at the identity.

The "Academicus Dialogues" are clearly representative of this additional cause of resistance to the inoculation project in that they highlight the anti-intellectualism, a change in traditional disciplinary practices, resentment of theocratic rule, a pushing back against the practice of medicine by some ministers, as well as the beginning of professionalization of doctors. This controversy highlights the way the health of the body was handled. The "machinery of power" was being fought over by two groups of power brokers, both laying claim to the human body; both groups wanted to own the body.

This change further contributed to the beginning of new disciplines. Such "disciplinary forces" would eventually result in the modern hospital, all the "disciplines" of the life sciences and medicine, as well as psychology and social sciences. According to Foucault, "[t]he historical moment of the disciplines was the moment when an art of the human body was born, which was directed ... at the formation of a relation that in the mechanism itself makes it more obedient as it becomes more useful, and conversely ... . The human body was entering a machinery of power that explores it, breaks it down and rearranges it."[6] One could insist, though, that the body had previously been owned by religion or the religious not only in the colonies but also in other countries. Foucault himself often referenced the military as an early owner of the body as it came under the power of warring rulers.

The First Academicus Dialogue: An Attack on Wm. Douglass and Mundungus

In the sequence of the inoculation project, the first "Academicus" dialogue, written most likely by Greenwood and C. Mather, appeared March 6, 1722, and parodies both Douglass's Scottish brogue and Mundungus's eccentric English spellings. Douglass had already distributed his: "The Abuses and Scandals Of some late Pamphlets in Favour of Inoculation of the Small Pox, Modestly obviated, and Inoculation further considered in a Letter to A—S, M.D. & F.R.S." composed as a letter.[7] The quotation on the title page makes plain the intention of the first dialogue written by the Inoculators: "Not since, we live in such a fulsome Age, When Nonsense loads the Press & choaks the Stage; When Blockheads will claim Wit in Natures spight, And ev'ry Dunce that Starves, presumes to write; ... "[8] Any parody is humorous and makes fun of or belittles someone by imitating him or her. The "Blockhead" was most likely Mundungus, but Greenwood and Mather can be implying both or either John Williams and/or Douglass. Although clearly Williams was a caricature, a butt of jokes, and even had been self-mocking in his own writings, he was clearly less learned and articulate than Douglass. That does not mean the authors of the first dialogue went easy on the Scottish physician. They had even positioned a so-called "Advertisement" as was frequently done in the front of pamphlets. The advertisement, which is reproduced exactly as it appeared in the 1722 text, was also pure mockery and showed the extent to which it ridiculed Douglass's first pamphlet:

> Whereas Dr. W. D. has lately published a *little vain Book, full of Can't and impropriety;* which *yet in Vanity he judges, would be acceptable* to A. S. M.D. and F.R.S. These are to inform the Reader, that the said W. D. is a *Credulous and Whimsical* Blade, a *Madman* and a *Fool;* and his Account is full of LYES *and* EQUIVOCATIONS. And *as a Caution to him (who has been troublesome* to Dr. A. S. *with his trivial Credulous Stories)* least by his *Communications Home, he may impose on our mother Country; he is to be advertised, that a true and faithful account of this Experiment, as least as far as can be learnt shall in due time be sent Home well vouched, and signed by some whose proper Business it is to make such Observations.* Together with a short History, of all the EXTRAORDINARY MACHINATIONS that have been devised against it; the *Ill Language,* and BRUTAL MANNERS it has been treated withal; together with the *Abuses and Scandals of some* LATE PAMPHLETS *modestly OBVIATED.*[9]

Although parodies can be used as rhetorical strategies to lessen the tension in the debate, these parodies perhaps succeeded in further heightening the tensions. At the same time, in each of the two dialogues there were moments that seemed to function as comic correctives. While much of the time the texts during the inoculation debate set up stark binaries, in the parodies we see some relief from that pattern. For Burke, his interest in the concept of comedy was to break through binarial thinking and avoid totalizing narratives; comic frames had not often been seen in the other inoculation texts in 1721 Boston. Burke seemed to see comic correctives as rhetoric that can help people to be observers of themselves, even while they are acting.[10] We can see ourselves as others or others as ourselves in each other's frames. For example, in the first parody, an Inoculator plays both roles of Inoculator (Academicus) and Anti-Inoculators: (Sawny) or (Mundungus). In the analyses below, there will be several points where the dialogues seem to break through the binaries.

There were other changes in the Boston area at the time, some coming in with new ministers, such as Benjamin Colman, who seemed to shine a light on the manners and literacy of the earlier Puritan arrivals. Although a son of Harvard, his wider travels had produced in him more of a cosmopolitan mix that combined what Shields calls a "politeness and Reformed Christianity ... for those embarrassed at homespun yet uncomfortable with courtly finery."[11] In addition, the curriculum at Harvard had also changed with seemingly more concentration on rhetoric as a subject and less on theology, presenting an opening for the entry of Colman's poetry that tapped into the sublime. The Harvard students turned their attention from producing only rational or logo-centric texts to also writing ones based on emotions. All of these changes created a crucible from which the "Dialogues" emerged. Emotions and humor were given freer rein.

In the advertisement above that was printed above the first dialogue, the authors clearly mocked Douglass's pamphlet, as well as alluded to the title of his second pamphlet. "Whimsical" and "credulous" were the terms Douglass used to refer to and ridicule Mather's adoption of the inoculation project. Both of Douglass's tracts were addressed to "A.S. M.D. & F.R.S. in London;" the Anti-Inoculator had sent both of these to the "Mother Country," England, to undercut the project and the Inoculators. Douglass took umbrage with Mather who claimed to also be a Fellow of the Royal Society (F.R.S.). Thus, he addressed both pamphlets to A.S. M.D., who is Douglass's friend in Britain *and* a Fellow of the Royal Society. The first letter addressed to Alexander Stuart, one that was written by William Douglass on September 25, 1721, regarding the smallpox inoculation project in Boston, had indeed been read by Stuart to the Royal Society in London on November 16, 1721. In the first letter, Douglass had lambasted the project as "rash" practice, asked what the English doctors thought of inoculation, and characterized Mather as a "certain credulous Preacher of this Place." The second tract was even more strident in tone; it had been published by James Franklin and was anonymous, but everyone knew it was written by Douglass.

This attack sent abroad to the learned group, whose favor Mather sought, enraged the minister and the other Inoculators. Thus in the advertisement, the Inoculators took Douglass to task for his actions that undercut Mather's reputation and authority, as well as the ethos of the project. They accused the Scottish physician of imposing his lies on the Mother country and announced that the actual documentation for the project, ("well vouched") by those who were actually conducting the inoculations, would be sent to the Royal Society in due time. In fact, Boylston and Mather documented all their efforts and results; they did not release the names of their patients to protect the inoculated citizens, since both the minister and the doctor had suffered attacks both in print and one physically. However, Mather had already published a good-sized extract (2/5) of smallpox inoculations in a London press, to prove that the project in the colonies was not out of line with current medical thinking abroad.[12]

The dedication of the dialogue was to Zabdiel Boylston, the doctor doing the inoculations in Boston. The discourse was at times epideictic, contained such phrases as the following: "Such has been your undaunted Resolution, and truly Heroic Courage, thro' the whole Course of your dangerous Enterprize; and such your Conduct and Wisdom, as merits our highest Regards, and most public Thanks."[13] Greenwood/Mather wrote that history would redeem Boylston and eventually find the physicians who resisted the life-saving technique in disfavor.[14] Given the predominance of the name Boylston on landmarks around Boston in the 21st century, this prediction proved true.

The dialogue then had begun with Academicus ("AC:") addressing Sawny ("Sa:"/ Douglass), in which he ridiculed the Scot's dialect. Greenwood and Mather can both claim the "Academicus" (AC) title given Greenwood's role at the time as a Harvard student and Mather's as alum.

Using satire, the Inoculators began to retaliate against their attackers. This spoof of Douglass's discourse, a brogue, which Greenwood attempted to represent phonetically in the text, was a rhetorical strategy to point out the Scottish physician's difference as an outsider and someone other than a Bostonian or Puritan. He could have been trying to appeal to a xenophobic attitude of his audience. Perhaps Mather and Greenwood also parodied Douglass for his use of the English language to paint him, along with his apparently semi-illiterate companion, Mundungus, as unschooled and ignorant, although Douglass had been well educated in Europe.

To get a taste of this strategy in the "Debate:"

AC: Prithee, *Sawny*, come hither, I want a little talk with thee.
Sa: *I'se come Maister, what plaise ye Sar?*
AC: Good now, don't beat my Ears with such a coarse Dialect; I am not used to Such Gibberidge; speak English.
Sa: *Maister, ye ken vary weel that I canno spak Englis?*
AC: I see, thou wilt never leave the old trade, *Sawny*.
Sa: *Ye mean Leasing, Maister.*
AC: Yes, I do mean in plain English, *Lying*.
Sa: *Why mon, co'd I spak Englis, wo'd I prent against* - EXTRAGROUNDLESS *Machinations?*
AC: I don't think, you can speak true *English;* but you have learnt *broad English;* and in *English* you shall talk to me.
Sa: *Indeed, Sar, I canno'.*
AC: Indeed, Sir, you can; for you have had a liberal Education at *Billingsgate;* the only place in the world to learn *Broad English* at. You have also just now published a Libel; which is all *Broad English;* Therefore speak *English* to me; be it never so broad, I care not.[15]

Billingsgate refers to an old gate in London and the fish market there, first referenced in 1652. However, thereafter it referred to verbal abuse, vituperation, invective, and/or vitriol. The gate itself lies in southeast of the City of London between two bridges: London and Tower on the north bank of the Thames; in this context it refers to coarse language.

Not only was Academicus ridiculing Douglass's dialect, but he had also derided his alma mater. In addition, he castigated the physician for publishing a libel in English, although Sawny claimed in the parody not to be able to speak English, thus positioning readers to question Douglass's credibility. This strategy could have cast doubt in the colonists' minds that not only was this degreed physician a "foreigner," but he might have been an imposter as well, since his schooling, according to Academicus, should have taught him how to speak English "correctly." Academicus could also have been implying that this dialogue was a ruse to connect this supposedly learned man to those with less education than the Mathers, that same audience usually addressed by Mundungus.

Following this first salvo, Academicus told Sawny he wanted to debate him. In the next part of the dialogue, Sawny boasted as to his education, his worldliness, and belittled his competition, the non-degreed, ministers practicing Physick, which also included the main surgeon and Inoculator, Boylston, as "*Illiterate Numbskulls.*"[16] Douglass had arrived in Boston with the expectation of close contact with the Governor of the colony, which would have immediately put the Scottish doctor in a privileged position, but that didn't happen after all; it had been a deeply felt disappointment to Douglass that the man he hoped would have been appointed Governor before he arrived, had not been so appointed. Before he initiated the project, Mather had included the Scottish physician in his efforts to reach all the doctors of Boston about inoculating the citizens and claimed that Douglass himself had lent him information about smallpox inoculation. Douglass finally had admitted that he had

> lent to a certain Reverend Gentleman of this Town [Mather] the *Philosophical Transactions,* wherein he found the Letters of *Timonius* and *Pilarinus*, from the *Levant* to the *Royal Society* in *London*, giving some Account of the Method and Success of this Practice in those Countries; *being a Man of Whim and Credulity [Mather], thinks this Juncture a fit Opportunity to make Experiments on his Neighbours, (which in Vanity he might Judge acceptable to the Royal Society), takes the Hint, sends circular Letters to all the Practitioners of the Place, (the Owner of the Transactions excepted [Douglass]),* inviting them to come into it.[17]

Douglass characterized Mather in an *ad hominem* attack as a gullible person who sought to impress the Royal Society. Also, the Scot had complained that he had not been invited to join the circles of interest Mather, as one of the leading scholars in the town, had created to discuss the natural world and medicinal lore, including inoculation. The earlier "slight" of Douglass by Mather was an ongoing point of controversy. Especially in the beginning of the inoculation project, Mather had sought support quite widely from the various physicians, ministers, and scholars in Boston.

Also in his text, The Abuses, Douglass *had characterized Cotton Mather as a "man void of candour," who promotes a "Medical Experiment, without the knowledge of, or taking any notice of him from whom he had the Communication."*[18] This statement followed up on the controversy and Douglass's having given the Royal Society texts by Pylarino and Timoni documenting the inoculation process to Mather. The Scotchman referred to his own credibility: " ... *whose M.D. is as good and more regularly acquired as his D.D. [Mather's], one not inferior to himself in Birth, Fortune, Education, and the good Opinion of his Neighbours; who [Mather] calls a Man that has resided several Years in this Country, and constantly paid Taxes and other Rates, a newComer, a meer Stranger.*"[19] This ethical appeal was an attempt to undercut the previous claims made by the Inoculators about him.

In the first long speech full of boasts by Sawny in the parody, the Inoculators characterized him as having had an attitude of intellectual superiority and bias toward the other physicians that he claimed were not as well trained as he had been. In his supposed monologue, he had also dropped the accent, notably, a rhetorical strategy that most likely had been written to support the charge of pretense by Academicus. Although by highlighting his own academic training as better than that of the resident Bostonian doctors, Douglass was positioned by Greenwood, in the group of Inoculators, as not after all a man of the "common people" represented by Mundungus and the other Bostonian physicians. Included in the text, was also a clever pun: "*And if any Man is so brazenly impudent, as to whisper a good word of any other Physician but my self, he shan't escape* Scotfree: *I'll be foul on him.*" Greenwood has Sawny (Douglass) say this line.

In Academicus's long answer to this supposed retort, he had spent some time in word play on *foul.* Then Greenwood had him make a key point in the otherwise often derisive Scottish physician's humorous discourse. It was an interesting admission that had been noted in an earlier work of Douglass. It could be read ironically, but Douglass had confessed in his own writing that in a few years hence he might then reconsider the inoculation technique. In his first letter, "Inoculation of the Small Pox as Practised in Boston, Consider'd in a Letter to Alexander Stuart," Douglass had written: "I impatiently wait for some further Account of its [inoculation's] Progress in London, their Cautions and Rules in the Procedures, I hope may be of use to Us. For my own part, *till after a few Years, I pass no positive Judgment of this bold Practice.*"[20] Such an admission, however, points to the strong possibility that this disagreement over inoculation may have been more about power and control over the body (individual, professional, and political) than about the practice itself.

> Greenwood's response via Academicus was: *But if it be possible for you once in your Life to speak a word of Truth,* prithee, tell me,what you further designed in your Letter. It can't be to oppose the *Inoculation of the Small Pox*; for you expertly declare, *Till after a few Years you shall pass no judgment on this Practice.* And indeed, this is the only Sentence that has so much as the least shadow of sense in it, for *Sawny,* you suspect that in a *few Months*, you shall find the Ablest PHYSICIANS in *England* and all *Europe,* to approve the Practice, (which to your Confusion, *we can assure you of already,*) and that Persons of Quality, *and great Numbers in the City and Suburbs,* are saved by it; and then you hop'd to have an *Hole* to creep out of. But, *Sawny,* why must the world wait a *few Years* for that profound *Judgment* of yours, by which you think all Mankind must be determined.[21]

This point was well made, if not widely accepted at the time. Although Douglass had in his first letter made the point himself, that concession could be seen as either a strength or a weakness in his own argument. He also had shown his willingness to accept the practice if more support came from abroad. Yet admitting a possible change of mind left him open to being ridiculed and challenged. He had already told the Inoculators, in this same letter, that their documentation and the researchers themselves ("vouchers") had been less than credible in support of the technique, because of their citing testimony from the enslaved, Turkish practices, etc. In this part of the "dialogue," it seemed as if Greenwood and Mather were suggesting there were other motives for Douglass's lack of trust in the inoculation project, alluding to his dislike of Mather and challenge of Boylston as a fellow physician. Which profession should have the right to introduce new medical techniques and what if a physician or a surgeon chose a practice that the others didn't support?

Another interesting aspect of the dialogue is Academicus's accusation of Douglass's harshness toward Dr. Boylston. Greenwood asked: "Hadn't enough damage to the Inoculators already been done by Mundungus? Why had he (Sawny) felt it necessary to enter in the attacks?" Douglass's reply was that Mundungus and other Anti-Inoculators had been much too "respectful" of Boylston.[22] Academicus next charged Douglass and John Williams with a conspiracy against the ministers to insert a wedge between them and their parishioners.[23] In fact, he accused the Anti-Inoculators of wanting to "destroy the Religion of the Country," a heavy and serious charge indeed.[24] This claim would be difficult to understand unless one contextualizes the debate and struggle as one over political power. The challenge is also to the dynasty of the Mathers and is rhetorically a metonymy, a substituting *religion* for the persons of the Mathers and the theocracy, especially the church's control over the body that the Anti-Inoculators led by Douglass were trying to disrupt.

After more dialogue over the infamous letter in June 1721 that Mather sent to all the physicians and whether or not it had been also sent to Douglass, Academicus returned to why the Scot would oppose the project. He asked at one point: " ... if thou hadst been advising with several Good *Old Women,* we have among us, how to handle the *Small Pox* in the *Common Way* [naturally], willst thou Opposed *Inoculation;* many a life might have been saved ... ?"[25] In other words, Greenwood made the point that had the knowledge of inoculation come from someone other than Mather (and perhaps other than the enslaved and Turks as the Scotsman had written), Douglass might not have been opposed. It is doubtful, though, Douglass would have honored a new medical practice by "Old Women" given the prejudice of the times. It was possible that a number of the Inoculators thought that the attack on Mather, Boylston, and the project, in general, had also been based on a personal enmity towards Mather and Boylston. Academicus might not have offered such a possibility if *that* view had not been shared rather widely. However, this interpretation might have been in retrospect a narrow one as there were clearly other larger issues of power and professionalism in play. The latter view highlights the beginning of changing medicine as a practice only for physicians and no longer perhaps in the domain of the clergy.

The dialogue continued with Academicus and Sawny debating various translations of the texts from Timoni and Pylarino. Then Academicus pointed out that by Douglass's raising the issue of possible future support of inoculation revealed the Scottish doctor didn't know what side of the "hedge" he was on. The physician wanted to have it both ways; he would want, most likely, to have come down on the correct side of such an important medical issue. Douglass's own first letter had actually undercut the physician's own position rather than that of Mather's.

The dialogue then addressed education and intellectual ability. Academicus brought up Mundungus, who also had so vigorously attacked Mather. Greenwood first defended the minister in this way:

> Tho' 'tis very probable that a Gentleman [Mather], that has published so much in the *Latin Tongue,* wants a little of your Instruction: Especially since *Mundungus*, too, (a Fellow who 'tis well known, could not spell a Common English Word; no not *Tobacco* if it were to save his life, tho' for the word *Pilfer* I will not say,) has found out that Dr. MATHER *wants Grammar Learning*. However, I hope, when you have taught him *Latin*, and your Brother has taught him *Grammar* and *Syllogisms,* (as he pretends to do), he may be something of a Scholar at last.[26]

This text represents a tug-of-war between who was a scholar, and who had credibility. Although the commentary was humorous and hyperbolic, there had been much trading of barbs about intellect. Greenwood, a student at Harvard, was doubly insulted that Mather should be so maligned. This debate showed not only the two men caught in the power struggle, but also asked a broader question. Should ministers or physicians be the knowledge brokers when it comes to medicine and power over the body politic/individual body?

Later in the dialogue, Academicus discussed with Sawny/Douglass the official threats made by the Selectmen against Mather and Boylston. Here the debate turned serious. This discourse concerned the meetings of the Selectmen and the beginning of charges that had been drawn up against Boylston and Mather. Here also Academicus hinted that the words of Mundungus and Sawny incited violence against the two Inoculators. Academicus opined to Sawny,

> Only I cannot but observe one odd expression of your malice toward him; you say … that if two or three men should be deposed, that *they*

> *heard a man* say, that *Somebody told him,* that *he heard a Report,* that Dr. MATHER had been guilty of a *Felonious Action;* ... : you declare it should be *worth his Neck,* in any Court of Justice, where you should go be *Foreman* of the Jury.[27]

Here he was quoting a threat of a death sentence against the two, Mather and Boylston, and if they were tried in court, Douglass would have wanted to be leading the jury. In the parody, Greenwood had Sawny admit to having said the above. That Douglass and the Anti-Inoculators, as well as the Inoculators, had heightened their verbal attacks on each other by this time was clear. However, the only violent actions or threats on record were taken against the Inoculators, particularly Boylston and Mather, and none against the Anti-Inoculators. Dalhonde's (the Frenchman's) narratives had inspired the Selectmen to announce there would be formal charges subsequently against any who would continue the practice of inoculation. Douglass had indeed upped the ante that such an action was "felonious" and suggested he would find Mather guilty, punishable by death if he were foreman of the jury.

Academicus continued to highlight the language Douglass had used to incite violence against Mather and actually accused him of having encouraged the firebombing of the minister's home in November 1721 (note the use of "*Sulfurious*" below.) "But stay, *Sawny*, that *Lark-time* [prank time] is not come yet; But thy Crew may use a more Sulfurious way to dispatch him, for I ought to know. In the mean time, *are not thou out of thy* LINE, *Sawny*?"[28] After Academicus expressed his (and most likely Mather's) outrage at the attacks against him, he had turned his attention to the attacks against Boylston:

> What but malice could inspire you to move that, Dr. BOYLSTON should be brought upon Tryal for his Life, as your Bloody Brother, and constant Friend *Mundungus* also does; whose Soul most certainly, if ever one Soul acted two bodies, has a full possession of yours. You say you would indite him for *poisoning* and *spreading Infection;* which you say is by the penal of *England*, a *Felony.*[29] Any felony then was considered a capital offense.

Greenwood then reverted to his earlier ridiculing of both Douglass and Mundungus for their scholarship (or lack thereof). "Now *Sawny*, be not angry, if we poor Scholars that must sit at the feet of such a *Gamaliel,* presume to Contradict you."[30] The reference to Gamaliel is to a scholar and wise man celebrated both in Judaism and Christianity. He was a grandson of Hillel and had been a noted rabbi in the first century CE and had apparently been instrumental in teaching Paul of Tarsus Jewish law. Some believe he argued to spare Peter's and other apostles' lives during the persecution of practicing Christians after Jesus of Nazareth's death.[31]

In the dialogue, Academicus then returned to using more logical argument strategies, such as the following: "You know, *Sawny,* that in *England*, 'tis a very common thing to carry Children into Infected Chambers, on purpose to give them the *Small-Pox;* because they judge their Childhood the best Time for them to have it in. But, was ever a *Spreading the Infection* prosecuted as a *Felony?* And is not *Inoculation* less dangerous and poisoning than this?"[32] When he had Douglass argue back that all medicines are poisonous, Academicus wanted to know if the physician himself shouldn't be brought up on felony charges, too.[33] Actually, in this period of time, many medicines were indeed poisonous: mercury, arsenic, etc. See C. Mather's medical compendium, *Angel of Bethesda* for a great wealth of such "cures."

In the last part of the dialogue, Greenwood continued to question Douglass's wisdom and even challenged his skill as a physician. He cited numerous instances in which Douglass purportedly was mistaken that a patient was near death and had not advised the family or friends. He had also intimated that Douglass was relatively unknown until he challenged the inoculation project, thus had insinuated that perhaps the doctor had another motive for writing and speaking so vehemently against the ministers and Boylston.[34] To add insult to injury, the author maintained that " ... you [Douglass] were one of the most unsuccessful PHYSICIANS in town."[35] At that point in his text, Greenwood (and perhaps Mather, too) had made most of the arguments against Douglass as representative of the Anti-Inoculators, even though the text also positioned Mundungus as one of the targets in the dialogue.

Attacks on Mundungus's Education and Writing Style

Toward the end of the hypothetical "debate," Mundungus was brought in by Academicus, and, although the pages devoted to him were fewer than those against Douglass, they were most interesting in their rhetorical strategies. Greenwood had begun with Mundungus even as he had begun with Douglass, with a critique of *his* language. This part of the parody bespoke of a criticism based on speaking in dialect (as he had shown toward Douglass). In immigrant communities (the early English colonists had indeed been immigrants to a land of another people, who were either indigenous or much earlier arrivals from another continent), there is often a key attention to language, both spoken and written. Such a tactic here serves to identify the more recent arrivals or else, in the case of Mundungus, the less well educated and less well regarded in intellectual circles. Greenwood's first addresses to Mundungus, then, were: " ... don't *speak* as you *spell*, [or] I won't hear a word you say."[36] This rhetorical strategy manages to make the two Anti-Inoculators more alike, by finding a common topic for each: their unusual or less than "standard" speech and writings.

The audience was then treated to a rendition of Mundungian spelling, which remains as obscure as it must have been at the time (thus was subjected to heavy, editorial assistance by the Franklins in the *Courant*). In light of who has credibility in colonial society, such illiteracy had been sufficient evidence of Williams not having been admitted to a culture marked by boundaries of education, class, and status. Such a tactic on the part of the Inoculators to discredit Mundungus, however, because he had been representing the "common people," could well have backfired. Some could argue that it did, since inoculation against smallpox was soon stopped for a number of decades. A few lines of Mundungian prose are featured below, and then my translation:

> *I cum to thell my Brether Sonni, that he is a foule. Becas he is so fouleche as to speke for hoomain invenecions in Fisecke. And, becas he dus not daddicut his Boucke to wurthy Seleket Men for them to be the Pattroones of his Abuseis on the Minesteres and Scakered Scripters. And becas he dus not imponeselly shay, that the best plase to gat Grammur Larning, and larn the Rols of Selegesem & studded Sempeti & Anthepeti, & solfe quescions & rigte tretes on Inokelacion is a Thobacko ciiler.*[37]

Mundungus had been represented as writing in the above lines that

> he come[s] to tell his brother, Sawny, that he is a fool. Because he is so foolish as to speak for human inventions in Physick. And, because he does not dedicate his book to [the] worthy Selectmen for them to be patrons of his abuses on the ministers and sacred scriptures. And because he does not especially say, that the best place to get grammar learning and learn the rules of Sydenham and study sympathy and antipathy and such questions and write treatises on inoculation is [from] a tobacco seller.[38]

This speech was Greenwood's set up of Mundungus to expose both his lack of education and vanity. The issue for Williams had supposedly been that Douglass's writings could have been dedicated in order to pay tribute to and flatter the Selectmen. The Anti-Inoculators had already involved the Selectmen of Boston in the debate, and that strategy had been a wise one, as they were the power brokers at the time and shared power in Boston (a tripartition of the clergy of the church, the crown-appointed Governor from England, and the Selectmen, a council of elected citizens of Boston). To further reinforce his derision of John Williams (Mundungus), Academicus next purported to have found an excellent manuscript in the Mundungian language. He listed on two pages, in two columns each, some eighty-five words with the erroneous spelling positioned across from the correct spelling he had put in (for the 1700s, when English/American spellings were still not so stable or standardized). Not all of the words in the brief text supposedly in Mundungian speech are in the vocabulary list. The fact that both speech and spelling were targeted in the dialogue was noteworthy, providing a real emphasis on class status, literacy, and education.

Before a further discussion of the various positions within this debate regarding the kinds of binaries (including use of "proper" language vs. dialect) set up between the Inoculators and the Anti-Inoculators on the part of both groups, it's necessary to complicate the notion of class differences in this fight for control of the "docile body." The constructs positioned by both sides in this struggle over influence on the body from a health or medical standpoint involve power.

" ... [T]he power exercised on the body is conceived not as a property, but as a strategy, that its effects of domination are attributed not to 'appropriation,' but to dispositions, manoeuvres, tactics, techniques, functionings; that one should decipher in it a network of relations, constantly in tension, in activity, rather than a privilege that one might possess; ... ."[39] For this chapter, although "class" and "privilege" are shorthand for what appears in the dialogues, it's important to keep in mind the concept of the apparatus. In the dialogues, we will see how the strategic positions were being challenged in fact by those who had been dominated and the way power had been "exercised" in the past had been disrupted. This change would ultimately affect and alter the immediate outcome of the inoculation project. Thus highlighted above are various rhetorical strategies and moves that had occurred: the "manoeuvres, tactics," and exercises.

Foucault goes to some pains in *Discipline and Punish* to lay out the interactions of power relations and suggest that the power extant in society "is not exercised simply as an obligation or a prohibition on those who 'do not have it'; it invests them, is transmitted by them and through them; it exerts pressure upon them, just as they themselves, in their struggle against it, resist the grip it has on them."[40] This understanding is what must undergird the debate in this chapter, because these "relations go right down into depths of society, that they are not [only] localized in the relations between the state and its citizens or on the frontier between classes."[41] These relations and operations of the apparatus are omnipresent and work, although I would argue we can see them better exposed in the discursive practices within such controversies as the inoculation project, and those operations do seem to be partially focused on class divisions.[42] While there certainly is continuity in these various practices, they cannot be regarded as univocal, because they are not stable, have their own contradictions, and even if they temporarily change the power structure, they are subject to their own risks and may fail ultimately or for a time.[43] Such an understanding could and can explain how voters, for example, can advocate or vote against their own best interests. In the following passage we see more evidence that does seem to invert the power relations, all the while remaining still part of the spoof.

Greenwood wrote the last pages of the Appendix in an epideictic spoof. Here are brief sections of that long monologue:

> And since he [Mundungus] has so honoured this part of the World, as first to impart it to *us;* we humbly conceive some *marks* of Honour ought to be conferred upon him: and we propose, that he be preferred *Professor* of *it,* among the *Sons of Harvard;* his language be inrolled into the Number of *learned Tongues,* and his *Manuscript* be preserved as a valuable *Curiosity* in the *Library*; ... "[44] [And], "further, *whither* he should not be constituted *Censor* of the Age and *Imprimator* of the Press? And be desired, to write a *Spelling-Book*, for the Use of the *Schools* ... ."[45]

The reference to the spelling book is an allusion to Isaac Watts, an English Dissenter, who wrote *The Art of Reading and Writing English* (London, 1721), a textbook on basic English usage widely adopted by schools in England and the American colonies. It included how words should be pronounced.

The authors then commented on Mundungus's rhetorical style: "And since it is so *Rhetorical* and *persuasive,* we move that, he be *Prolocutor* in all public Assemblies ... we can't pass by his profound skill in *Logic,* particularly, in the Art of *Syllogising.*"[46] The Inoculators are making fun of the tobacconist's attempt to emulate the rhetorical style in the higher education of the time, which included study in syllogistic reasoning. Because Williams's own syllogisms were quite crude as seen in the chapter on religion, he had left himself open to this attack for his style. With much sarcasm, Greenwood (and most likely, Mather) put Williams forward as an equal with them, even proposing that he write a spelling textbook, take a position as editor of a press, and serve as prolocutor at assemblies. The rhetorical move here created a stark division between the two classes, between the literati and the merchant of tobacco and apothecary, and between those with advanced education and those without. These status markers were indicators of power and privilege, as well as knowledge.

Greenwood's willingness to highlight Mundungus's style and education indicates that this split was already apparent in the culture, or it would have found no toehold within audience members. And there was some evidence that Mundungus, as a spokesperson, was highly effective among some facets of the society, or else why would he have come under attack? If the tobacconist's writings were largely ignored, why would it have been necessary to parody him? Evidence of resentment of the Bostonian elite, the Harvard ministers, particularly the Mathers, could be found throughout many writings over the inoculation period. Some have been included in the previous chapters, in this chapter, and in those that follow. The Anti-Inoculators had chosen well when they selected John Williams as a mouthpiece, one who appealed successfully to at least one sizeable audience, while Douglass had been more persuasive with the physicians and other more formally educated Bostonians.

One last volley that ended this parody concerned the prank played on Boylston and his horse that had turned out to be the wrong horse. This joke had been attributed to the tobacconist. Greenwood thus wrote,

> Mundungus has also discover'd so great a knowledge in *Divinity* that we move he be elected CONSCIENCE-KEEPER-GENERAL of the Country; and all Cases of difficulty be referred to him; and if any MINISTER shall meddle without his Liberty, it shall be deemed *a going out of his line,* and he shall be oblig'd to pay fourfold for the *tarr'd* Breeches.[47]

"*Going out of his line*" in the *Friendly Debate* was a reference to many of the Anti-Inoculators' charges against Mather, that he had meddled in "Physick" as a minister, rather than having respected some emerging professional boundaries, i.e., of the physicians of Boston. In the meantime, Mundungus, Douglass, and others against inoculation had spent much time publishing arguments using the Scriptures, so the charge of not respecting boundaries could well have been leveled (and sometimes had been) against both sides. Paying "fourfold for the *tarr'd* Breeches" was of course a reference to the tar on the saddle of some poor unknown victim's horse.

The reference to "going out of his line" represented an important aspect of the debate. Minardi, Silva, Sivils, and Schmotter have argued that this time in American history marked the beginning of modern American medicine. In addition to noting how the inoculation texts and their rhetorical moves worked in the debate itself, it is important to highlight how the issue of professionalization began to emerge. This issue emerged at the end of the first dialogue, but it was much more prominent in the *Abuses* letter written by Douglass. He had argued for clearer boundaries between the professions:

> The ministers, I mean those that have the Oversight of a *Flock,* in this great Town, should cease pretending to *Physick*, there being Practitioners sufficient in Number and Qualifications to supply the Place. Further, we find in great Towns, where there is Variety and Multitude of Business, that the Practitioners may be the better qualified for their *particular Professions* … .[48]

The Scottish doctor then noted how the various divisions within medicine were also quite specialized and quoted Hippocrates as a reliable source: "*Physick* itself is divided into distinct Branches, as *Physicians, Surgeons, Apothecarys, Chymists,* etc., each keeping within his bounds. How then can we suppose, a Man of a *Vocation,* which requires all his Time, conscientiously to discharge the same, should pretend to a Business of so great Extent?"[49] The Anti-Inoculators also made the point in the same Douglass tract that "A very eminent modern Physician, says, That many *Gentlemen* of universal Reading, and *old Women* by long Nursing, know as much of Physick as to kill themselves and Neighbours when sick, by the preposterous indiscreet Use of some noted Medicines."[50] Mather was known as a prodigious reader, so the passage could again have referred to him, but it also referenced others, including "old Women." That claim set up the next part of the argument, that "To be more or less *Book learned*, is not a sufficient Qualification for a *Physician;*" there needed to be more, including much exercise (practice) of the art.[51] Douglass continued in his letter to make other strong claims against the procedure being a "regular" one as the Inoculators had insisted. Instead, he noted that Boylston had begun inoculating before the physicians had had enough time to consider the question. The Selectmen had later called the physicians in for their opinion, which had been a negative one, resulting in the procedure being forbidden by the Selectmen. The Selectman had justified this decision by saying that the contagion was past, and many had escaped without inoculation and that in England only prisoners had been inoculated in a carefully controlled experiment.[52] This claim turned out not to be true. After each recitation of evidence, the author would ask, "How is this a regular procedure"? This epistrophe was used very effectively in this part of Douglass's letter.

The Second "Academicus Dialogue": The Response from Rusticus

The Anti-Inoculators' response to the first parody/dialogue had then followed swiftly; it was advertised in the *New-England Courant* the week before it appeared as a text from the Franklins' print shop on March 19, 1722 (13 days after the first "dialogue" appeared). The date of authorship was within days of the first salvo's publication. In the timeline of the smallpox epidemic itself and the series of variolations, Boylston continued to inoculate somewhat frequently until February 24, 1722. The inoculations in January and February had taken place in Charlestown and Cambridge, not in Boston proper. The disease temporarily waned in the city, so much so, that on February 26, 1722, the Selectmen had published in the *New-England Courant* that there were no longer any known cases locally. On April 14, the same body contradicted a rumor in Boston that the disease had returned in force, and many Bostonians had become infected, a number of whom had died. Instead, the Selectmen had continued, " ... the Report is false and groundless, there being but three Folks known to have the Small-Pox."[53] However, smallpox came back with a vengeance in a forceful new wave of infection.

Douglass, himself, made a brief reply to the release of the first Academicus "debate," but by far the more interesting text was that of "Rusticus," who many believe was John Williams (Mundungus), one of the targets of the first "debate." His *A Friendly Debate, or, A Dialogue between Rusticus and Academicus about the Late Performance of*

[A]cademicus followed much of the same form as Greenwood's with a similar tone, true to the earlier *tour de force*. The voice, however, does not sound like Mundungus's writing. One source suggested that this second farce had been written by Samuel Mather, son of Cotton Mather.[54] This was not possible, because such a text would not have been printed at the Franklin press, nor would it have made such reasoned arguments (at times) against inoculation. Mather's son was an adamant defender of his father, had been born in 1706, so at the time the tract came out, he was a 15-year-old Harvard student, who later became a clergyman. It's possible that a later cataloguer of the *Dialogues* confused Samuel Mather and Samuel Checkley, Jr. Both were born in 1706, both later became clergymen at Second Church in Boston. Most likely, the text would have been written by another Checkley, John. As a friend of James Franklin and an Anti-Inoculator, he had written an essay for the first edition of the *Courant*, in which he had written a salvo against the Puritan clergy accusing them of "teaching and practicing what's Orthodox, pray hard against Sickness, but preach up the Pox!"[55] John Checkley had been Oxford-educated.[56] Samuel Mather and John Checkley would have been at opposite ends of this debate, as John Checkley had had a feud with Cotton Mather over Calvinism in 1719 or 1720.[57] Checkley had also been the Anti-Inoculator who had tried to cast a shadow on Cotton Mather's claim that he was a Fellow of the Royal Society. In the very month smallpox broke out, C. Mather wrote to England, begging Edmond Halley (Halley's Comet), the famous astronomer, "to send him a certificate as to 'Mr. Mather's being a Fellow or not a Fellow.' Such a document, he protests will 'capacitate me to defend myself from these Sons of Strife, Schism and Sedition.'"[58]

As Academicus had begun, so, too, did Rusticus, with an "Advertisement":

> *Whereas Mr.* I. G. [Isaac Greenwood] *has lately publish'd* a little Friendly Debate *full of* broad English, broad Scotch, broad Latin, broad Mundungian, *and* good Billingsgate; *which yet in Vanity he may judge be acceptable to* C.M. D.D. *and* F.R.S. *These are to inform the Reader, that the said* I.G. by broad panegyricks *has satirized the said* C.M. (who has justly merited the Honour of being a Member of the ROYAL SOCIETY) *as well as many eminent and superior Persons among us.*

At first blush, this advertisement seems to be for quite a different text, but again, it was part of the spoof. Rusticus made fun of the fact that Greenwood had foregrounded language issues in his tract, such as "Billingsgate." Because of the unverifiable nature of authorship, Williams (who is best represented by Rusticus) will be used here. He suggested that Greenwood had "satirized" Cotton Mather, perhaps trying to drive a wedge between the two "Inoculators" or perhaps returning like for like. To have been a Fellow was one of the largest honors in European and colonial

Society, for it signaled a contributor on the cutting edge of Natural Philosophy. It had been an Achilles heel for Mather and thus a vulnerable spot for the Anti-Inoculators to harass the minister again and again by saying he was *not* a member.

The Dedication was another matter. Unlike Greenwood who seriously dedicated his defense of the Inoculators and his attacks on the Anti-Inoculators to Zabdiel Boylston for his courageous work, Rusticus dedicated the tract not to Douglass or another physician, as one might expect, but to Cotton Mather, addressing him as "Very Reverend and Learned."[59] If one did not know better, and most likely the cataloguer of the Digital Book Index did not, just reading the dedication would lead to the assumption that the book had been written by an Inoculator. The only departure from what looked like a serious dedication was the place of origin: "from the South Side of My Haystack."[60]

The text itself, like Greenwood's, contained serious, more reasoned arguments, pure farce, and liberally sprinkled insults. Early in the text, the author positioned the clergy and Inoculators as the elite versus the hard-working Bostonians. Rusticus asked what it was Academicus intended in writing the first dialogue. The author of the second parody then put the following words in Academicus's (Isaac Greenwood's) mouth: *I intended to let you know that I am a Man of Letters, and that not only* Sawny *but all the illiterate Scribblers of the Town,* (the Leather Apron Men) *are* proud and vain Fellows, and that 'tis not possible for them once in their Lives to speak a Word of Truth." Rusticus (Mundungus) brought up territorial claims early in the parody: "*I hope you don't think to take the same Liberty with me that you did with* Sawny and Mundungus: *This is boldly to invade the Province of another.*"[61]

The next part of the debate was devoted to discrediting the Inoculators by attacking the role of ministers and how the clergy had become not "healers" of rifts in a culture but rather the sowers of discord and unhappiness. To mount his attack, Rusticus chose to quote a Mr. Baxter:

> It is a dreadful Instance of the sottish deceivableness of Mankind, that one of the most happy Kingdoms on earth, should be almost consumed by their own hands, in Divisions infamous through the World, and that to this very day the *Cause* and *Matter* of them is not known (except to the contrivers, among ourselves) by such who madly continue the Divisions ... . And it's one of the saddest notices of the World, that studious, Learned Pastors that have grown old in Studies, and profess all to be devoted to Truth and Love, are so far from having *Skill or Will to heal us,* that they are the Men that *cause the Wound,* and keep it open, and are greater hinderers of our Concord and Peace, than Princes, Lords, or any Seculars. And both sides confess while they lay it on each other, that it is the Clergy that are the deadliest Enemies of Peace.[62]

For a number of generations, the Puritan clergy had been the ruling power of this colony, even though the Governor sent from England had been the nominal head. Within the theocratic society, the group that had kept the people together and had led them in the interpretation of life's vicissitudes had been their religious professionals. The clergy, especially the Mathers, who also had helped to establish and command the institutions of learning in addition to the churches, had come to be resented over time certainly by some Bostonians, partly perhaps because of mistakes made in the past and partly from what had been a tight control over a relatively long period of time. Walter Isaacson noted this schism and praised the initiation of the *Courant* "as America's first fiercely independent newspaper, a bold anti-establishment journal that helped to create the nation's tradition of an irreverent press."[63] Perry Miller noted, "It was the first open effort to defy the norm."[64] The *Courant* was established at the beginning of the inoculation controversy and most likely because of it. In addition, leading up to the Revolutionary War period itself, a number of Bostonians had been restless for a new chance at leadership and had also been resentful of any authority which purported to make the decisions for them regarding their futures. Add the fears generated by a cruel epidemic, and the society had begun to foment for a changing of the guard.

Rusticus punctuated his heavy indictment of the clergy with a straight-on attack of academicians and education as well: "I might likewise add the Opinion of Mr. *Daille*, formerly Minister of the Gospel in the Reformed Church of *Paris, in his Treatise concerning the right use of the Fathers*, p. 155, which may also shew you that an ACADEMICAL Education is often lost on those who are favour'd with it."[65] This quote is further evidence of educational and class differences having been conflated with anticlerical views, since not all members of the colony had opportunities for higher education. Most who did have the opportunity were the future clergy at Harvard. Rusticus continued this lengthy monologue suggesting that the clergy had grievously erred in their judgment and gone away from the truth. He also had written that it was indeed the parishioners themselves who had held the accurate views. He had maintained this thesis was especially applicable to the inoculation project.[66]

This Rusticus, although pointed in his rebukes of the clergy and "learned" men, was arguing from a more reasoned position and did not rely on name-calling. He even wrote in the dialogue a decent rebuttal for Academicus, that using Baxter was taken out of context, because his treatise had been written as an attack on the clergy of England and France, and could not have been applied to colonial clergy on this continent. [67] The two discussed this claim for a time, and then Rusticus set up Academicus for the next attack via this question:

> "[W]ho do you take to be the *Principal* Ministers of Religion in *New-England*?"[68]

Academicus replied, "*Who!* Dr. Increase Mather *and his Son.*"[69]

Rusticus, having known how effective an attack would be on Cotton's respect abroad, continued to work on this theme by having Academicus again rehearse the status of Mather in Europe by highlighting his membership in the Royal Society. Then, using the argument style of academic criticism (as differentiated from clerical claims backed by Biblical texts), Rusticus again quoted a supposed expert source: "Right again, 'Demicus, he has certainly a *great Name* abroad for *Something*. Tho' many Authors mention him with *great Veneration,* yet as I am now conversing with an *Academical* Brother, what Mr. *Oldmixon* says in his *History of the British Colonies,* Page 108, 109, is most to my present Purpose."[70] This introduction set up an argument for a well-known historian to challenge another academic. This move also enhanced "Rusticus's" ethos. This was the opposite tone of what Academicus had written in the first dialogue, practicing a more "rustic" vernacular in order to parody Williams. The Anti-Inoculator then cited a harsh review by Oldmixon of one of Mather's works:

> The *History of New-England* written by *Cotton Mather* ... is a sufficient Proof, that a Man may have read hundreds of Latin authors, and be qualifi'd to construe them, may have spent his Youth in a Colledge, and be bred up in Letters, yet have neither Judgment to know how to make a Discourse perspicuous, nor Eloquence to express his Sentiments so that they may please and persuade the easiest way to Conviction.[71]

John Oldmixon, 1673–1742, had written two volumes on the British colonies and islands of America.[72] He was the most preeminent historian and writer about the colonies at the time.

Again, as in the first dialogue/debate, both sides of the inoculation project are debating styles of writing and speech. They were using rhetorical analyses to challenge each other repeatedly, examining the ability to persuade, but not using scientific fact nor doctrinal law/proofs in these texts. Their appeals were more to ethos than logos. These particular dialogues served to challenge directly the knowledge base of each, too, arguing about education, class, and professionalism. The question can be titrated as to who is able to talk about medicine, and who has the *bona fides* of an intellectual.

Next Rusticus attacked Mather's history further via the critic, Oldmixon:

> For all the Books that ever came from the Press with venerable Title of a History, it is impossible to shew one that is so confus'd in the Form, so trivial in the Matter, and so faulty in the Expression, so cramm'd with Punns, Anagrams, Acrosticks, Miracles and Prodigies, that it rather resembles School Boys Exercises Forty Years ago, and *Romish* Legends, than the Collections of an Historian bred up in a Protestant Academy."[73]

Thus Rusticus treated the Boston community to the harshest remarks on Mather's text. The Anti-Inoculator continued in this vein at length, having pointed out that this atrocious style of writing was the use to which New England clergy had put their education. In many ways, the Anti-Inoculator writing the Rusticus dialogue was claiming that the powers-that-be, or had been, were now out of date, no longer relevant, and that their education had been at best idiosyncratic. Additionally, he had made some comments denigrating Harvard, but later said that the design of the university had not been at fault but rather the running of the school and execution of its curriculum (in certain years in the hands of Increase Mather, of course.) Rusticus claimed, too, that the teachings had been popular some one hundred years ago, but were no longer valid. Instead, the religious teachings needed only be backed up by Biblical texts, instead of out-of-date "cant."[74]

Academicus's very brief reply following this prodigious monologue was to suggest that Rusticus could not profit, then, from Mather's words from the pulpit. To this charge, Rusticus had replied that he wished the town could just keep him in the pulpit, implying that many would have preferred keeping him out of the inoculation and medical treatment arena: "I like him *best* in the Pulpit Mr. '*Demicus,* and believe it would be much for the Peace of the Town and Country if he could ever be confin'd to it."[75] This part of the argument addressed the boundary issues once again, as the disciplines of religion and medicine had started to formulate themselves as separate when it came to controlling public health as well as controlling the "docile" bodies of the populace.

But what is a "docile body" and why is it an important concept to consider throughout this debate? "A body is docile that may be subjected, used, transformed and improved."[76] The smallpox inoculation project had indeed presented itself as a way to transform and ultimately "improve" the "docile body," because it could protect the actual body against fatal and acute cases of smallpox, as well as ultimately protect the social body, the parishioners of the ministers and the citizens of Boston and its surroundings by hypothetically stopping a major epidemic. But again, one must consider the wider implications of control and the power relations that were in play at this time not just in America but throughout Europe as well. Foucault maintained that there was a new aspect to the way the body was considered: "What was so new in these projects of docility that interested the eighteenth century so much? It was certainly not the first time that the body had become the object of such imperious and pressing investments; … ."[77] Foucault suggested what was new was the "modality." By modality in this case, he meant an overarching surveillance method or supervisory lens that implied constant coercion, that is not interrupted, and that oversees not the results but the processes itself.[78] We see such a modality coming into play via the Selectmen and the Anti-Inoculators on the one hand, in their efforts to stop the inoculation of Bostonians and, on the other hand by the Inoculators, who were instituting a method not just of disease control, but social control of the operations of the body, often necessary in the midst of an epidemic.

Of course some "social control" had already come into play in Boston, as mentioned earlier in the text, in the use of quarantines, which had waxed and waned depending on the various epidemics that had made their way into Boston harbor. The disciplinary foci are also of issue, as shown in the textual evidence above. This difference may seem subtle, but in the smallpox controversy, one sees the early stirrings of the set-up of a new machinery of power. As Foucault had suggested, human bodies can enter machineries of power that take over and rearrange all aspects of our human functions.[79] Here one can think on the microscopic level of the inoculation itself when a powerful substance has entered a body and rearranged its immune system; on the social or political level, one can think of a group of people being inoculated or, in this case, the society refusing such a medical technique. "A 'political anatomy,' which was also a 'mechanics of power,' was being born; it defined how one may have a hold over others' bodies, not only so that they may do what one wishes, but so that they may operate as one wishes, with the techniques, the speed and the efficiency that one determines." Thus discipline produces compliant or "docile" bodies subject to control. While being within a discipline of medicine (or protocols, as modern medicine has every action within a hospital, for example, controlled and dictated by a "protocol"), there are more forces on the body, especially in terms of social utility and economics. At the same time, there are fewer forces in terms of "obedience" of the individual and the individual's body than those found in strict church dogma, which also dictated what one could and couldn't do vis-à-vis the body. Because of this rupture in the power system, then, there was in some ways more freedom in saying "No," to the clergy, even if it meant saying no to inoculation. The theocracy had early on through sermonic and Biblical injunctions dictated a spiritual body or ideal use of the body dissociated from an actual body, which had created their social control over the parishioners. While such control formulates a body, whether social or individual with some ideal in mind, on the one hand, it also changes the energy flow or power dynamic into a relation of subjection, in this case by the clergy.[80] At the same time, while the clergy had also been in charge of "Physick," it had also garnered power over the actual health and illness processes of the physical body.

Early Attempts at Re-Organizing a Political Anatomy

These two parodies during the controversial project highlighted the workings of these changes that are more easily seen at certain times than at others. Such shifts work in tidal fashion, a systole and diastole of movement and action over time, not just in one dramatic moment. Foucault also maintains that any reconfiguration of a political anatomy is not suddenly present but takes place for a period through many smaller events or discursive practices in different places that like waves can repeat themselves, verge together, or imitate and support one another until they eventually converge into a new *modus operandi.*[81] The changes, however, were not at any completion stage yet, but instead this analysis acts as an x-ray of the early movements in that direction. In the dialogues, we see other power moves, especially vis-à-vis the Selectmen of Boston.

In the next part of the parody, Rusticus questioned Academicus as to why he had so vigorously attacked the Scottish doctor; Williams maintained that the patient who had so complained about Douglass's practice of medicine recanted his attacks. Then he challenged Academicus again by asking him why he had upbraided Douglass for not dedicating his recently published tract to the Selectmen.[82] The author has Greenwood admit that it was for revenge because the Selectmen had demanded the ministers appear before them to account for the inoculations. In the first dialogue, Greenwood thought that the Selectmen were supporting the Anti-Inoculators too much, undercutting the success of the inoculation project, and denying the chance to protect the town from a surfeit of death and suffering.[83]

Not to be outdone by Greenwood, the author of this text also included appendices. These are part of John Williams's text: *Several Arguments, Proving, That Inoculating the Small Pox Is Not Contained in the Law of Physick, Either Natural or Divine, and Therefore Unlawful: Together with a Reply to Two Short Pieces, One by the Rev. Dr. Increase Mather, and Another by an Anonymous Author, Intituled, Sentiments on the Small Pox Inoculated: And Also a Short Answer to a Late Letter in the New-England Courant,* all of which were written earlier in response to Mather's text: *Several Arguments*. The last part concerned itself, like Greenwood's appendices, mostly with the language issue, indicative again of them as powerful markers of class and literacy. Answering the first dialogue in kind in which Greenwood or Mather had satirically suggested that Williams be made professor, editor, and spelling/pronunciation/grammar textbook author, Rusticus had written in response:

> Yet we presume the *Mundungian Language* can afford us a Name for it; (tho' probably the word *Therebal* [terrible] in the *Vocabulary* lately publish'd may do for the present: And therefore, we propose, that at least Two Thirds of the *Sons of Harvard,* who write in this Stile, may be doomed to the *Cellar of Mundungus,* to perfect themselves in his Language. We likewise propose that instead of scattering Scraps of *Latin* and *Greek* in their Writings ... they use now and then a Phrase in the Mundungian *Language,* the very sound of which is *rhetorical* and *persuasive.*[84]

Rusticus next continued with the topic of public speaking (having addressed writing style):

> And since all illiterate Men are forbid (by the Learned) to speak in *Publick Assemblies,* we move that all *Town-Meetings,* and Associations

> of the *People,* a *Mundungian Scholar* may be the *Prolocutor:* and that he not be lost in the crowd, we propose, that his Head be neatly bound with a roll of *Tobacco;* and that this Neck cloth be made of WILLIAMS *best Virginia in the leaf.*[85]

This last part of the text clearly aped the lines of the Greenwood tract, even to the point of agreeing that indeed Mundungus should be "Prolocutor" and lead assemblies, as Greenwood had satirically asserted. Williams (or Checkley) joined in the joke and added the tobacco plant to signify the tobacconist's role. This last part of the published tract was much more clearly a response to Academicus in tone and spirit, while the previous and main part of the responding track had been in a more serious vein.

The author(s) ended with a poem, most likely written by Williams. The rhymes were poor; there's an attempt to write an elegy. This part of tract turned a bit sinister, because of Greenwood's status as a Harvard student at the time he wrote the Academicus piece. The elegy by the Anti-Inoculator was titled "On the Death of a Young Schollar."[86] There was no record of any serious attempts on Greenwood's life or welfare, as well as could be determined. However, as mentioned above, there were threats against Mather and Boylston, one of which had been carried out only months before. The poem reviewed the youth's bright wit and knowledge (in Mundungian "Noleg") and then said he was "as learn'd a Youth as e'er was bred at Coleg."[87]

Other Commentary on Education

Other young scholars, perceiving the attacks on their senior alums and mentors, as well as their institution, had joined the fight. Greenwood was not the only student involved in the smallpox inoculation debate. Samuel Mather also figured prominently in the debate. There were numerous accounts and editorial letters going back and forth between the newspaper editors of the *New-England Courant* (the Franklins), the young Samuel Mather, Increase Mather, and others who had entered the fray. A number of editions carried this controversy, so it continued for some length of time with refutations, denials, accusations, corrections, and contractions in great numbers.

The young Samuel Mather, Cotton's son, had apparently brought news to the *New-England Courant,* which of the three Bostonian papers was the one most against the inoculation project, about large numbers of smallpox inoculations being carried out in London and having been reported in the *London Mercury* from September 16, 1721. One of the editors, either Benjamin or James Franklin, had written in response to some question regarding how the ill will between the grandfather, Increase Mather, and the paper, had begun. In detailing how the controversy began, the editor wrote a letter that centered on the reportage: "*Great Numbers of Persons in the*

City and the Suburbs are under the Inoculation of the Small Pox [London and its suburbs]. Among the rest, the eldest Son of a noble Duke in Hanover Square, had the Small Pox inoculated upon him."[88] When the *Courant* editor later examined that issue of the London paper, he said he had been unable to find the information: "About Noon on the Day that the *Courant* came out, I saw the Four first Pages of the *London Mercury of Sept. 16* and found nothing in them, but that *the eldest son of a noble Duke in Hanover Squares, had the small Pox inoculated upon him* INCOGNITO."[89] In other words, according to Franklin, there were no large numbers of people inoculated, and the son of the Duke had been inoculated without having identified himself as the Duke's offspring. The editor said the word *Incognito* had been left out of Samuel Mather's letter.

The editor then had reprimanded the young Mather, "Here our young Spark was detected in a downright Falshood, and lost his Credit with *New-England Courant*; and I had great Reason too to believe that the Part of the above Paragraph was not in the other Half-sheet of the *Mercury*, together."[90] The grandfather, Increase, however, had maintained that he himself had transcribed the passage citing the numerous inoculations word for word and included "Incognito."[91] Then ensued further discussion that the passage had been included instead in a "Weekly Mercury."[92] After that debate, much was made over whether or not Increase Mather had been a subscriber of the *Courant* and then ceased his subscription, instead asking that the letter be published in the *Gazette*, a newspaper much more friendly to the smallpox inoculation project.

Samuel Mather, having read the various editorials that attacked his grandfather and father, had already been insulted in print by the *Courant* about an earlier letter he had sent to the *Gazette*. The editor, Franklin, had questioned the youngster's schooling:

> a young scribbling Collegian, who has just Learning enough to make a Fool of himself, has taken it in his Head to *put a Stop to this wickedness* (as he calls it) by a Letter in the last Week's *Gazette*. Poor Boy! When your Letter comes to be *seen in other Countries*, (under the Umbrage of Authority,) *what* indeed *will they think of* New-England![93]

Franklin voiced concern for how the colony might be perceived. Also, he and other Anti-Inoculators had often in print referred to Cotton Mather as a "scribbler," suggesting the grandson/son was a "chip off the old block." The editor answered his own question:

> They will certainly conclude, *There is bloody Fishing* for Nonsense *at* Cambridge, *and* [Illegible] *Work at the* Colledge, [Illegible] Wretch, when he [the young Mather] calls these [Anti-Inoculators] who write the several Pieces in the Courant, *The Hell-Fire Club of Boston*, and finds a *Godfather* for them, [which is a Hellish Mockery of the Ordinance of Baptism, as administered by the Church of *England*].[94]

The "Hell-Fire Club of Boston" refers to the Hell-Fire Club in London, a scurrilous hangout of high society "gentlemen." In Boston, this name was given by the Inoculators to the Society of Physicians the Anti-Inoculators had begun in August 1721 after the smallpox inoculations had begun.[95] Both sides had intensified the rhetoric over the controversy, but it is noteworthy here that class and education issues had again risen to the fore.

In another letter Samuel sent to the paper on the same issue, the following language about the grandson of I. Mather and his relation to the school appeared:

> It is, that no Man except his Head were made of *Butter*, and in *a melting Posture*, would ever publish such a *Diabolical Medley of Nonsense,* as scarce any Age or Country can parallel. And in my Opinion, it will be a lasting Repoach [sic] to *Cambridge,* that such Poysonous and more than Humane Malice from thence should Issue.[96]

Again there is another allusion to the boy's parenthood: "It Seems the *Venomous Itch of Scribbling* is Hereditary; a Disease transmitted from the *Father to the Son.* Our Young Scribbler has made a very fine Beginning, and given the World a wonderful Specimen of what they may expect hereafter."[97]

Other mentions regarding the education had figured earlier in the debate, including in the following unattributed letter in the first issue of the *Courant* in August 1721. The first column makes fun of questions that might be asked before an author was entitled to publish in Boston: "Was you bied at Colledge Sir? And can you (like some of them) square the Circle, and cypher as far as the Black Art? &c."[98] The author sought to conflate college education with the practitioners of the black arts, i.e., witchcraft, another allusion to Cotton Mather and a put-down of Harvard.

That letter was followed in the same issue by another. "At the Request of several Gentlemen in Town: A Continuation of the History of Inoculation in *Boston*, by a Society of the Practitioners in Physick." Apparently, though, the author of the "History," probably an Anti-Inoculator, was answering an earlier letter in a different venue that had attacked the people of Boston opposed to the inoculation project, calling them ignorant, etc.

> At first reading of this Composure, many were persuaded, that it was only a piece of Humour, Banter, Burlesque, or Ridicule on the Inoculator, &c. in treating a Character of low Life with a sort of strain'd Sublime, in a P—t manner; but were surprized [sic] to find two Gentleman, not in the Question, having given no Shadow of Offence, called Illiterate, Ignorant, & c. This (as they prophesied) *the Town takes very much amiss.*[99]

This quotation is confusing today, but in fact was at first supposed to fool readers into thinking they were reading in favor of inoculation, suddenly to find the meaning in fact was that those against inoculation had been targeted as "Illiterate" and "Ignorant." Thus in the statement above, two gentlemen, most likely Dr. Douglass and John Williams, were treated the same way as the "Character of low Life." "P—t in the quotation was "Papist," a slur meaning the two men had been treated poorly like those who practiced Catholicism.

The author, presumably a physician in the "Society," also wrote: "B—n was represented in a soft Manner, as illiterate, ignorant, rash, &c. only with respect to the Small Pox, and the dubious, dangerous Practice of Inoculation; these Gentleman [sic] are called so in gross."[100] "B—n" probably stood for Boylston and suggested he had come in for a bit softer handling and called all names only in regard to the inoculation project, while the Mundungus and Douglass were called by Greenwood *illiterate* "in gross," or overall characterized in this way, not in just one area. Because this letter was most likely written by a physician, it's possible that Boylston had been attacked more mildly than the other men, although Douglass had not held back in a similar way. Physicians in the colony, except for Douglass, at the time had trained with other physicians as apprentices, but that training had taken place at patients' bedsides, not in a college or university. The point here is that learned men who had "idled" away for four years were not worthy of the respect that they deemed fit. The author believed that the Anti-Inoculators had been insulted on the basis of their lack of education in a letter that had said, "Because they [the physicians except for Boylston] did not *idle away four Years at Colledge, as some of our learned Men have done?"*

The Silence Dogood Letters

The most damning attack on the education of the elite and on Harvard itself was Ben Franklin's Silence Dogood letter #4 of May 7–14, 1722 in his and his brother's paper. Not even James knew the authorship of the Silence Dogood letters at first, as the younger brother used only the name Silence and slid the letters under the door of the weekly anonymously.[101] "James Franklin and his friends knew that 'Silence Dogood' was a pen name and not a 'real' woman ... and concluded that the writer using the pseudonym was a clever and well-read man of town; they had no idea that the real author was James's younger brother."[102] When later the younger brother admitted his authorship, then perhaps had begun the alienation that was to take place between the two; Ben had received considerable attention as a result of the 14 Silence Dogood letters. James had become more and more resentful of his younger brother's success.[103] In B. Franklin's *Autobiography*, he recalled that James had cautioned [him] against being too vain because of the reception the Dogood essays had received."[104]

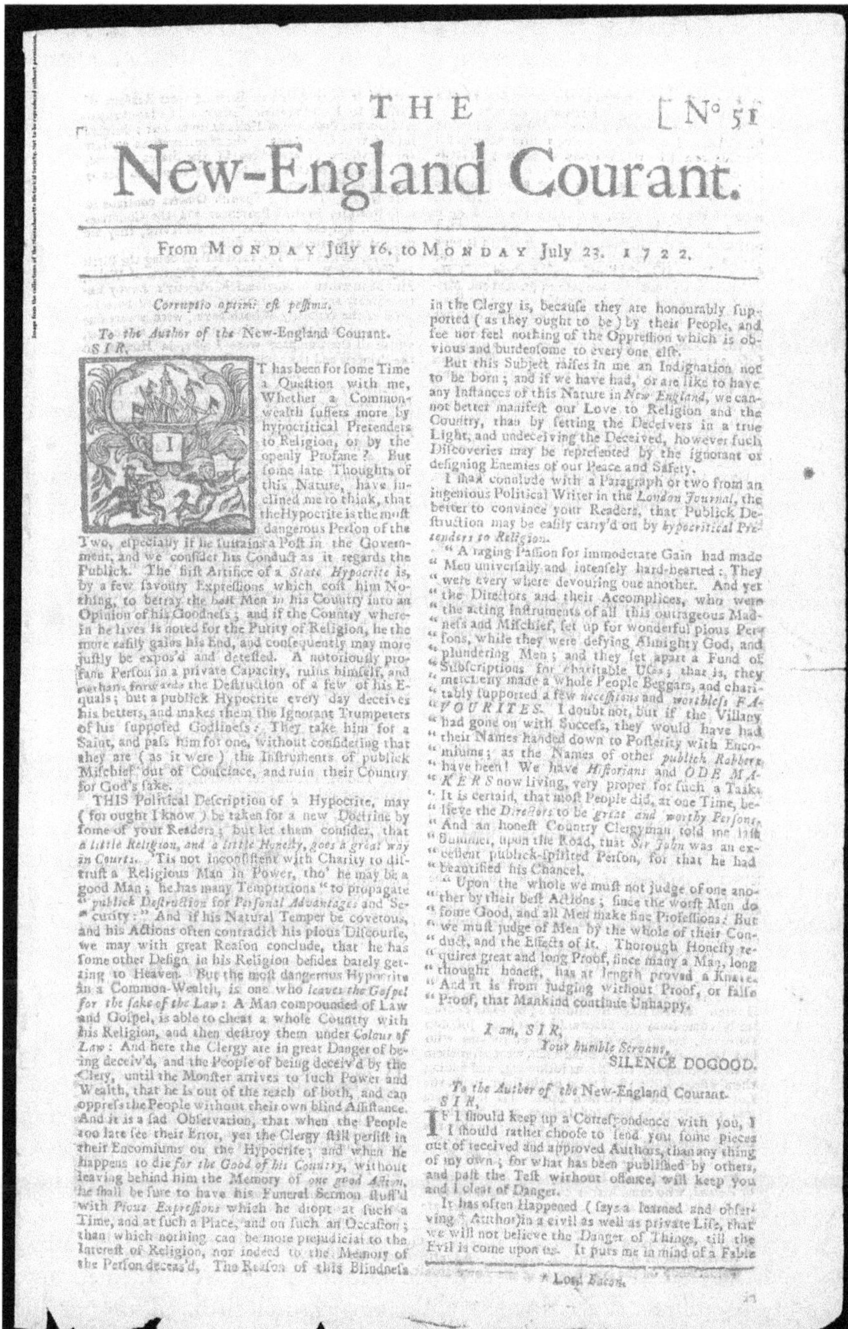

THE [Nº 51

New-England Courant.

From MONDAY July 16. to MONDAY July 23. 1722.

Corruptio optimi eſt peſſima.

To the Author of the New-England Courant.

SIR,

IT has been for ſome Time a Queſtion with me, Whether a Commonwealth ſuffers more by hypocritical Pretenders to Religion, or by the openly Profane? But ſome late Thoughts of this Nature, have inclined me to think, that the Hypocrite is the moſt dangerous Perſon of the Two, eſpecially if he ſuſtains a Poſt in the Government, and we conſider his Conduct as it regards the Publick. The firſt Artifice of a *State Hypocrite* is, by a few ſavoury Expreſſions which coſt him Nothing, to betray the beſt Men in his Country into an Opinion of his Goodneſs; and if the Country wherein he lives is noted for the Purity of Religion, he the more eaſily gains his End, and conſequently may more juſtly be expos'd and deteſted. A notoriouſly profane Perſon in a private Capacity, ruins himſelf, and perhaps forwards the Deſtruction of a few of his Equals; but a publick Hypocrite every day deceives his betters, and makes them the Ignorant Trumpeters of his ſuppoſed Godlineſs: They take him for a Saint, and paſs him for one, without conſidering that they are (as it were) the Inſtruments of publick Miſchief out of Conſcience, and ruin their Country for God's ſake.

THIS Political Deſcription of a Hypocrite, may (for ought I know) be taken for a new Doctrine by ſome of your Readers; but let them conſider, that *a little Religion, and a little Honeſty, goes a great way in Courts.* 'Tis not inconſiſtent with Charity to diſtruſt a Religious Man in Power, tho' he may be a good Man; he has many Temptations "to propagate "*publick Deſtruction for Perſonal Advantages* and Se"curity:" And if his Natural Temper be covetous, and his Actions often contradict his pious Diſcourſe, we may with great Reaſon conclude, that he has ſome other Deſign in his Religion beſides barely getting to Heaven. But the moſt dangerous Hypocrite in a Common-Wealth, is one who *leaves the Goſpel for the ſake of the Law*: A Man compounded of Law and Goſpel, is able to cheat a whole Country with his Religion, and then deſtroy them under *Colour of Law*: And here the Clergy are in great Danger of being deceiv'd, and the People of being deceiv'd by the Clergy, until the Monſter arrives to ſuch Power and Wealth, that he is out of the reach of both, and can oppreſs the People without their own blind Aſſiſtance. And it is a ſad Obſervation, that when the People too late ſee their Error, yet the Clergy ſtill perſiſt in their Encomiums on the Hypocrite; and when he happens to die *for the Good of his Country*, without leaving behind him the Memory of *one good Action*, he ſhall be ſure to have his Funeral Sermon ſtuff'd with *Pious Expreſſions* which he dropt at ſuch a Time, and at ſuch a Place, and on ſuch an Occaſion; than which nothing can be more prejudicial to the Intereſt of Religion, nor indeed to the Memory of the Perſon deceas'd. The Reaſon of this Blindneſs in the Clergy is, becauſe they are honourably ſupported (as they ought to be) by their People, and ſee nor feel nothing of the Oppreſſion which is obvious and burdenſome to every one elſe.

But this Subject raiſes in me an Indignation not to be born; and if we have had, or are like to have any Inſtances of this Nature in *New England*, we cannot better manifeſt our Love to Religion and the Country, than by ſetting the Deceivers in a true Light, and undeceiving the Deceived, however ſuch Diſcoveries may be repreſented by the ignorant or deſigning Enemies of our Peace and Safety.

I ſhall conclude with a Paragraph or two from an ingenious Political Writer in the *London Journal*, the better to convince your Readers, that Publick Deſtruction may be eaſily carry'd on by *hypocritical Pretenders to Religion.*

"A raging Paſſion for immoderate Gain had made "Men univerſally and intenſely hard-hearted: They "were every where devouring one another. And yet "the Directors and their Accomplices, who were "the acting Inſtruments of all this outrageous Mad"neſs and Miſchief, ſet up for wonderful pious Per"ſons, while they were defying Almighty God, and "plundering Men; and they ſet apart a Fund of "Subſcriptions for charitable Uſes; that is, they "mercileſly made a whole People Beggars, and chari"tably ſupported a few *neceſſitous* and *worthleſs FA*"*VOURITES.* I doubt not, but if the Villany "had gone on with Succeſs, they would have had "their Names handed down to Poſterity with Enco"miums; as the Names of other *publick Robbers* "have been! We have *Hiſtorians* and *ODE MA*"*KERS* now living, very proper for ſuch a Task. "It is certain, that moſt People did, at one Time, be"lieve the *Directors* to be *great and worthy Perſons.* "And an honeſt Country Clergyman told me laſt "Summer, upon the Road, that *Sir John* was an ex"cellent publick-ſpirited Perſon, for that he had "beautified his Chancel.

"Upon the whole we muſt not judge of one ano"ther by their beſt Actions; ſince the worſt Men do "ſome Good, and all Men make fine Profeſſions: But "we muſt judge of Men by the whole of their Con"duct, and the Effects of it. Thorough Honeſty re"quires great and long Proof, ſince many a Man, long "thought honeſt, has at length proved a Knave. "And it is from judging without Proof, or falſe "Proof, that Mankind continue Unhappy.

I am, SIR,

Your humble Servant,

SILENCE DOGOOD.

To the Author of the New-England Courant.

SIR,

IF I ſhould keep up a Correſpondence with you, I ſhould rather chooſe to ſend you ſome pieces out of received and approved Authors, than any thing of my own; for what has been publiſhed by others, and paſt the Teſt without offence, will keep you and I clear of Danger.

It has often Happened (ſays a learned and obſerving * Author) in a civil as well as private Life, that we will not believe the *Danger of Things*, till the Evil is come upon us. It puts me in mind of a Fable

* Lord *Bacon.*

Figure 4.2 The New-England Courant, Wikimedia Commons.

B. Franklin's "Silence Dogood Letter No. 4" took higher education and Harvard itself to task. In his own parody in the *Courant*, he had "Clericus" give Silence advice on the education of her son, and Ms. Dogood claimed that "the information which he gave me, was neither pleasant, nor such as I expected."[105] Dogood (B. Franklin) then told the reader he had napped and dreamt about a "Temple of LEARNING: Every Peasant, who had where-withal, was preparing to send one of his children at least to this famous Place; and in this Case most of them consulted their own Purses instead of their Children's Capacities: So that I observed ... the most part of those ... were little better than Dunces and Blockheads."[106] The young journalist/apprentice editor had given detail that clearly marked the target as Harvard, describing the "large and stately Edifice" and the statuary with "Antique Figures ... Latin, Greek, Hebrew, &c. and that ... most [at Harvard] ... pretended to an intimate acquaintance with them."[107] In the dream, after her tour of the Temple of Learning, Silence insisted that "I saw nothing worth mentioning, except the ambitious and fraudulent Contrivances of Plagius, who ... was diligently transcribing some eloquent Paragraphs out of Tillotson's Words, &c. to embellish his own." In this parody, the nap is interrupted by Clericus and after the dreamer related the odyssey to him, he had concluded and interpreted the dream as being " ... a lively Representation of HARVARD COLLEGE."[108] That such a letter had found wide acceptance and popularity indicates the extent of hostility toward higher education and its theocratic founders, Harvard specifically, and intellectualism in general. The irony was that Franklin not many years later was known for his erudition. Young Franklin himself had been forced to give up his own schooling when his father needed an apprentice, and yet he had very much valued books and practiced his writing skills. In the text above, he had made clear the hypocrisy and pretense had been the culprits he had been targeting. The Silence Dogood letters add more evidence of the resistance to the old regime building up in the Boston Puritans.

Reflecting on the Power Relations Revealed

In the above texts, it should be clear that there is a convergence of power and knowledge in the context of the inoculation project as the two sides debated where education should be produced, and what kind of learning should be valued. Should it be issued through colleges, professions based on experience, politics, or religion? Foucault maintained that power produces knowledge and vice versa, that there is no true power relation without at the same time epistemic work.[109] Thus knowledge about any discipline, even medicine, becomes intertwined and implies the power to learn, practice, and disseminate that knowledge; the two are married and inseparable. What counts as knowledge runs through all the texts of the inoculation project, but it was perhaps most naked in the texts attacking higher education, "mother wit," or common sense, and who had the power to decide which of these was more valid. The power system does need to be analyzed in tandem with the modalities of knowledge.[110] The process of reconfiguration can be seen in those subjects who "know," even though they are challenged again and again; in what techniques are to be known, such as vaccination; and in the modalities of knowledge. We see the early domains here of current and future knowledge forming, dissolving, and forming again. The power itself and/or the resistance to power in the end determine what domains of knowledge will be possible..[111]

The set of two dialogues, letters to the editors, and Franklin's Dogood columns were remarkable in a number of ways. First, their humor had been sometimes quite effective and yet somewhat hard to imagine in the midst of a smallpox epidemic, although that wave had started to wane at that particular point in time. Given the seriousness of the antagonism between the two camps and the number of letters, newspaper columns, and pamphlets that had been published, to take a new tack of approaching the argument through humor, albeit at times very biting and even cruel, seemed a surprising departure from the other texts. Secondly, the emphasis on language itself and also in relation to education and class made it evident that discourse and the attendant education had been major markers of status. Even more importantly, language was used to determine who might be sanctioned to acquire the power/knowledge and how and where that power/knowledge might be gotten and used. One's ability to use language in a certain manner also seemed to determine who had authority to speak at this time in the colonies, perhaps particularly in Boston, just as it had been, and continued to be in the colony, in England, and other European countries. Education was the privilege of the wealthy and those who had a legacy of status. The extended discussions of "Mundungian" language and the sport the author (s) had made with it had made it very clear how important not only speech was (dialects were also graded in England at the comparable time) but also the written language. Those who could write were rewarded with higher status. Even at a time when spellings were still not standardized, close attention was paid to how words were spelled and how important literacy was.

Thirdly, what surfaced even in the midst of a smallpox epidemic and the introduction of a vaccination against the disease was the resentment toward Harvard, the institution of higher learning presided over for a number of years by Puritan ministers, including Increase Mather; the fatigue with the Mathers as a ruling family; and the anger toward those colonial men, most of whom were destined to be ministers, who were able to attend that institution. Close to the surface of the discussions of language, the resentment of those in the educated class by the less educated had begun to erupt as was seen, for example, not only in the "Academicus Dialogues," but also in the letters and editorials in the *Courant,* as well as the "Silence Dogood" series.

This resentment of the Mathers' continued elevated status and leadership over several generations had grown. Even as the Mathers and their colleagues and compatriots were attempting to change a scientific and medical paradigm, so were a large number of the colonists trying to change the status quo. This resistance to traditional power holders was beginning to proffer a new paradigm in terms of class, education, and intellectualism in the colonies. This represented an impending new political structure, disciplinary practice, and forecasted still more revolutionary changes in the formations of power relations in 18th-century America. For many generations in the past, the ministers had ruled the roost. Their word had not only been a comfort to people who struggled in a new climate with diseases both endemic and epidemic, but also their rhetoric in the pulpit as interpreters of the word of God had gained them and retained for them much power.

As seen in the various letters and editorials in the *New-England Courant,* there had been a real currency in upbraiding citizens on one side for not having a college education and on the other side for having one. Clearly, there had been a split at this time, and it was one of the frames that had an impact on the debate about the inoculation project. Those who had a Harvard education were for the project and those without often were against variolation. There had of course been some exceptions on both sides: Boylston on the side of the Inoculators, and Douglass (with a European university education, not one at Harvard) on the side of the Anti-Inoculators.

Ruptures could be particularly generative, not just in this case of an attempt to interject an inoculation against a disease, but also generative of other changes. From the texts examined so far, it was clear that disruptions were occurring in many arenas, often, it would seem, instigated by the fact that the Mathers and other ministers were supporting "new" interventions in the lives and safety of the colonists. This combination of the highly educated, influential clergy, and aging leadership with the anti-intellectualism and celebration of a popular tobacconist had combined to further enrage the populace against smallpox inoculation. At the same time,

> [L]et there be no misunderstanding: it is not that a real man, the object of knowledge, philosophical reflection or technical intervention, has been substituted for the soul, the illusion of the theologians. The man described for us, whom we are invited to free, is already in himself the effect of a subjection much more profound than himself. A 'soul' inhabits him and brings him to existence, which is itself a factor in the mastery that power exercises over the body. The soul is the effect and instrument of a political anatomy; the soul is the prison of the body.[112]

But another power relation must be considered: still another element in the apparatus. C. Mather's sources in addition to microscopy for the inoculation had also come under scrutiny. These groups had been framed by the

Inoculators as the sources of the procedure in addition to the microscope: enslaved Africans, Royal Society members writing about Turkish inoculators, and both Greek and British women who either practiced or advocated for the vaccination. In examining those texts containing challenges to the received wisdom, the next chapter will offer evidence of how their voices had also played a role in the debate. Again, who had the power to speak, and whose cultural body had been considered valid to inform the body politic of Boston in the 1720s?

Notes

1 Kenneth Silverman, *The Life and Times of Cotton Mather* (New York, NY: Welcome Rain Publishers, 2001), 3, 15, 18, 46.
2 George L. Kittredge, "Introduction," Increase Mather's and Anonymous's [Cotton Mather's] *Several Reasons for Transplanting the Small Pox, Is a Lawful Practice, and That It Has Been Blessed by God for the Saving of Many a Life. Etc.* and Cotton Mather's *Sentiments Written on the Small Pox Inoculated* (Cleveland, OH: 1921), 27.
3 Kittredge, "Introduction," 65.
4 David S. Shields, *Civil Tongues and Polite Letters in British America* (Chapel Hill, NC: University of North Carolina Press, 1997), 211.
5 James Franklin, ed. *The New-England Courant* (Boston: J. Franklin, No. 32, March 5–12, 1722).
6 Michel Foucault, *Discipline and Punish* (New York: Pantheon, 1977), 137.
7 J. Franklin, *Courant,* No. 32, March 5–12, 1722.
8 Academicus (Greenwood), *A Friendly Debate, Or, A Dialogue, Between Academicus, and Sawny & Mundungus, Two Eminent Physicians, about Some of Their Late Performances* (Boston: J. Franklin, 1722), title page.
9 Academicus, *A Friendly*, title page.
10 Kenneth Burke, *Attitudes Toward History* (Oakland, CA: University of California Press, 1984), 171.
11 Shields, *Civil Tongues,* 224.
12 Kittredge, "Introduction," 41.
13 Academicus, *A Friendly Debate,* 2.
14 Academicus, *A Friendly Debate,* 2.
15 Academicus, *A Friendly Debate,* 1.
16 Academicus, *A Friendly Debate,* 2.
17 Academicus, *A Friendly Debate,* 1–2.
18 William Douglass, *The Abuses and Scandals of Some Late Pamphlets in Favour of Inoculation of the Smallpox* (Boston: J. Franklin, 1722), 6.
19 Douglass, *Abuses*, 6.
20 William Douglass, *Inoculation of the Small Pox as Practised in Boston, Considered in a Letter to A[lexander] S[tuart], M. D. F. R. S., in London,* (1722), 26.
21 Academicus, *A Friendly Debate,* 2.
22 Academicus, *A Friendly Debate,* 3.
23 Academicus, *A Friendly Debate,* 3.
24 Academicus, *A Friendly Debate,* 3.
25 Academicus, *A Friendly Debate,* 6–7.
26 Academicus, *A Friendly Debate,* 8.

27 Academicus, *A Friendly Debate*, 16.
28 Academicus, *A Friendly Debate*, 16.
29 Academicus, *A Friendly Debate*, 16.
30 Academicus, *A Friendly Debate*, 16.
31 Solomon Schechter and Wilhelm Bacher. "Gamaliel." *Jewish Encyclopedia.* 2002. Accessed June 19, 2009. https://www.jewishencyclopedia.com/articles/6494-gamaliel-i
32 Academicus, *A Friendly Debate*, 16.
33 Academicus, *A Friendly Debate,* 17.
34 Academicus, *A Friendly Debate*, 20.
35 Academicus, *A Friendly Debate*, 20.
36 Academicus, *A Friendly Debate*, 20.
37 Academicus, *A Friendly Debate,* 20–21.
38 Academicus, *A Friendly Debate,* 20–21.
39 Foucault, *Discipline,* 26.
40 Foucault, *Discipline*, 27.
41 Foucault, *Discipline*, 28.
42 Foucault, *Discipline*, 28.
43 Foucault, *Discipline*, 28.
44 Academicus, *A Friendly Debate,* 23.
45 Academicus, *A Friendly Debate,* 23.
46 Academicus, *A Friendly Debate,* 23.
47 Academicus, *A Friendly Debate*, 24.
48 Douglass, *Abuses and Scandals*, 8.
49 Douglass, *Abuses and Scandals*, 8.
50 Douglass, *Abuses and Scandals*, 8.
51 Douglass, *Abuses and Scandals*, 8.
52 Douglass, *Abuses and Scandals*, 9–11.
53 *The Boston News-Letter* in *18th Century American Newspapers in the Library of Congress,* (Boston: Bartholomew Greene,1722), no. 950.
54 "History of Medicine, Epidemics: 1721 Boston (Smallpox) in *Digital Book Index* (New York: Burt Franklin and Sons, 2000–2015).
55 Walter Isaacson, *Ben Franklin: An American Life* (New York: Simon and Shuster, 2007), 23.
56 Isaacson, *Ben Franklin*, 23.
57 The author is still contested but thought to be a collaboration of Mundungus, Douglass, and the Franklins. "Rusticus" is credited here, which is how it is listed in early *American Bibliography*: "Rusticus, pseudonym).
58 "Lost Works of Cotton Mather," *Proceedings of the Massachusetts Historical Society,* 3, no. 45 (Oct 1911–Jun 1912), 422.
59 Rusticus (John Williams [Mundungus], William Douglass, James and Ben Franklin), "Dedication" to *A Dialogue Between Rusticus and Academicus about the Late Performance of* Academicus.
60 Rusticus, *A Dialogue between Rusticus and Academicus*, 1.
61 Rusticus, *A Dialogue between Rusticus and Academicus*, 1.
62 Rusticus, *A Dialogue between Rusticus and Academicus*, 3.
63 Isaacson, *Ben Franklin*, 22.
64 Perry Miller, *New England Mind, From Colony to Province* (Cambridge, MA: Harvard University Press, 1953), 344.
65 Rusticus, *A Dialogue between Rusticus and Academicus*, 3.
66 Rusticus, *A Dialogue between Rusticus and Academicus*, 4.

67 Clark, Ruth, *Strangers and Sojourners at Port Royal* (Cambridge: Cambridge University Press, 2014), 309, 324, 335; Geoffrey F. Nuttall, *Richard Baxter* (London: Nelson, 1965); Rusticus, *A Dialogue between Rusticus and Academicus,* 4.
68 Rusticus, *A Dialogue between Rusticus and Academicus*, 4.
69 Rusticus, *A Dialogue between Rusticus and Academicus*, 4.
70 Rusticus, *A Dialogue between Rusticus and Academicus*, 5.
71 Rusticus, *A Dialogue between Rusticus and Academicus*, 5.
72 John Oldmixon, *The British Empire in America: Containing the History of the Discovery, Settlement, Progress and Present State of All the British Colonies on the Continent and Islands of America* (2 volumes; London: Printed for J. Nicholson et al., 1708), illust. by Herman Moll.
73 Rusticus, *A Dialogue between Rusticus and Academicus*, 5–6.
74 Rusticus, *A Dialogue between Rusticus and Academicus*, 6.
75 Rusticus, *A Dialogue between Rusticus and Academicus*, 6.
76 Foucault, *Discipline*, 136.
77 Foucault, *Discipline*, 136.
78 Foucault, *Discipline*, 137.
79 Foucault, *Discipline*, 138.
80 Foucault, *Discipline*, 138.
81 Foucault, *Discipline*, 138-139.
82 Rusticus, *A Dialogue between Rusticus and Academicus*, 7-8.
83 Rusticus, *A Dialogue between Rusticus and Academicus*, 8.
84 Rusticus, *A Dialogue between Rusticus and Academicus*, 11.
85 Rusticus, *A Dialogue between Rusticus and Academicus*, 11–12.
86 Rusticus, *A Dialogue between Rusticus and Academicus*, 12.
87 Rusticus, *A Dialogue between Rusticus and Academicus*, 12.
88 James Franklin, ed. *The New-England Courant,* no. 27 (Jan. 29, 1722,) 1.
89 J. Franklin, ed., *Courant,* no. 27, 1.
90 J. Franklin, ed., *Courant,* no. 27, 1.
91 J. Franklin, ed., *Courant,* no. 27, 1.
92 J. Franklin, ed., *Courant,* no. 27, 1.
93 J. Franklin, ed., *The New-England Courant,* no. 25 (January 15–22, 1722).
94 J. Franklin, ed., *Courant,* no. 25.
95 Kittredge, "Introduction," 16.
96 J. Franklin, ed. *Courant,* no. 25.
97 J. Franklin, ed., *Courant,* no. 25.
98 James Franklin, ed. *The New-England Courant,* no. 4 (August 7–14, 1721).
99 J. Franklin, *Courant,* no. 4.
100 J. Franklin, *Courant,* no. 4.
101 Massachusetts Historical Society, *Benjamin Franklin in the New-England Courant* (2015). Accessed March 30, 2015. https://www.masshist.org/database/viewer.php?item_id=55&pid=15
102 Massachusetts Historical Society, *Benjamin Franklin.*
103 H. W. Brands, *The First American: The Life and Times of Benjamin Franklin* (New York: Knopf, 2010), 32–33.
104 Massachusetts Historical Society, *Silence Dogood: Benjamin Franklin in the New-England Courant* (2015). Accessed March 30, 2015. https://www.masshist.org/online/silence_dogood/essay.php?entry_id=203
105 James Franklin, *The New-England Courant* May 7–14, no. 41 (1722).
106 J. Franklin, *Courant,* no. 41.
107 J. Franklin, *Courant,* no. 41.

108 J. Franklin, *Courant,* no. 41.
109 Foucault, *Discipline and Punish,* 30.
110 Foucault, *Discipline and Punish,* 30.
111 Foucault, *Discipline and Punish,* 30.
112 Foucault, *Discipline and Punish,* 30.

Bibliography

Academicus (Samuel Greenwood, Cotton Mather?). *A Friendly Debate, Or, A Dialogue, Between Academicus, and Sawny & Mundungus, Two Eminent Physicians, about Some of Their Late Performances.* Boston: J. Franklin, 1722.

Brands, H. W. *The First American: The Life and Times of Benjamin.* New York: Knopf, 2010.

Burke, Kenneth. *Attitudes Toward History.* Oakland, CA: University of California Press, 1984.

Clark, Ruth. *Strangers and Sojourners at Port Royal.* Cambridge: Cambridge University Press, 2014.

Douglass, William. *The Abuses and Scandals of Some Late Pamphlets in Favour of Inoculation of the Smallpox.* Boston: J. Franklin, 1722.

Douglass, William. *Inoculation of the Small Pox as Practised in Boston, Considered in a Letter to A[lexander] S[tuart], M. D. F. R. S., J. Franklin Press, Boston.* 1722.

Foucault, Michel. *Discipline and Punish.* New York: Pantheon, 1977.

Franklin, James, ed. *The New-England Courant.* Boston: J. Franklin, nos. 4, August 7-14, 1721; 25, January 15–22, 1722; 27, January 29–February 4, 1722; 32, March 5–12, 1722; 41, May 7–14, 1722.

"History of Medicine, Epidemics: 1721 Boston (Smallpox)" in *Digital Book Index.* New York: Burt Franklin and Sons (2000–2015).

Isaacson, Walter. *Ben Franklin: An American Life.* New York: Simon and Shuster, 2007.

Kittredge, George L. "Introduction" to Increase Mather's and Anonymous's [Cotton Mather's] *Several Reasons for Transplanting the Small Pox, Is a Lawful Practice, and That It Has Been Blessed by God for the Saving of Many* a *Life. Etc.* and Cotton Mather's *Sentiments Written on the Small Pox Inoculated.* Cleveland, OH: Printed for Private Distribution, 1921.

Massachusetts Historical Society, *Benjamin Franklin in the New-England Courant* (2015). Accessed March 30, 2015. https://www.masshist.org/database/viewer.php?item_id=55&pid=15

Mather, Cotton. "Lost Works of Cotton Mather" *Proceedings of the Massachusetts Historical Society,* 3(45) (Oct 1911–June 1912).

Miller, Perry. *New England Mind, From Colony to Province.* Cambridge, MA: Harvard University Press, 1953.

Nuttall, Geoffrey F. *Richard Baxter.* London: Nelson, 1965.

Oldmixon, John. *The British Empire in America: Containing the History of the Discovery, Settlement, Progress and Present State of All the British Colonies on the Continent and Islands of America.* 2 volumes; London: Printed for J. Nicholson et al., 1708, illust. by Herman Moll.

"Rusticus" (John Williams [Mundungus], William Douglass, James and Ben Franklin), "Dedication" to *A Dialogue Between Rusticus and Academicus about the Late Performance of* Academicus. Boston: J. Franklin, 1722.

Schechter, Solomon and Wilhelm Bacher. "Gamaliel" *Jewish Encyclopedia*. 2002. Accessed June 19, 2009. https://www.jewishencyclopedia.com/articles/6494-gamaliel-i

Shields, David S. *Civil Tongues and Polite Letters in British America*. Chapel Hill, NC: University of North Carolina Press, 1997.

Silverman, Kenneth. *The Life and Times of Cotton Mather*. New York, NY: Welcome Rain Publishers, 2001.

The Boston News-Letter in *18th Century American Newspapers in the Library of Congress*. Boston: Bartholomew Greene, 1722. no. 950.

5 The Discrediting of African, Levantine, and Women's Experience

Introduction

It's now obvious that in order to fully understand the variolation controversy, the analysis must include the reactions toward the Inoculators' sources that they used as the foundation for the vaccination project. As Mather wrote in his medical compendium, the inoculation was first introduced to him by the enslaved man, Onesimus. Kelly Wisecup argued that his presenting Africans' testimony regarding variolation against smallpox during the controversy gained him ethos as "as an authoritative collector and evaluator of medical knowledge useful in the Americas and in Europe."[1] While today that is very true, this particular source, an enslaved African, drew reactions from the opponents of the project at the time who sought to discredit the knowledge on that basis. Thus far, a number of different rhetorical frames for the project have been discussed. This chapter shows the already present discrediting views toward African, Turkish, and female (the Greek woman inoculator's and Lady Montagu's) experience, knowledge, and customs. That discrimination also played an important role in the debate. These particular sources highlight not only the cultural attitudes at that time but also elucidate what Foucault, Clifford Geertz, and Paolo Freire referred to as "local knowledge" or "subjugated knowledge" and the resistance it can engender.[2] The African, Turkish, and Greek knowledge is from other locations, but it is in the context of the colonies that the knowledge is brought into a locale in which for the most part these peoples and gender were not respected. Clearly, the scene was Boston, but the *local* knowledge of Africans and others in Boston, who brought their own knowledge with them, is the meaning of *local* knowledge here. The opposition to variolation on that basis helped to enhance the physicians' arguments.

The analysis reveals that this particular colonial population believed enslaved individuals, Muslims, and women were not capable of providing credible information on the subjects of health and disease, except for some of the female herbalists and midwives operating in just those areas of healthcare in Boston. Truth claims were weighed within the light of *ethos:* who the speakers were and were they credible speakers on certain topics

DOI: 10.4324/9781003312369-6

within the rhetorical framework of colonial American discourse. Mather's various texts clearly indicated that he believed the narrative regarding inoculation based on African testimony would be taken as truth. His assumption seemed to be that because a number of Africans believed in the method and seemed to have benefitted from the practice and not contracted smallpox, the colonists would be persuaded to adopt it, also. In his medical compendium, Mather wrote:

> I was first instructed in it by a Guramantee-Servant of my own, long before I knew that any *Europeans* or *Asiaticks* had the least Acquaintance with it; and some years before I was Enriched with the Communications of the Learned Foreigners, whose Accounts I found agreeing with what I received from my Servant, when he showed me the Scar of Wound made for the Operation; and said, That no Person Ever died of the *Small-Pox,* in their Countrey that had the Courage to use it.[3]

Onesimus's exact words regarding his own experience in his English dialect that Mather used in another text are in the Introduction.

While it's tempting to cast the opposition to African truth claims as "racial," a recent article by Margot Minardi challenges that descriptor. Although she posits the resistance in terms of enslaved people only because they were "dependents," but rather than her either/or approach, a both/and stance can also be adopted. Africans and other cultural groups were discriminated against both as dependents and also racially. She suggested that scholars have viewed the inoculation controversy itself in numerous ways: (1) historians of medicine have viewed it as evidence of the beginnings of medical profession in North America; (2) other historians have been more interested in the incident as a possibly emergence of the concept of race based on a complicated structure in which bodily characteristics were combined with social and intellectual worth. Minardi wrote that a concept of race was not yet fully formed for colonials, who thought of others only in terms of *dependents.*[4] She further suggested that sometimes an "unintentional" documentation of an incident like the smallpox inoculation of 1721 can provide a lens through which rich cultural developments can be viewed. While that suggestion can easily be agreed with, it is not within the scope of this text to explore the construction of race in the colonies or in America in the 1720s. Nor is it in the scope of this analysis to show how being labeled a "dependent" would later morph into, among other things, a concept of race. Her view simply complicated the picture, which helps provide a more accurate reading. Thus, for the purposes of this text, both racism and the enslaved's dependent status militated against many of the colonists' accepting this source of knowledge.

Other evidence points to concepts of race that must have influenced colonists along with many others of European heritage and ancestry. Londa Schiebinger's work in the 90s remains highly respected by contemporary scholars of race in this period. She focused more on the development of a concept of race in the second half of the 1700s, and yet many documents dating back to the 1600s have specific commentary on racial identity and characteristics. In *Nature's Body,* Schiebinger noted that it was in the 1700s that scientists and early anthropologists began using racist descriptions not only to stereotype groups of people but also to insist they could not have been able to complete the epistemic work credited to them in Egypt, for example.[5] She also wrote that as the male medical profession began to consolidate in various European countries,

> it also coincided with the revolution in definitions of race and the attempts to ground scientifically the exclusion of men of color from science. In France, the traditional exclusion of people of color from European professions was codified in 1763 by a royal ordinance that among other things forbade any man of African origins, whether slave or free, to practice medicine or surgery. Thus women stood at the center of a debate concerning race at a time when both women and peoples of color from science was being formalized.[6]

Although the formalization took place later in the 17th century than the inoculation in Boston, those attitudes formed before then, and as Schiebinger also maintained, "European men, dominating ... science, increasingly tightened the reins on what was recognized as legitimate knowledge and who could produce that knowledge."[7] Clearly such attitudes were already culturally integrated in the American colonies.

Martin Bernal argued in his controversial *Black Athena* that the focus shifted to Ancient Greece as the cradle of science to wrench credit away from the African continent. Even earlier in 1575, Ambroise Parè had successfully put forth the idea that "Ethiopians, Egyptians, Africans, Jews, Phoenicians, Persians, Assyrians, and Indians have invented many curious sciences, revealed the mysteries and secrets in Nature."[8] The inoculation project takes place in a liminal zone between those two world views.

Foucault, who did not dwell at length on the construct of "race," did address it in his 1976 lectures, 11 of them devoted to the history of racism, modern constructions, and racial discursive practices. His *History of Sexuality* contains a few references to race as well, but for him, he was more interested in racial history as a set-up for the more rigid yet varied racisms of later years of the 18th and particularly the 19th century. He wrote about the emphasis of moral cleanliness and vigor of the social body, "And in the name of a biological and historical urgency, it [the supreme authority] justified the racisms of the state, which at the time were on the horizon."[9] Boston colonials, having been Europeans until a relatively short time ago, were very much influenced by the attendant racial attitudes.[10] As Stoler argues,

> … racism was not a colonial reflex, fashioned to deal with the distant other, but part of the very making of Europeans themselves. 'Internal colonialism' … was not a peculiar form of empire building … but, according to Foucault, its earliest and enduring incarnation.[11]

For the theorist, racism was also a "complex subtext" of his more over-arching concept of power.[12]

In addition, in urban slavery in cities such as Boston, where poor whites, indentured servants, Native Americans, and Africans often socialized together, there was often a lack of clear social difference, causing more anxiety, especially among the dominant class of religious people who sought to convert them all.[13] At the same time, the Africans were regarded as "non-Christian heathen," and in a colony so deeply rooted in religious belief, the religion of the enslaved was used to further marginalize them. At the same time, they were subject to intense proselytizing so that they would adopt the religion of the colonists. Although they were often forced to attend Christian church services, in the 1720s the beliefs and utterances of the Africans, both because of their dependent status and their racial difference, were still regarded with suspicion. Rather than being "absent from the colonial stage … they were people precariously poised, economically vulnerable, and socially askew. Effaced from view and then pushed to center stage at strategic moments, these were people about whom colonial officials virulently disagreed."[14] As Mather had written in response to criticism of his sources in *Some Account …*,

> It is *Cavilled* … that this *New Way* comes to us from the *Heathen*; and we *Christians* must not *Learn the Way of the Heathen*. I Enquire whether our *Hippocrates* were not an *Heathen*? And Whether our *Galen* were not an *Heathen*?[15]

As Minardi argued, much of this suspicion toward African testimony might be more attributable to the distribution of their status to the bottom of the social hierarchy *and* the lack of common, religious beliefs rather than toward the racialized body, "because inferiority had not yet been indelibly written onto the bodies of Africans."[16] Yet others have complicated Minardi's view of race. Even if race had not yet been fully formalized in the 1720s, this fluid identity could have accounted for the intellectual space of Mather and a few others to seriously consider Onesimus's methodology for protecting people from contracting a lethal case of smallpox. One can legitimately question why Mather did believe the experience and wisdom of his enslaved African. Was he more free of prejudice than many others in Boston?

Onesimus's Testimonials

Mather had written about his slave, Onesimus, in *Angel of Bethesda* as well as in his diary entries, crediting him with being his very first source for the procedure to prevent smallpox. Even though the entire compendium was not published until the 1970s, the 17-page chapter about variolation had been published in 1722.[17] In addition, Cotton Mather had recorded the exact speech of Onesimus, which might represent the first time the dialect was recorded in Boston or perhaps in the colonies. Even though Bostonians were very much interested in their language and its various presentations, when other authors wrote about African testimonials about the smallpox vaccination, they did not write in the dialect. Like many of his era, especially those who read the Royal Society *Transactions*, Mather was a collector and documenter. The *Transactions* continue to be published to this day and began in the 1600s. In other texts by supporters of the inoculation project such as Benjamin Colman and Daniel Neal, when they wrote about African testimonials, they did not quote the exact words, but reported African stories in third person. Kathryn S. Koo and Minardi have both commented on Mather's use of Onesimus's dialect or pidgin in his medical compendium and found his report

> helped to reaffirm prevalent ideas about the Africans living among them. With their childlike diction and unquestioning faith in a medical procedure that was surely beyond their comprehension, the Africans that Mather 'ventriloquized' on the printed page only reaffirmed the notion of a simple-minded people who would helplessly perish 'like Rotten Sheep' without the good graces of the Maker.[18]

Both authors had read Mather's use of the exact language as counterproductive. With English as their second language, Africans were blamed for their diction, and their speech only reaffirmed for colonials that the Africans were childlike and unable to understand medical procedures. This emphasis on critiquing dialects was also pointed out in the "Academicus Dialogues" in the previous chapter. At the same time, the Bostonians also considered enslaved people as hapless unless they adopted the religion of the Puritans.[19] Minardi wrote that Mather's capturing of the dialect in his compendium had given Cotton a "strange mix of humility and condescension," claiming that the minister had framed Onesimus's speech as "precious or even deviant."[20] Minardi further suggests that one of the supporters of Mather, Benjamin Colman, had made his own comments regarding his willingness to listen to African testimonials based on Biblical terms:

> I believe I shall be scoff'd at for telling this *Simple* story, but I think it very pertinent & much to the purpose here; and whosoever seeks the Truth & desire to be informed will not despise it. And he that has learnt any thing as he ought, has this—to be willing to learn of the poorest *Slave* in Town.[21]

While Minardi's and Koo's interpretations are helpful, there is another possibility. In addition to quoting Onesimus's dialect, Mather also used Indian language and Spanish in his various texts, even translating some Biblical works into Native American languages; there wouldn't be such interpretations over those efforts. However, that's not to say these authors are wrong; scholars cannot determine intent, but Mather *was* known for "reporting" everything. He considered himself a researcher and faithful recorder of his surroundings and experiences. Koo herself wrote that the writing was not as important a skill as being able to read in the colonies at that time. Jennifer Monaghan confirmed that writing was more typically used to take notes in business or education (or in Mather's recording many of his father's long sermons) and was not seen as a reflection of one's personal expression or identity, although conversely, Mundungus was taken to task for his spelling.[22] Individuals were, however, taken to task then as speakers; their speech and rhetoric were very important.

In the previous chapter, much of the fictional dialogue in the *Academicus* parody was supposedly from spoken language, although the dialogues had been written down as if transcribing the speech Greenwood claimed to have heard. Academicus even attempted Mundungus's spelling and Douglass's Scottish brogue. However, Mather valued writing above all, perhaps because of having had a stutter. In his writing he could be fluent. He also used his prodigious productions to further his personal ethos in the Royal Society. Minardi also argued that Mather, in quoting Onesimus, was trying to make his story "as authentic as possible" to his audience, which would undoubtedly have been made up of mostly white readers.[23] Still it was possible that Mather had simply been recording the dialect of Onesimus, as he was known to do in other situations.

Mather, who had been given Onesimus by his parishioners in 1706, must have learned about the variolation before he freed him in 1716, most likely in 1714. Robert Tindol questioned why in Mather's June 6, 1721 diary entry in which he had noted that his "African servant," who was preparing for baptism, was worried about getting smallpox, if this servant was Onesimus, why he was not very confident he would not get it?[24] Clearly Tindol was not aware that Onesimus had been given his freedom by Mather in 1716.[25] Mather was talking about another servant who replaced Onesimus named Obadiah. Proof for this also can be found in the fact that the servant in question was getting ready for baptism, and Onesimus was never baptized. Mather often agonized in his diaries that much to his chagrin and in spite of his vigorous efforts, Onesimus was never converted. Thus, he was not eligible for baptism. Mather owned only one servant at a time over a number of years.

Winthrop Jordan pointed out that the first Africans had come to New England in 1638, when Puritan settlers exchanged Indian Prisoners of war for African slaves from the West Indies.[26]

There's been a consistent myth that New England's slavery was a "passing and curious anomaly," but there had been steady slavery and indenture even if the percentage of the enslaved to freemen was small throughout the decades. Africans and the indentured had helped greatly in growing the economy,[27] and the period of time that included the controversy (between 1700 and 1750) saw significant growth of this region.[28] The enslaved and indentured servants included kidnapped Africans, captured Native Americans, and impoverished whites (including children sent overseas in times of famine in their own countries), all of whom were serving in somewhat but not entirely interchangeable positions. The 1619 project pointed out that the very first enslaved Africans landed first in Virginia in a similar exchange. Ben Franklin had been indentured to his older brother James when his printing business began; families could indenture their own children.

Mather's Attitude toward Africans

Silverman's characterization of Mather as "ambidexter" also fits his relationship with Onesimus, whom he credits at times and about whom at other times he complains. He goes back and forth on the value of Onesimus, and of enslaved Africans in general. Koo called Mather "a public advocate," as he funded a school for those Africans who wanted to learn to read.[29] Mather did this even though he was known throughout most of his life as having some financial problems, as his minister's salary had never been generous. In addition, Mather had a religious society for Africans, and they met in his home. Two of Mather's many books were written regarding the Africans in Boston: *Mather's Rules* (1693) and the *Negro Christianized* (1706). The titles alone speak as to his perspective. In these works, Mather does not quote dialect. On the one hand, he had respect for a knowledge brought from Africa regarding medical preventatives, and on the other hand, he anguished over the unwillingness of Africans in Boston to embrace his religious beliefs and dictates. Robert Tindol addresses this seemingly contradictory mindset of Mather.

> With his promise that scientific discovery must be compatible with the will of God, Mather seemingly had a constitutional aversion to the type of dogmatic backwardness ... but if the errand in the wilderness had any validity at all as a God-fearing enterprise, then the scientific enterprise must generally work in its favor.[30]

In his "Rules" for the society he had started in 1693, there's a clear coercive and controlling purpose on his part and on the part of colonial society regarding behaviors for the enslaved. In the community, they were to come on time to the Sunday evening meeting at seven o'clock and stay till nine o'clock for what sounds like a church service complete with hymns, prayers, and a repeat of the sermon from the morning.[31] No absences were tolerated, nor was any lying, cursing, drunkenness, swearing, stealing, "notorious" disobedience, or unfaithfulness. Unfaithfulness was included because people like Onesimus, for example, had a wife and a family. If one had indulged in any of these practices, he or she would be barred from the meeting for one week. Everyone was required to learn the catechism. Without learning the catechism, a person could not be baptized and become a proper member of the church. At the same time, there had been some concerns on the part of colonists regarding baptism and church membership, because then the enslaved would have been able to participate in local politics.[32]

Yet Mather had never been able to get Onesimus to learn the catechism and be baptized, even though he not only had made sure that he could read, but also made sure he could write. In a 1712 entry, Mather asked one of his children to "hear the Negro-Servant Say his Catechism."[33] It is not known whether they did so, however.[34] Although the minister granted Onesimus freedom after ten years, he had at first thought to put many restrictions and demands on him as to what he must be willing to do, for example, keep the Mathers' firebox full of cut wood, and in a bad winter shovel the snow, etc. The document in which he had written up these conditions for this so-called freedom begins here:

> My servant, Onesimus, having advanced a Summ, towards the purchase of a Negro-Lad, who may serve many occasions of my Family in his Room, I do by this instrument, Release him so far from my Service (and the claims that any other or after me might make unto him), that he may Enjoy and Employ his whole Time for his purposes, and as he pleases.

It's believed that his new "servant" was Obadiah. The first part of the document makes it sound as if this was true freedom, but Mather then contradicted himself. He was apparently concerned that his new enslaved man should be at first somewhat supervised by Onesimus even after gaining his own freedom, in case the new arrival was not up to all the tasks the former had accomplished. In addition to keeping the wood supply up and shoveling, if necessary, Mather continued:

> Secondly, when the Family shall have any Domestic Business more than Daily affairs, he shall be ready upon being told, of it so far to Lend an helping Hand, as he will go no Large nor Long Interruption to the Business, of his own, to which I have dismissed him; As particularly, to carry corn unto the mill, and help in the fetching of water for washing, if we happen to be destitute. And in the piling of our wood, at the season of its coming in. Whereas also, the said *Onesimus* has gott the money (which he has advanced as above-mention'd, from the Liberties he took, while in my Service, and for some other Considerations), I do expect, that he do within six months pay me the sum of Five Pounds, wherein he acknowledged himself indebted to me.[35]

In that original document, it was clear that Mather had a change of mind because he had crossed through many of the restrictions and obligations above.

Smallpox in the Slave Trade and Other African Testimonials

Larry Stewart, in his article published on slavery and smallpox, found differing opinions on how widely spread the practice of inoculating against smallpox (or "engrafting") was in Africa.[36]

> [I]t has been suggested that the practice may have been indigenous to some parts of Africa, although the evidence, especially for the west coast, is not remotely conclusive before the nineteenth century. The exception appears to be on the Barbary Coast, as the Boston Minister informed Dr. John Woodward after having read a report in the *Philosophical Transactions* of 1714 and subsequently questioned his own slave.[37]

Stewart's research, done predominately on the slave trade, discovered a number of different opinions and reports as to the enslaved's mortality from smallpox during the Middle Passage. What is also clear is that inoculation was known to the traders and discussed during the 1720s, and, of course, in subsequent decades until it became accepted practice. The historian agreed, though, that Mather had relied on Onesimus's testimony, as well as on those from other Africans, and the Royal Society's publications.[38]

In addition, Eugenia Herbert questioned that although Mather's report of inoculation in Africa was the first mention in her experience, had it been common practice there or not?[39] This author has extensive information regarding early African inoculations, including sites of the inoculations in Africa, the location of the inoculation on the body, which varied, and which part of the pox itself was used (fluid, scab, powder, etc.). She acknowledged, though, that the various and earliest reports of inoculation, not including those of Mather and his colleagues, but based on travel diaries, naval officer reports, and anthropologists' notes could have been unreliable.

As have others who have researched this question, she found it difficult to answer if one relies only on the rare medical reports from the colonial era and ship captains' travel journals. Cadwallader Colden's later account (1753) seemed to confirm the use of inoculation in West Africa and Ethiopia.[40] Elizabeth Donnan documented a number of Boston advertising flyers that mentioned Gold Coast "slaves" had been both procurable and desirable because they were not vulnerable to smallpox.[41] However, that could also mean that those persons had already had smallpox naturally. Boston's captains enjoyed an active trade with the Gold Coast and preferred that area themselves because of the especially lucrative market for their rum.[42]

CHARLESTOWN, *April* 27, 1769.

TO BE SOLD,

On WEDNESDAY *the Tenth Day of* MAY *next*,

A CHOICE CARGO OF

Two Hundred & Fifty

NEGROES:

ARRIVED in the Ship COUNTESS of SUSSEX, THOMAS DAVIES, Maſter, directly from GAMBIA, by

JOHN CHAPMAN, & Co.

⁂ THIS is the Veſſel that had the Small-Pox on Board at the Time of her Arrival the 31ſt of March laſt: Every neceſſary Precaution hath ſince been taken to cleanſe both Ship and Cargo thoroughly, ſo that thoſe who may be inclined to purchaſe need not be under the leaſt Apprehenſion of Danger from Infection.

The NEGROES *are allowed to be the likelieſt Parcel that have been imported this Seaſon.*

Figure 5.1 Sale of the Enslaved, Charleston, "Courtesy of the American Antiquarian Society".

While Mather acknowledged other sources in addition to Onesimus for the procedure, it is significant that he situated the African American lore first in support of the technique. Another supporter of the inoculation project had used the African American source as secondary. Kittredge believed "Mather was ... the first person to call the practice of inoculation in Africa to the notice of Europeans in a formal or public way."[43] There was, however, an entry in the *Philosophical Transactions* of the Royal Society in London indicating that Sir Hans Sloane had heard of the African practice three years before Mather, as well as the 1714 source mentioned above.[44] Sloane was a well-known Anglo/Irish physician educated at a university in France, a member of the Royal Society, and inducted into the Royal College of Physicians in England. Although Mather does not give a detailed chronology of his acquaintance with the procedure, he did write that he knew about it from Onesimus "long before" the European/Turkish connection, and it had been "some years" before communication regarding the European reports from the *Transactions* had reached him from abroad.[45]

Smallpox "variolation" had been introduced to Europe by Lady Mary Montagu after living in Turkey for several years. She had her own children inoculated and on her return to England in 1718, enthusiastically promoted the procedure informally to her social circle. The medical establishment in England wanted no part of variolation possibly because it was "Oriental" and because of Montagu's gender. In spite of this opposition, a member of the royal family, Princess Caroline, had her children inoculated: her daughters in 1722 and her sons in 1724.[46] And even though

> The Royal College of Physicians vehemently opposed smallpox inoculation, ... the members of the Royal Society, the premier scientific institution in Britain, endorsed the practice and published instances of its success in their journal ... [Also,] the crown itself supported inoculation on several Newgate prisoners and the results were published in various British newspapers—to mixed response.[47]

However, regardless of the timeline of Mather's knowledge and the similar practices of smallpox variolation adopted by a few in England, the minister had chosen to highlight the knowledge of the Africans as his first source when he initiated the practice of inoculation with Boylston and in the medical compendium he wrote before or possibly during the epidemic. Mather's mention of the African source, however, was not the only African testimonial alluded to during the inoculations. In Colman's text, *A Narrative of the Method and Success of Inoculating the Small-pox in New England*, he refuted many of the charges being made by the Anti-Inoculators in Boston at the time. This text was published in Dublin with a "Historical Introduction" written by Daniel Neal, M.A. who sought to acquaint the people of Europe with the happenings in Boston from a positive viewpoint. While this text was published in Ireland, it circulated in America, too, although under a different title.

In the introduction, Neal recorded that in a recent letter from "New England, published by Mr. Dummer, the author acquaints us, that he had met with several *African Negroes*, who assur'd him" that the method was practiced "so generally."[48] Neal then cited a trader off the West coast of Guinea who reported putting ashore those captives he had rounded up for trade in the West Indies to be inoculated before he sold them, because they would bring much higher prices if the cut marks left by inoculation were visible on their arms.[49] Even the physician, William Douglass of the Anti-Inoculators, in his 1722 *Inoculation Considered,* admitted that such a practice took place for other, similar contagions and might have been useful to traders:

> It [inoculation] is then a palliative Prevention of the Small Pox for some time, and then not *very mortal,* and consequently may be of great Use to the *Guinea Traders,* when the Small Pox gets among their Slaves aboard to inoculate their whole Cargo, and patch them up for a *Market,* as is already the Practice of them in the other Pox or *Yaws,* by some *slight, palliative* Cure to fix them up for quick Market, tho' to the *great Damage* of the next *Purchasers.*[50]

In this passage, Douglass's willingness to see inoculation's value for some purposes is interesting. However, he had then demurred because if the captives had still been contagious, they could have spread the pox to the new owners. He clearly differentiated between short-term, successful medical interventions for Africans, but then had discounted it for long-term or future protection of Bostonians. Stewart suggested another possible reason for Douglass's reluctance to see the value of inoculating for smallpox: "Perhaps Douglass was afraid that inoculation might merely mask symptoms of smallpox. ... Douglass had also suggested that slavers were making use of inoculation for their own profit, whatever the dangerous consequences might be."[51]

The Scottish physician's many tracts against the inoculation project focused partly on the credibility of truth-claims of those not regarded by Bostonians as credible due to their status as dependents or race. All of them would have been regarded as lacking knowledge and as being inferior by many of the Colonials. In short, dependents would have had no *ethos,* no credibility. In the eyes of most Bostonians, including Douglass, the status of Onesimus as an African *and* a dependent made him incapable of knowing and interpreting the natural world.

With newly arrived captives, the question of smallpox was one that figured importantly in the slave market. The enslaved had been asked if they had had smallpox, or their arms had been examined for evidence of the inoculation.[52] Some captives carried the scars of natural smallpox itself, although their essential health as survivors would have had to have been good enough to survive the horrors of the Middle Passage. Severe cases would have left the survivors of the disease in a weakened condition, and slavers and kidnappers picked the healthiest and most able-bodied in order to make good profits.

Stewart, however, in examining the British records from the slave trades found less conclusive evidence of inoculation and also some controversy regarding the use of inoculation among those who captured and transported them. However,

> There can be little doubt that the enthusiasm in the Royal Society for inoculation and the public debate about it [in England in 1721] encouraged the African Company [major slave trading company] to hope smallpox could at least be controlled in the slave trade.[53]

Traders were well known to complain about the loss of their captives during the Middle Passage from various diseases, including smallpox.[54] According to Stewart,

> the instructions of the Company to their factors in Africa were quite specific. The Court of Assistants, ... was of the opinion that inoculation 'would be of great advantage to Us, could it [inoculation] be put in practice by saving the Lives of great Numbers of Slaves, amongst whom the Small Pox is very fatal, especially, when it seizes them on their Voyage.'[55]

One of the traders, James Phipps, who served in the African Trading Company on the Gold Coast (Guinea) from 1703 to 1722, had written numerous letters about his voyages. He claimed that the rates of mortality from numerous causes across the Atlantic had been horrendous although not just from smallpox. Phipps had remarked that "natives of the Gold Coast 'were not much subject to the Small pox.'" It was possible they had already been vaccinated as youth.[56] Overall, the data presented in various documents were not consistent. There were many different tribal groups, and the slavers preferred to not just kidnap Africans from one tribe. Especially on the large plantations in the Caribbean and the American colonies in the South, keeping the enslaved from a number of areas of the African coast meant that they shared no common language or culture, and thus were more easily controlled.

Returning to Neal's support, he championed Colman, Mather, Boylston, the project, and the testimonials from the Africans. He added to his introduction, another source for the method: the traders' practices following the introduction of African testimonials. Thus he, like Mather, created a hierarchy of claims. Bruno Latour and Steve Woolgar in *Laboratory Life* suggested that science, as in multiple academic areas, advances by means of claims, and particularly in terms of a certain hierarchy of claims.[57] In their ethnographic work in a scientific laboratory, the co-authors theorized a hierarchy of claims arranged 1–5, with a Number 5 claim being a most easily accepted claim by a broad audience and one that could be unsupported by evidence as it would be broadly assumed.[58] Then, as the claims advanced into areas of newly discovered data, they became more difficult even for a specific and educated audience to accept without extended and multiple proofs over time. The last description applies to a Number 1 claim.[59] Thus, throughout academic work or intellectual arguments, a claim's status is reflected in a certain hierarchy staged for utmost persuasion. Here in the arguments advanced by the Inoculators and particularly Mather, their hierarchy of claims shows a flawed understanding of a Bostonian audience. Neal was more effective in his placement of claims, at least acknowledging that the claim featuring testimonials from the enslaved may be a weak one and fall short of persuading the intended audience. He had been direct in his qualms about the first claim situated by Mather: "But the Truth of this Relation depending chiefly upon the Testimony of *Negroes*, I should think it worthwhile to consult some of our *English* traders to those parts, before we give entire Credit to it."[60] In addition, he could have been giving some quarter to those who had raised objections to the project on the basis of the status of the enslaved. As a highly regarded Puritan minister and historian, he had been known for his ability to avoid narrowness and sectarianism in his texts.[61] Also, Neal gave some ground to Douglass's argument, perhaps seeing an opening in the doctor's willingness to see inoculation as valuable in some instances. In that time, claims were valued more coming from an English trader's testimony than that of a dependent and African. In other words, Neal could have been a more persuasive advocate for inoculation because of the way he structured his arguments.

Daniel Neal was one of the most important Puritan ministers in colonial Boston, as well as one who played a large role in the politics of that era. His *The History of the Puritans* was not only a standard 18th-century source for more modern scholars, but also, according to Laird Okie's biography, "prefigured nineteenth-century Whig conceptions of Puritanism."[62] Neal's four-volume work was published after the inoculation debate, but he had made his mark earlier as someone who had a large stake in it. His work is believed by some scholars to be "an official Dissenting history of England, one which glorified the role of Puritanism in fostering English liberty."[63] In addition, Neal had made such rhetorical moves as mentioned above by giving some credence to those arguments against inoculation, although he clearly favored the Inoculators.[64]

Although seemingly fair in his approach, like all authors, Neal's critics had other views on his text. His *History of the Puritans* dealt with the time between the Protestant Reformation and 1689; the first volume appearing in 1732, and the fourth and last in 1738. The first volume was attacked in

1733 for unfairness and inaccuracy by Isaac Maddox, afterward bishop of St. Asaph and bishop of Worcester, to whom Neal replied in a pamphlet, *A Review of the Principal Facts Objected to in the First Volume of the History of the Puritans*; and the remaining volumes were attacked by Zachary Grey (1688–1766), to whom the author made no reply.[65]

In Benjamin Colman's text, he told another story of an African connection to the practice of inoculation. The clergyman had apparently visited a home where the owner of the house suggested that the enslaved man there had also been inoculated in his own country.[66] Colman then questioned the older African. The man told him that smallpox had come to his village in Africa and after a few deaths, the rest of the townspeople who did not yet have the disease were inoculated, and the disease was stopped.[67] The African had declared that

> when the sickness gets into five or six houses, so that when people begin to despair of being able to stop it, then all who had not had it went presently and receiv'd it in the way of Inoculation ... and that not one more died of it in the whole town.[68]

In In addition, the African man told Colman that if young men in a village were planning to go on a trading trip several hundred miles away and had not yet had smallpox or been inoculated, they would get inoculated before leaving on their trip to insure immunity from the disease.[69] When asked if he knew where the inoculation had come from, the African had answered: "[H]e knew nothing of those things; he suppos'd it was long before he was born; and no doubt but God told it to poor Negroes to save their lives; for they had not Knowledge and Skill as we have."[70] In this statement, the "we" refers to the white formerly English Bostonians. Whether this statement accurately reflected what the man actually said or had been rhetorically styled by Colman to acknowledge the reigning mindset of detractors or reflect the obsequiousness expected of the enslaved by the colonists is not known. In several places in the text, Colman disclosed his own vulnerability to those attacking the inoculation; his credibility could have been enhanced by his honesty, but he was unable to escape scorn from the Anti-Inoculators. Mather had not shown this self-consciousness or give indication of the awareness of his own vulnerability in *Angel of Bethesda* when discussing the role of Onesimus. He had, of course, reacted to the firebombing of his home.

Opposition to the Sources by Doctors and Other Bostonians

When the Mathers' folio, *Several Reasons* ... was published, the Anti-Inoculators responded in force. One writer in the *New England Courant* of November 27, 1721 parodied Mather's *Sentiments on the Smallpox* in a string of syllogisms. Mather's actual quote, for example, was:

> But the Method of managing the Small Pox in the way of Inoculation, is a most successful and allowable Method of preventing Death, and many other grievous Miseries by this terrible Distemper. Therefore, 'tis not only lawful but also a Duty to make use of it.71

The opponents' syllogism making partial use of the quote had become: "Several Arguments, proving, that inoculating the smallpox, is a lawful and successful practice; and not only so, but a Duty. Made plain and familiar to the meanest Capacity, but withal, so strong as to convince all Gainsayers, but such as want a Purge of Hellebore"—the traditional remedy for the insane.[72] Mather did mention in "Sentiments" a "Purge of Hellebore," but this phrase occurred several pages later in the text and was in relation to another example he gave. He asked: "Will any scruple the taking of this Artificial Purge? Surely, None but such as want a Purge of Hellebore."[73] Mather's example was that if a terrible "Bloody Flux" had come to town and hundreds had died, would anyone be reluctant to take a purge offered by a doctor that protected them from the disease? He suggested that only those who were crazy (needing a Purge of Hellebore) would refuse to take the herbal purgative and not the smallpox variolation, as charged by his opponents. In today's medicine, it would be counterintuitive to purge when one had bloody diarrhea, but in the medicine of Colonial America in 1721, it was the traditional treatment.

The anonymous opponent, thought to be Douglass, continued his sarcastic and inaccurate quoting with "A Method of preventing Death, which an Army of Africans have given us all the Assurance which rational Mind can desire, that it is used in Africa with success, is not only lawful, but a Duty."[74] The Anti-Inoculator had put two sentence parts together from Mather's text. One was the phrase about "Duty." In addition, Mather did use the phrase "an Army of Africans," there but in a different context. Mather had offered two sources in this tract: the learned men of the "Levant" and "an Army of Africans." He used both as evidence for his advocacy for inoculation. He wrote, "Men of Honour, and Learning, and of Incontestible Veracity, not one or two, but a considerable Number of them, agree in the Relation they give us, of its being used with constant Success in the Levant."[75] In this tract, unlike in *Angel,* he listed the Turkish evidence first, before that of the African knowledge. In between his positioning of the two-pronged evidence, he accused the Anti-Inoculators of bringing no evidence to their own argument against inoculation. The reference to Africans followed that accusation, as further bolstering of the veracity of the effectiveness of inoculation. "And we have an Army of Africans among our selves, who have themselves been under it [variolation], and have given us all the Assurance, which a Rational Mind can desire, that it has long been used with the like success in Africa."[76] There was no actual "army" of Africans in Boston who had received inoculations, nor did Mather say there were. He used the term in a slightly different context than that of what Douglass elided here. Even so, it was not unusual for

Mather to use terms and commit slips of the tongue that would give fodder to those who then used his words against him. Approximately 1000 Africans dwelled in the Boston area; the town itself was one of the largest port cities at that time. To feel confident enough as a writer from the opposition to parody "Sentiments" so closely is an indication how widely recognizable the phrase and text would be to the readers of the *Courant*. Also, although the *Courant* was well known for its opposition to Mather and the inoculation project, the tone indicates confidence in the widespread view of the Bostonians that the knowledge of the enslaved was not valued.

In the Boylston tract, which Gordon Jones and Kittredge believed was probably co-written with Mather, Mather and the surgeon had described those who had been interviewed as a "considerable number of Africans in this town."[77] It simply indicated that Mather had made more inquiries of other Africans after talking to Onesimus, as had Boylston and Colman. Another unsigned letter in the *Courant* had another mention of African knowledge: that a certain pastor received testimony "viva voce from some scattered members of the good people of Guinea."[78]

In December 1722, William Douglass mocked Mather's words in his *Inoculation*. I quote the passage in its entirety to further illustrate his attitudes and those of the Anti-Inoculators still attacking Mather's claim:

> Their second voucher is an army of a dozen or half a score Africans, by others called negro slaves who tell us now (tho' never before) that it is practiced in their country. The more blundering and they tell their Story, it is the more credible, says C.M.'s *a paradox in Nature* for all they say true or false is after the same manner. There is not a Race of Men on Earth more false lyars, etc. Their Accounts of what was done in their Country has never been depended upon till now for Argument's sake. Many *Negroes* to my knowledge have assured their Masters that they had the Small Pox in their own Country or elsewhere and have now had it in *Boston*. Some of Dr. *M.'s Inoculated Army* has had the same fate, which might serve as an Argument that the *Inoculated* may have the Small Pox afterwards in the common way but such weak Arguments our cause not require. To confirm this, you have at length in two of their little Books a silly Story or familiar Interview and Conversation between two *black Gentlemen* and a couple of *Reverend Promoters*, concerning Inoculation. *O Rare Farce!*[79]

Douglass clearly had not valued the Africans' testimonies and had regarded Mather's use of African narratives as further evidence of the absurdity of the project. The Scottish doctor had discounted the Inoculators' belief in the veracity of their experience and had said that no one else had considered African practices in their ancestral home as a warrant in arguments supporting inoculation. It is possible that if the slavers captaining the ships were very familiar with the practice, one might assume that buyers and owners might also have been aware of the importance of inoculation among the enslaved. Stewart's work supports the notion that at least some traders were very much aware of the technique.

However, Douglass's lack of knowledge of variolation's role in conversations between slavers and their captives was surprising, especially in light of the other statement attributed to him regarding this topic. His verbiage regarding having had "it" in Africa or elsewhere and then having "it" in Boston is confusing because of the undifferentiated pronoun. If he had been talking about having inoculation in Africa or elsewhere and then having smallpox in Boston, then that was doubtful and even impossible if the variolation had been successful. However, given language difficulties, perhaps newly arrived Africans had been unable to ascertain what the traders and buyers had been asking, although the pox scars or the variolation marks would have been visual testimonies. Even if not much was known about smallpox, Mather and many of his cohort had also noticed that those enslaved persons who nursed others with the smallpox seemed less susceptible to the disease. Slavers, sellers, and buyers considered a disease preventative a major factor in favor of buying someone who would not die in the next epidemic. In fact, one company sent a surgeon, a Dr. Houstoun, to Africa to inoculate the kidnapped people prior to sailing, as "... [i]t was the doctor's responsibility to insure that the captives put aboard the company's vessels were merchantable."[80] In the early 18th century, the literature shows that discussions among England and British and American trading companies often centered on the slave trade and particularly on the health or lack of disease, as well as smallpox among the captives. Douglass himself had been dismissive of his own argument as "weak" in the quote above, although in the list of arguments he made, he had felt it necessary to reinforce his attack on African testimonials.

Boylston, in his *Account of the Small-Pox Inoculated in New England*, presented a table in which he charted the various outcomes of those he had inoculated. There were cases in which some patients "had an imperfect small-pox by inoculation," and one could take this description to mean perhaps the person had not broken out in more than a one or two pocks following the inoculation or perhaps had already had smallpox because the inoculation had not taken.[81] Because the procedure was not perfected, and because there was still quite a debate regarding its efficacy, those who did choose to use inoculation were often judged by opponents based on the cases in which the procedure had offered only partial immunity or none after all.

When it came to opposing the variolation project on the basis of dubious sources, it was clear that the Anti-Inoculators knew their audience of Bostonians better than the Inoculators. Although some like Boylston, Mather, and other ministers in their alliance may have regarded African narratives as valuable and trusted them as people one could indeed learn from, many Bostonians had not been so inclined. The argument opposing inoculation based on that knowledge source would have appealed to many, particularly those Bostonians not Harvard-educated and distrustful of Mather. The Anti-Inoculators seemed bent on mobilizing this particular group of citizens against the minister. Individuals of little means saw doctors and clergy as the privileged class, as seen in the tracts, letters, and dialogues in the previous chapter. Many poor white Colonists inhabited Boston and eked out livings in manual labor in the city itself or on hard scrabble farms surrounding Boston as they learned to adapt to a new climate, soil, and topography. In contrast, the privileged whites had an enslaved person or two to do their hard work for them. Thus, resentment toward the privileged could be transferred onto the Africans whose knowledge of the procedure had been valued by the Inoculators.

Douglass could have had many different reasons for denying the validity of African knowledge, not the least of which were his views regarding the professionalization of medicine in the Colonies and his acting as gatekeeper of Physick. Douglass's arguments delegitimized those not having his education and rejected, therefore, any disease preventative procedures based on African narratives. One does need to be cautious, though, in interpreting the past through today's lenses. Douglass was a product of his time, but how, then, does that explain Mather and his followers who had seemed to get beyond the time's construction of race/dependency, status, and/or religion?

> To see ourselves as others see us can be eye-opening. To see others as sharing a nature with ourselves is the merest decency. But it is from the far more difficult achievement of seeing ourselves amongst others, as a local world among worlds, that the largeness of mind, without which objectivity is self-congratulation and tolerance a sham, comes.[82]

As a recent immigrant from Scotland, Douglass was also an "outsider," even as the Africans had been outsiders who did not elect to be in the Americas. The Scot was a European university-educated physician practicing in Bristol, and when he discovered his friend may become Governor of the Colony of Massachusetts, readied himself, and set sail for the city of Boston. Because his friend had not been chosen governor and that he had no immediate and powerful supporter within the colony and port town, he was on his own to build what he hoped would be a lucrative career.[83] Some of his later detractors thought that he may have even been jealous of the Mathers, as they had been part of the elite of Boston society. Still he could have so resented the forays into his medical field that that resentment took on a valence of its own.[84] While some of his antagonism toward Mather was fueled undoubtedly by his drive for professional legitimacy, his hostility toward African testimonials was the harshest published during the debate. This belligerent rhetoric toward African testimonials was very effective among Bostonians of this era.

Reverend Peter Thacher also weighed in on the rhetoric Douglass employed:

> The greater part of the physicians in town & those of most eminence reprobated inoculation in the strongest terms. Douglass placed himself at the head and did not hesitate to use any weapons lawful or unlawful to destroy his antagonists.[85]

Thacher, also a prominent pastor who was part of the Inoculators, wrote that Douglass had tried to ruin Boylston's medical practice.[86] The pastor was quoted as saying about Douglass: "This man, who had in perfection the hungry penetration and the unrelenting bitterness of his native country, left no method untried to load Dr. B with obloquy and prevent the success of his practice."[87] Peter Thacher, born at Salem in 1651, had been graduated from Harvard College in 1671. After traveling to England and visiting the preeminent ministers there, he received his first Massachusetts church in 1680. His brilliant sermons were apparently "greatly enhanced by the peculiar suavity and sanctity of his deportment."[88] Like his father, Rev. Thomas Thacher, he ministered to the body as well as the soul and spent part of his salary every year to purchase medicines and supplies for the sick and poverty-stricken. The physical healing was a legacy from his father, the Rev. Thomas Thacher, who had published the first broadside on disease in 1677 in the Boston colony: *A Brief Rule to Guide the Common People in the Smallpox and Measles*, which was published in a second edition in 1702. An even earlier work, according to Michael Flannery, was "a famous holograph 'Receipts to Cure Various Disorders for My Worthy Friend Mr. Winthrop,' written in 1643, probably by a Dr. Stafford."[89]

Douglass also continued to berate Mather twenty years after his death.[90] However, Douglass's motives might have been somewhat unique. His need for professional legitimacy alone might not explain the large appeal to the majority audience in Boston of all oppositional claims against the project, especially his antagonism toward the African testimonials. Perhaps his outsider status had played a role as well.

In addition to rejecting people's testimonials on the basis of their class, "dependency," race, or difference, there is additionally the rejection of knowledge of one minority group of people from a distant and unknown culture. Both were using the local knowledge from their own familiar contexts. A number of theorists have addressed the importance of local knowledge in different ways, but the combination of their epistemes can perhaps also help explain the rejection of African narratives in the time of the inoculation project. *Local knowledge* has long been a research term and practice among anthropologists because of Clifford Geertz's work in the 70s and the more recent essays in his 2000 text. In *Local Knowledge,* Geertz writes that "To an ethnographer sorting through the machinery of distant ideas, the shapes of knowledge are always ineluctably local, indivisible from their instruments and encasements."[91] Geertz argued that even what people thought was common sense (like the idea that it doesn't make sense to give someone a case of the disease one was trying prevent) "*was* a cultural system; a loosely connected body of belief and judgment, rather than just what anybody properly put together cannot help but think ... Common sense is not a fortunate faculty, like perfect pitch; it is a special frame of mind ... ."[92] The anthropologist worked to deconstruct social edifices of knowledge as privileged and argued that both wisdom and expertise within any discipline needed to be interrogated.[93]

What is known is that local knowledges, when cultures had clashed as they had in Boston, should be examined within new contexts. Although someone like Douglass is clearly confident about his choices and decisions within familiar medical cultures of Europe, Mather was equally confident in his willingness to examine others' experiences of the disease. Another of Geertz's comments is apropos regarding the fact that people are uncomfortable accepting another "local knowledge," different from their own:

> To turn from trying to explain social phenomena by weaving them into grand textures of cause and effect to trying to explain them by placing them in local frames of awareness is to exchange a set of well-charted difficulties for a set of largely uncharted ones.[94]

Human nature seems reluctant to give up one set for another.

In addition to Geertz, Foucault also addressed the use of local knowledge in *Power/Knowledge*. Foucault defined it as *subjugated knowledge*, that of persons not in positions of power, as the "whole set of knowledges ... disqualified as inadequate to their task or insufficiently elaborated: naive knowledges, located low down on the hierarchy, beneath the required level of cognition or scientificity."[95] This category is useful for the analysis because Africans and their families' and cultures' knowledge, understandings, and experiences were subjugated and disqualified in the smallpox inoculation project. In the hierarchy of knowledges within the colony, the constructions of science, religion, logic, and common sense were privileged and also familiar and circulated widely among the citizens.[96] Douglass clearly believed the role of his own academic medicine as scientific knowledge was the most valid episteme and that the episteme of African experience should be dismissed.

In Paolo Freire's (1993) *Pedagogy of the Oppressed*, he also worked with and theorized local knowledge in the context of his own country. . Freire's 1993 work can be used to hypothesize both about Mather's research methodology and his mindset. He makes it clear that in each generation and culture, *certain* people find it possible to include the knowledge of those who have not been given privileged status. When the role of the classical/academic/Platonic systems of knowledge is privileged over other epistemes, it mirrors the power structure between privileged knowledge holders over those whose knowledge is not acknowledged, and then their input and experience are purposely (then habitually) discounted and misrecognized. Those without power often internalize the hierarchy as in the case above of the older African man who told Colman that "... no doubt but God told it to poor Negroes to save their lives; for they [the enslaved] had not Knowledge and Skill as you [white Bostonians] have."[97] In the case of the inoculation project in Boston in the 1720s, some accepted the local "knowledge" (as defined by Geertz, Foucault, and Freire), and some clearly did not. It is known that Mather consulted many sources, including those of Onesimus, other Africans, and scholars of the "Levant" found in the *Philosophical Transactions* of the Royal Society in London. Others of the Inoculators also accepted other knowledges as valid. If Mather and his allies had been successful in winning acceptance of the Africans' knowledge in Massachusetts about smallpox, many lives could have been saved. In addition, although Mather had believed in the different sources, because his credibility had already been in question, those sources proved less persuasive to many.

More specifically, knowledge about disease was key. Wisecup, quoting Humphreys Warner, suggests on the other hand that historians of medicine saw the controversy as arising from the different interpretations of disease, with the Puritan belief that natural phenomena pointed to spiritual causes while Douglass and others Anti-inoculators only believed in only natural causes.[98] Those views, however, represent only one of many reasons and minimize the Puritan interest in science, Mather's correspondence with the Royal Society, and his own, if somewhat erroneous, use of the microscope and beliefs in a fledgling germ theory. After all, it had been the physicians, except for Boylston, who had used religious arguments in the debate, a rhetorical strategy that had been calculated to appeal to the public Puritan audience. Warner and Wisecup also believed Mather promoted inoculation because he "hoped to improve his own position as a figure of importance in New England society" and to defend ministers' influence in both religious and political affairs.[99] Physicians had used an effective appeal to religion for the majority of Bostonians; Mather's appeal to the educated privileged fell short for all except for the other ministers, and this ironic situation continued to make a difference in acceptance. In England at about the same time, some of the physicians had tended to support inoculation but not all. The opposite was true of ministers there, who had tended *not* to support the procedure because of their religious views. Mather had hoped to redeem his status and reputation, which had continued to suffer because of his earlier history.

Regarding the language Mather used to bring forward African testimonials, numerous literary scholars such as Wisecup, David D. Hall, and David S. Shields regarded the plain language Mather and other Inoculators usually used to further their argument conflicted with the more satirical prose of Douglass, Mundungus, and other Anti-Inoculators.[100] Hall, in particular, argued that the *Courant* created a new space for the mapping out of both public and private zones for insider/outsider language and various new forms. However, close examination of pamphlets and two of the other Bostonian papers at the time revealed that the satirical writings of both sides were often featured, including parodies from both sides. One of the papers clearly championed the Inoculators and the other two papers the Anti-Inoculators. The *Courant,* initiated in the time of the smallpox inoculation, continued to politically challenge Mather, his father, and the other ministers (the weakened theocracy) supporting the intervention. Wisecup and D. Hall both argue that the *Courant* formed part of a "politics of culture" that sought to "create a sphere that was liberated from the pulpit."[101]

Samuel Grainger, another of the Anti-Inoculators, noted that the physicians who had been asked their view of inoculation had also rejected it because they were not supportive of the value of the African claims.[102]

> Neither will I *pretend* to Examine, how far agreeable and consistent it is with *Rules of* Physick ..., I should perhaps have been *as little regarded,* as *our most eminent professors of that noble Science* were ... when their *Opinion* of this *Practice* was publickly desir'd, and rejected perhaps by some, for no other reason but because not agreeable to the *New Scheme* of those *Judicious people* called *Africans* ... .[103]

One could expect that among the Bostonians there would be some resistance to African and other cultural knowledges being imposed on them in the midst of a great threat to their health. Many felt they had little in common with enslaved people and foreigners. Particularly with their religious beliefs infusing their reactions to many if not all life's events, an imposition of alternative cultural views would have created cognitive dissonance, threatening their tenuous hold on life in the midst of great fear of another devastating smallpox epidemic. Stewart acknowledged that smallpox and other epidemic diseases had "held the eighteenth-century public frozen in perverse fascination and often bewilderment."[104] Frightened people often revert back to and become more entrenched in dogmatic ideas. The perception of many Bostonians was that *their own* knowledge was supreme. There was, in addition, an unusual struggle over power: efforts to remove the Mathers from the heights as well as to remove the British Governor, and to raise the status of Anti-Inoculators like Douglass, Grainger, and Mundungus among others. It's also helpful to briefly contextualize this resistance to African wisdom within the larger context of New England slavery.

Slavery in 1700s New England

In addition to contextualizing resistance, it's important to also contextualize acceptance. Slavery in New England at this time was not identical to slavery everywhere in the colonies, and it looked very different from the slavery in

Southern plantations, for example. Ira Berlin maintained that most enslaved in New England were Atlantic creoles, more acquainted with European culture and languages, who had established roots in port cities such as Boston.[105] Instead of coming directly from Africa, it was thought that many in the northeast came from the Caribbean Islands or the mainland South in small numbers. The colonists in Boston still had identified the enslaved as "Africans," though, no matter how they had gotten to their city. There were no large slave markets in the north, as in the southern ports, so those who had been rejected for plantation labor were sometimes shipped to New England and the Middle Colonies.[106] A Rhode Island merchant had told one of the captains to bring some of the West Indies rejects, traders contemptuously referred to them as "refuse," to the northern ports.[107] There, those unable to be sold in the South could find homeowners that, depending on the time period and individuals, appreciated their abilities. Yet, in the middle 1600s, the New Netherland governor complained with other northern slave owners about getting slaves who were "old and rejected," and who one Massachusetts official had said were "usually the worst servants."[108] The Rhode Island colonial legislature declared that such enslaved people from the Islands were no longer welcomed because they were runaways, lame, and/or had bad temperaments.[109]

However, in the 1700s it seemed as if many households appreciated the people with more experience, who had knowledge of European languages and habits, better resistance to disease, and more familiarity with other customs after having been in the West Indies for a decade or so.[110] It's possible Onesimus could have been one of these more experienced men, and one who also had been known to have clashed with his owner at times. His dialect could indicate he was an Atlantic creole with some capacity for English, but we don't have enough of his language to tell. He was definitely part of the Charter generation of those enslaved (under colonial charters) as distinct from the Plantation generations. Onesimus already had other trades and skills, and he and some others were allowed to make money outside of their servitude in Boston homes. Onesimus had a wife and at least two children, early deceased, who had lived off site in a small shack, while he frequently stayed in the Mather house or in a lean-to in the alley in back of it. Berlin asserted that the enslaved and their owners in the shared environment had enabled them to learn trades and to spend time with white journeymen, apprentices, and other servants in small taverns around the wharves of northern ports.[111] Mather had freed Onesimus to work in a money-making job based on the craft he had learned while still enslaved. Berlin also maintained that the upper classes of colonists thought the social cleavage was between non-free and free rather than black and white, since so many white men, women, and children were also servants.[112] This further context may have made the respect for African knowledge by some Bostonians such as Boylston, the Mathers, and other ministers more possible.

Other Disqualified Knowledge Fueled Resistance

Yet, Douglass and his Anti-Inoculators had fertile ground for appealing to the audience by rejecting divergent epistemes. Interestingly in Douglass's *Inoculation* (1722), it was not only the local African knowledge that had been discussed but also that of the Native Americans, but with a very different tone and point of view. Douglass had otherwise gone point for point with one of Mather's text, yet there is no mention in Mather's text of the Native example the Scot chose to highlight. The doctor had refuted a point Mather had made and had suggested that his [Douglass's] own example would have been a more appropriate one to have chosen. Douglass in the following passage commented on another disease, malaria, and the use of a natural quinine source (cinchona or Peruvian bark): "The Comparison of the Cortex Peru or Jesuits' Powder, favours this practice most, being a true Specifick in the case of intermittent Fevers or Agues. We learned for some considerable time the return of *aguish Fits*."[113] His point was the cleric should have used the example of Cortex Peru *because* it is a true specific, meaning a medication that addresses just one disease and not many problems. The Scottish doctor recognized the South American Indian source as valid and maintained that it was effective at preventing the fevers and flu-like symptoms of malaria, although the length of its effectiveness was not known. While it did not prevent the disease, it at least lessened the symptoms of malaria and held it off for a time.

In his next claim about malaria, Douglass raised the subtler point that medical interventions can have serious side effects, although he does not specifically mention vaccination here. It can be assumed enthymematically.

> At its first Entrance into *Europe* not having by Experience (and to the Cost of the first Tryers) learnt the doing and timing of it, and what Constitutions would bear it, instead of the intermitting Fever which it prevented, it left many chronical and fatal Ails, which did not appear but in Process of time; So that People were very shy of it, and rather chose the Ague should take its natural Course, or usual Method of Cure, tho' a few did die of it; than be liable to those *After-Claps*, of which in Process of Time many died.[114]

The Scottish physician suggested that without more complete knowledge of the process and timing of a smallpox inoculation, there were great risks. Inoculators could end up violating the Sixth Biblical Commandment, "Thou Shalt Not Kill," if patients died as a result of the variolation. Thus, he had used a strong, logical claim in the quoted passage and followed up with a religious one.

In response to Mather's text, Douglass further asked the Inoculators "whether at that time they who would not use the Cortex *were* Breakers of the Sixth Commandment [a point made by Mather]."[115] If doctors had chosen not to use the Peruvian bark for malaria or other fevers, and sufferers of malaria died, would they have broken the commandment?

> Even at this time, tho' the Use of the Cortex has been improved upon by the most polite Nations over some Scores of Years, some eminent *Physicians* and a great many Patients chuse rather to omit the Use of it, because of its suspected Consequences; are they Breakers of the Sixth Commandment.[116]

Douglass continued with this argument, one that was clearly relying on familiarity with other types of medical treatments that were used to intervene in, interrupt, prevent, or even cure a disease that had been common in the colonies.

This passage is fascinating on a number of fronts. Douglass recognized the efficacy of the Cortex Peru (quinine) in the intermittent fever/ague (malaria). He was accepting of the local knowledge (of the Americas and Native Americans) here and even suggested a possible key to changing his own rejection of the inoculation project: "... then the salutary use of it was not known." Because Mather had used the Sixth Commandment to justify use of an effective method to prevent smallpox, Douglass responded in kind. In directly debating each other, the two, Mather and Douglass, had sometimes used both religious and medical discourses.

Truth Claims of "Mohametans" Challenged

Another example of the debate's hinging on certain power relations of who was allowed to speak can be seen in a pamphlet titled "The Imposition of Inoculation As a Duty ..." published January 1, 1722 by one of the Anti-Inoculators, Samuel Grainger. This pamphlet was adorned with the following Latin phrase, "Aliquid Monstri semper profert Africa," which had been cited as Pliny's, but had been slightly altered from a passage in his Natural History,[117] "where, after speaking of strange creatures there produced, he adds: 'Unde etiam vulgare Graeciae dictum simper aliquid novi Africam adferre.'"[118] Samuel Grainger had written that "to bring armies of Africans, and troops of Mahometans, to prove it is lawful by their success in it, is like proving their religion of Mahomet, as true religion, because successfully propagated, and maintained by the sword, and protested by vast numbers, which fill whole nations of the Eastern World."[119] There were no "armies" of Africans being "brought" but only consultation with some of the Africans in Mather's and other Inoculators' households and of their acquaintance.

However, in this text the use of the term "Mahometans" or practitioners of Islam signaled another group whose knowledge about the medical preventative of inoculation had no familiarity in Puritan Boston. This reference was perhaps to some African slaves but more certainly to the Turks, whose practice of variolation was cited in the Royal Society's *Philosophical Transactions*. Mather had referred to their experience in his published writings on smallpox. Some Africans were also Muslim, but because they had been forced to practice the Christian religion in the colonies, it's unclear whether Bostonians knew that some enslaved African could have shared this religion with the Turks. Silva also agrees that "The anti-inoculators had already made much of the fact that procedure described by Timoni and Pylarino was a 'Mahometan' one, hoping that suspicion about a foreign religion would lead to apprehensions about inoculation."[120]

Concern about the religious beliefs of supporters of the inoculation project was also increased by the writings of Mundungus (John Williams), who further attacked inoculation through his "firm conviction that the Devil had devised inoculation to destroy the bodies of Christians and ensnare their souls."[121] Like the gravedigger in Hamlet, he still disported himself in syllogistic reasoning: "If inoculation of the small pox be not of God, then it is of the Devil. But, It is not of God. Therefore, It is of the Devil."[122] According to Mundungus, inoculation was a plot against the Christians to exterminate them in the New World by giving them smallpox. In *Angel* and *Some Account of What Is Said of Inoculating or Transplanting the Smallpox*, Mather's references to both Timoni and Pylarino, who wrote from Constantinople and Smyrna, gave rise to the fear of outsiders, especially those with other religions. Because both sources referred to Turkish and then Greek practices, the Protestant reaction against them was heightened. Even though they had been quoted in the Royal Society's *Transactions* and held in great regard among several in the colony, many others would not have found such evidence convincing. Mather and others often sent discoveries of new plants, animals, and other objects for categorization of the findings in the New World. Thus, the *Transactions* could cause some reasonable doubt, because Mather's entries had included both valid descriptions of specimens, while others had been products of his imagination.

Mundungus's audience heard him rail against the "Mahometans" without acknowledgment of where the sources had been published. In *Several Arguments* ... Mundungus had dismissed the use of any sources such as the *Transactions* out of hand: "The Practice of *Smyrna* and *Constantinople* is not a rule either of Faith or Manners, therefore I shall dismiss that Paragraph."[123] In rejecting truth claims because they come from an area of the world not sharing the same faith or culture, Williams had used reductive claims, collapsing all the accounts into a single term: *Mahometans*, even though Pylarino and Timoni both studied medicine at Padua, one being of Venetian ancestry and the other Greek. The anti-Islamic prejudice means that Westerners did not recognize the indebtedness of much of European medicine, science, and mathematics to scholars from that part of the world. Thus, the Inoculators' argument had been weakened and not strengthened by this evidence.

Douglass further debunked the project in his *Inoculation* tract by suggesting that Mather in a "late" paper had posited that Timoni and Pylarino advocated for the project, when they had reported it as mere observations. Douglass also wrote that "If all that was written in *Philosophical Transactions,* viz. Amusements, Projects, credulous Relations Etc. ought to be put into practice, the World would soon be turn'd upside down."[124] This statement was true. The proceedings from the Royal Society were known to be a creative assortment of oddities, curiosities, urban legends, carnival freak show items (two-headed calves, etc.), as well as major discoveries in science, and good documentation. Douglass then reported on an account of a blood transfusion in the *Transactions* that was well researched and applied, citing eye-witness and second-hand accounts, which made the invention of transfusion much more trustworthy even in his eyes.[125] The physician had also pointed out that Mather received the news of the Levantine methods third-hand through Dr. Woodward's account in the text of the descriptions from Timoni and Pylarino, which was a valid argument on Douglass's part. The original letter from Timoni, for example, had not been printed in the *Transactions.*[126] In addition, he pointed out that there were discrepancies between where Timoni gained his knowledge; at one point it was from Asia, and at another time Greece, which was also true.[127] Douglass himself had done a very close reading of Timoni's other texts in the *Transactions* and had found many discrepancies and inaccuracies in the details of his descriptions of the variolation. Douglass's points were accurate, and his detailed analysis had been thorough and convincing. His argument was much stronger in this part of the text when he had moved from *ad hominem* attacks to verifiable and carefully analyzed data. In doing so, he undercut some of the strength of the evidence on which Mather and the Inoculators had begun the project.

The use of the term "Mahometans" (Mohammedans or Muslims) was used strategically in other tracts by Anti-Inoculators. In *A Letter from One in the Country* ..., an anonymous author, who claimed to be neither an Inoculator nor an Anti-Inoculator, had written: "A certain *Clergy-Man* [C.M.] (by the way of *Europe*) received advice of the Practice among the *Mussel-men* & faithful people of the prophet Mahomet; also more immediately and *vive voce* from some of the scattered Members of the good people of *Guinea*, who communicated it to Physicians in your town."[128] This author went on to tell this hypothetical friend, presumably Dr. Francis Archibald, in a conceit often used in those times in such political/social tracts about the introduction of the smallpox inoculation as a disruptive and dangerous practice. After the introduction of the terms and berating of the practice, he also wrote the following: "To spread a mortal Contagion, What is it but to cast abroad Arrows and Death? If a man should willfully throw a Bomb into a Town, burn a House, or kill a man, ought he not to die?"[129] Not long after this publication, Mather's home was firebombed.

As the anonymous author[130] continued his argument, he used rhetorical questions such as,

> Suppose then again ... that of those many who are lately slain by the *Small-pox,* some few have taken it by their *Inoculated* Neighbours, who might otherwise have escaped it. How shall we excuse our *Mahometan* Missionaries, from being truly, tho' not designedly the cause of their death?"[131]

Most of this particular "letter" does not contain the religious discourse of Mundungus nor is it written in William Douglass's style. The writer ended with a suggestion that those who wish to infect themselves be quarantined in "proper Pest Houses in solitary places." Those inoculated the next year were sent to Spectacle Island for quarantine. In addition, he added once more: "or else to banish the Practice to the *Turks* and *Pagans*, whence it came."[132]

Women's Knowledge of Inoculation

The mention of the Greek woman inoculator gave a hint of what any attempt of support for inoculation by women in Boston might face. Timoni's and Pilarino's description of the Grecian "Inoculatrix" who had so successfully inoculated others had been the most convincing source for their advocacy of inoculation in their letters in the Royal Society's *Transactions.* In the Boston controversy, there had been little information regarding the attitudes the women might have faced, and, in fact, for the most part their voices were conspicuous by their absence. In an earlier chapter on the witchcraft debacle, young girls' voices were "respected" as they joined together to implicate a woman of color as well as numerous other women of practicing Satanic rituals. What is known is that women took some part in the healthcare practices of the community, particularly in herbal medicines, midwifery, and, of course, caregiving. Not only were ministers' wives active with their kitchen gardens of herbs that they grew, dried, assembled, and used for healing, but also other female herbalists practiced throughout the colonies.

The role of women during the introduction of vaccination in Britain, and especially London and surrounding areas, had been more robust, yet the texts of this same time, 1720 through 1722, revealed the necessity for low profiles for the most part, often hiding their identities and roles in inoculations behind their husbands or other men rather than being in the public eye. The single woman most associated with smallpox inoculation had been Lady Mary Wortley Montagu, who had survived smallpox herself in 1715 and found protection for her son from the dread disease later while in Turkey.[133] Her husband had been appointed ambassador there in 1716; she returned to England from Constantinople in 1719.

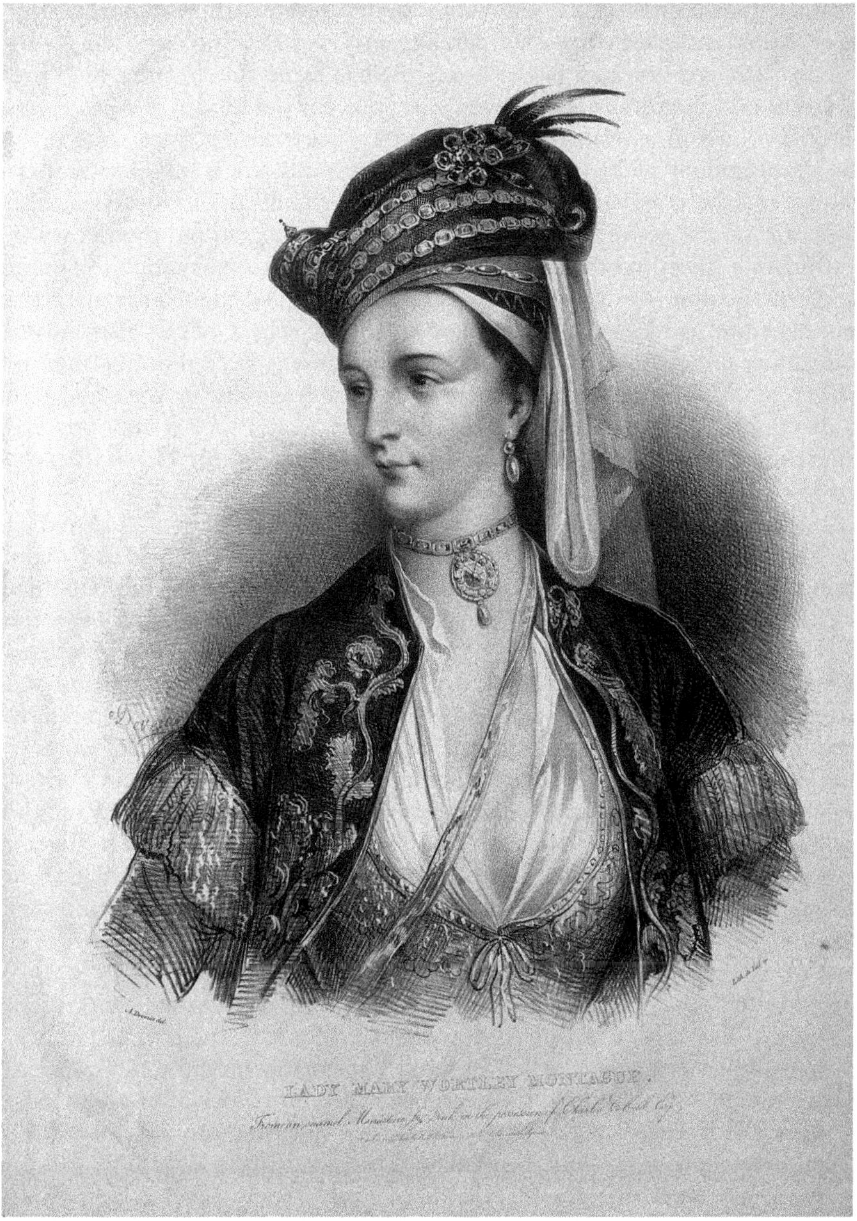

Figure 5.2 Lady Mary Wortley Montagu, Wellcome Commons.

When she had arrived back in London, she found a vehement smallpox outbreak that had forced Londoners indoors, limited all visits, except for the servants, many of whom had already survived smallpox and thus were the most desired workers in the home. At the same time, rather than just ministers and doctors in contention, the medical practitioners were themselves involved in a serious power struggle. The warring sides were often also separated by class with the apothecaries and some surgeons/barbers who served the poor versus the Royal Society's College of Physicians who took care of the wealthier patients. While Mundungus, an apothecary in Boston, was prized by the physicians for his ability to persuade the poorer people in Boston, the two groups in London argued vigorously over the treatment and possible prevention of smallpox. The College also moved against any unlicensed practitioners, and that move affected both classes of caregivers, who were charged with "Quacking about in the Office of Physicians."[134] The vehemence over this issue caused such a vigorous and dangerous dispute, that physicians John Woodward's, Sir Hans Sloane's, and John Freind's disagreement had included a duel.[135]

Another deadly outbreak or a further wave of smallpox occurred in England, as in Boston, in 1721, and Lady Mary had begun losing many friends and a few relatives to the disease. She decided to get her daughter inoculated and had written to Dr. Charles Maitland, who had been the surgeon at the embassy and was then practicing in Hertford. He had refused to perform the inoculation at first, because he feared for his reputation and career, because as a "mere surgeon" his doing an "engrafting" would have gone up against the powerful university-educated and wealthier doctors in the College of Physicians.[136] Maitland had done the vaccinations in Turkey, but in London he would only perform them if two or three doctors from the College would be his witnesses and confirm that he had not been negligent. That three from the prestigious group agreed to attend the inoculation of Lady Mary's child was an indication that the approval had come from very high up in the government.[137] Lady Mary's daughter was

> 'ingrafted ... in both arms, in the usual Manner'. On the tenth night after this she was 'a little hot and Feverish'. An 'Ancient' neighbourhood apothecary was called to see her; next morning the pocks began to emerge, and Maitland's observers were sent for 'one after another, to visit the young Lady.' They found her 'playing around the room, cheerful and well, with the Small Pox rais'd upon her.' The official witnesses were not alone. Friends of Lady Mary 'Several ladies and, other persons of Distinction,' saw the child during the few days before she [the daughter] was back to normal.[138]

Two of the three doctors/witnesses had positive views of what Maitland had recruited them to witness. One had already lost two sons to smallpox and wanted his only remaining son inoculated. A third physician/witness

> betrayed not only such incredulity as to its success, but such an unwillingness to have it succeed, such evident rancour and malignity, that Lady Mary ... said she would never leave them alone with the child one second, lest they should do it some injury.[139]

The warring over smallpox continued, but this time only over vaccination and with some different sides entering into the fray. This time the bitter media battle involved ministers, journalists, and some physicians and other practitioners against it, while a number of physicians from the College were supporting it. Lady Mary had begun to more openly but cautiously support the practice, and also had her son inoculated. Still she had to hide behind her husband's name for this child's preventative and also for the soon-to-follow Newgate experiment that involved using the technique on prisoners. If she had been at that time advocating for it, she would have had to endure anti-women rhetoric from those against the practice. This problem was certainly bound to be repeated in Boston during the same epidemic or pandemic had more use been made of the testimonials about the Greek woman's practice, or had women been comfortable advocating for it, which is most likely one of the reasons we hear no women's voice in the debate in Boston.

According to reports, a small group from the Royal College of Physicians "made a case" to the King (George I) for experimenting on condemned criminals at Newgate prison by inoculating them with smallpox. The inspiration for such an experiment had come from none other than Princess Caroline of Wales. Lady Mary had written that "the princess 'was her firm support and stood by her without quailing.'" As Isobel Grundy wrote:

> In the heated debate at the time, those papers and pamphlets, which supported inoculation found it expedient to suppress the heavy female involvement (which would only give an opening for misogynist bile) and to mention authoritative males in their stead.[140]

Princess Caroline had nearly lost a daughter to smallpox, wanted to protect and thus inoculate her other children, and others had wanted the King to experiment on the prisoners. Many reports still state to this day that Ambassador Wortley Montagu and George I were the initiators of the Newgate project. Maitland had again been called upon for inoculations, but again put forward conditions, especially given the terrible recriminations that he certainly would have had to endure in the troubled time. Ministers accused those who participated of meddling with God's will, and others suggested black magic was involved, much like in the Boston controversy. He asked Sloane to find a doctor with Turkish experience who could accompany him because his partner would then be "ranked above ladies, or foreigners, or a surgeon such as himself."[141] Timoni's article on the Turkish variolations, originally printed in the Royal Society's *Proceedings*, was reprinted in a London paper at around the same time in August 1721. Sir Hans Sloane had also been in attendance during the inoculations. All six prisoners, three men and three women, lived and were freed from their sentences of death; all six were petty thieves, except for one man who had stolen a horse, a theft not considered "petty."[142]

By 1721, Lady Mary was a very active promoter of the process, and in the continuing furor heard both extravagant praise as well as cruel excoriation. Some of the feedback had been more implicit than explicit; her rank had protected her among some in her class, but others were blatant with their scorn. Servants were covert with theirs, yet when she was in public, she had faced terrible harassment by passersby. Because the royals had been for variolation, oppositional and independent media had been against it. One of the royals was vaguely identified in the *London Mercury* as the "Eldest Son of a Noble Duke," the one that the *Courant* in Boston had had such a dispute over with Increase Mather.[143] The media

> struck a purposefully paranoiac tone, laying on prejudice not merely against the new science but also against foreigners and women. (Current [then] military events in eastern Europe provided a quite rational basis for anti-Turkish feeling: a gift to anti-inoculators.) Advocates for inoculation found it practicable to defend scientific advance, but not the female and oriental origins of the new process: these could only be concealed.[144]

Although the Newgate experiment on the six thieves had been proof of the inoculation process, much like the newspaper battles in Boston, the papers had continued to line up vigorously on different sides and spur on the debate. For example, the *Post Man* and the *St. James's Evening Post* had made opposite claims about a child's death in November 1721, one saying that the child had died as a result of the variolation, while the other wrote that it was attributable to natural smallpox.[145] Maitland continued to perform variolations with many royals by his side in spite of the disputes. After the success of Newgate, one of the prisoners, Ruth Jones, had been released to him in his Hertford practice where smallpox continued to rage, and he had her share a bed with a patient in full-blown smallpox to prove that the prisoner was still immune to the disease.[146]

By early 1722, vaccinations had "spread like wildfire."[147] Again, many of these were among the upper class friends and relatives of Lady Mary and Princess Caroline. Every spring for a few years until the epidemic abated, there continued to be inoculations. That didn't mean some inoculates didn't die; however, often the symptoms seemed to be other than those of smallpox such as convulsions and high fevers with no signs of pustules. It seems that unlike in Boston, where those who were newly vaccinated were kept separate from anyone who had not been inoculated or already had smallpox, in England friends and relatives would often visit the person, and especially children, who had undergone the procedure. As those recovering had some pustules and lower fevers, they were still contagious, so that quarantine behavior seemed to have been less well known in England or perhaps just not well practiced. Smallpox was contagious from the time the first pustules appeared in the mouth and throat until the last scab on a pox fell off.

Especially in the media, inoculators continued to be looked upon with mistrust. Two powerful anti-inoculators had teamed up, especially after the deaths of two small, royal children and played upon the general fears. Reverend Edmund Massey, a well-known and powerful minister, had preached a particularly persuasive sermon on the current "plague" as a judgment on sin, while a doctor from the College of Physicians, William Wagstaffe, issued pamphlets against inoculation because it was dangerous. He had used as his warrant his own superiority as a physician against surgeons/barbers, nurses, and apothecaries. Wagstaffe railed against those "inferior" to him and, in Grundy's words, "was racist, antifeminist, and orientalist."[148] He had also targeted Lady Mary as "some *sanguine* Traveller from *Turkey*."[149]

With the leadership of those two English anti-inoculators, Massey and Wagstaffe, the rhetoric became more polarized and stylized into two types. The political factions followed suit, with the Whigs for inoculation and the Tories firmly against, except for an occasional outlier. Not surprisingly, Maitland was one of the main voices *for* the procedure, as was Lady Mary, and Drs. James Jurin, and even John Arbuthnot, one of the few Tories with a positive view toward the procedure. Mather and others supporting inoculation in Boston had been aware of and had read Jurin's work in the Royal Society's *Philosophical Transactions*. Jurin was a well-educated M.D. who served as Secretary of the Royal Society under Isaac Newton as President. He had done a very careful and resourceful study that included gathering data from a large correspondence network in order to track the mortality from inoculated smallpox compared to what was referred to as "natural" smallpox. Before becoming an M.D., Jurin had studied mathematics at Cambridge, and is credited with having brought mathematics and statistics to Western medicine. He began his study after having read a letter from a Dr. Nettleton in Halifax who had inoculated about 40 in his town and the surrounding area in which his data showed that about 20% of those infected naturally died of smallpox, in contrast to 0% of those who had been inoculated. The study was obviously small, so Jurin set up and then reported out a much larger one. His report in the *Transactions* included the following:

> The Result … Of these Computations is, that, if the same Proportions should still continue, as have hitherto been determin'd by Observation, we must expect, That of all the Children that are born, there will, some time or other, die of the Small Pox, one in fourteen. That of Persons of

> all Ages taken ill of the natural Small Pox, there will die of that Distemper, one in five or six, or two in eleven. That of Persons of all Ages inoculated, without regard to the Healthiness or Unhealthiness of the Subject, as was practised in New England, there will die one in sixty. That of Persons inoculated with the same Caution in the choice of the Subjects, as has been used by the several Operators one with another, here in England, (if we allow in the two disputed Cases above mention'd, that the Persons died of the inoculated Small Pox) there will die one in ninety one.[150]

In the meantime, Boylston in Boston also kept very careful track of all the patients he had inoculated, the dates, and their results, in which inoculation had a 2.4% mortality rate.[151]

With the volleys flying back and forth between the two sides in England, the rhetorics were markedly different, although each side accused the other of a "violent tone."[152] Wagstaffe's and Massey's rhetoric fostered panic and paranoia, while Maitland, Jurin, and their allies appealed to reason and science. The paranoia among the supporters of the Anti-Inoculators had to do with fears about the Turks, women, and even plantation owners in the British colonial islands and of their possible strategies of eliminating troubling workers, heirs, and Christians by injecting or scarifying them. Although the Drs. Maitland, Jurin, and Arbuthnot had used facts, dates, statistics, good manners, and reason, Arbuthnot had suggested that the writings from the other side hinted at Satanic possession and witchcraft among the leaders and their followers.[153]

It was also at that time that Lady Mary, who had played such a strong role as a promoter of variolation behind the scenes, had publically entered the fray with her only written work of advocacy in print: "A Plain Account of the Inoculating of the Smallpox."[154] Her piece had begun by blaming doctors in the most strident tones, claiming that many of them cared more about their reputations and incomes than about their patients. Her attack was surprising considering the many doctors who were pro-inoculation, but she apparently felt that the procedure had already proven itself valuable and that it should not be left only to physicians to administer. Lady Mary had insisted in her article that the Turkish system of variolation was the best because it involved a tiny needle prick and a small amount of virulent matter rather than slashing huge wounds and using a large amount of fluid from the pustules. She also had advocated for fewer bleedings, purges, and other methods pre- and post-inoculation, all the while insisting doctors had badly compromised the best method she had brought with her from Turkey.[155] After her opinion was published, she had returned to shrinking back behind the scenes, but still had encouraged and visited those who had recently had vaccinations. She herself had been rendered immune by a natural course of smallpox before an inoculation had been available. The immunizations proceeded among some citizens well into 1725, although they always dipped when a small child died of what looked like natural smallpox after having had a smallpox inoculation earlier. In time, the role Lady Mary Wortley Montagu had played in England in the 1720s was recognized.

More Analysis of Boston

Given all the other arguments brought out in the previous chapters, it cannot be argued that attitudes toward African, Greek, Turkish, and female knowledge had been the only reasons that colonists exhibited apprehension about the new technique of variolation. Smallpox was a horrific disease, and the experience of the disease itself would have directly or indirectly affected every family in the port town of Boston at some point. It can, however, be argued that the texts framed their arguments based on some rhetorical strategies that did not serve to open up the debate but instead to disallow certain claims and allow others. As noted, Douglass had included some more logical arguments as had some others. But often the strategies had further separated rather than drawn the best minds together to combat a destructive disease in the midst of an epidemic.

More importantly, there continues to be a need to develop better understandings of what scientific, in this case medical, knowledge came from sources that have not been acknowledged, and how it could change our understanding of medicine in the Atlantic world. Claire Gherini's text on James Kilpatrick's work in "rationalizing" smallpox inoculation in Charleston, South Carolina 17 years later noted continuing difficulty in sorting out whose truth claims were to be accepted and whose were not. Unlike the opinions of physicians toward inoculation in Boston, Kilpatrick was a physician who advocated for variolation. But in that Southern colony, physician knowledge of inoculation had been challenged. However, Kilpatrick successfully argued the validity of his own view of inoculation and acknowledged Lady Wortley Montagu as well. As Gherini claims, in 1738 in the South Carolina Lowcountry during a smallpox epidemic, Kilpatrick was able to leverage "the circuits of information that defined the town in order to promote the practice of inoculation and to create a medical and scientific persona that fit the expectations of Lowcountry audiences."[156] In 1721 in Boston, the most influential Puritan ministers of the time were not able to enact the same leveraging, although Mather and particularly Boylston enjoyed success for their arguments later in London. The experience of controversy and failure on the British periphery continued to be a refrain until the practice of smallpox inoculation was finally accepted in that colony in 1775. In Boston, in the 1763 epidemic (there was no major epidemic between 1722 and 1763), acceptance in the colony was more widespread, although detractors remained. Thus, frames for the same "procedure" can vary, even in colonies on the same continent and not so far removed from each other. African, Turk, or Greek medical wisdom had been rejected and delegitimized. Even Royal Society texts had been rejected by Anti-Inoculators and many Bostonians after being framed as elitist.

To complete this analysis, the following chapter concludes with a comparison between the 1720 and 1722 with a much more recent resistance to vaccination for a novel virus that appeared exactly 300 years later. This chapter examines both differences as well as more and very surprising similarities between the two controversies.

Notes

1 Kelly Wisecup, *Medical Encounters* (Amherst, MA: University of Massachusetts Press, 2013), 100.
2 Michel Foucault, *Power/Knowledge* (New York: Pantheon, 1980); Paolo Freire, *Pedagogy of the Oppressed* (New York: Herder, 1971); Clifford Geertz, *Local Knowledge* (New York: Basic, 1983, 2000).
3 C. Mather, *Angel of Bethesda* (Barre, MA: American Antiquarian Society, 1972), 107.
4 Margot Minardi, "The Boston Inoculation Controversy of 1721–1722" *William and Mary Quarterly,* 61, no. (2004), 48.
5 Londa Schiebinger, *Nature's Body: Gender in the Making of the Modern Body* (Boston: Beacon Press, 1993), 185.
6 Schiebinger, *Nature's Body*, 142.
7 Schiebinger, *Nature's Body*, 142.
8 Quoted in Schiebinger, *Nature's Body*, 184.
9 Foucault, *The History of Sexuality*, trans. Robert Hurley (New York: Random House, 1978), 54.
10 Ann Laura Stoler, "A Colonial Reader of Foucault: Bourgeois Bodies and Racial Selves" in *Foucault and Beyond*, ed. Vernon W. Cisney and Nicolae Morar (Chicago: University of Chicago Press, 2016), 339.
11 Stoler, "A Colonial Reader," 330.
12 Stoler, "A Colonial Reader," 334.
13 Ira Berlin. *Many Thousands Gone: The First Two Centuries of Slavery in North America* (Cambridge, MA: The Belknap Press of Harvard University Press, 1998), 59.
14 Stoler, "A Colonial Reader," 337.
15 Cotton Mather, *Some Account of What Is Said in Inoculating or Transplanting the Smallpox, By the Learned Dr. Emanuel Timonius, and Jacobus Pylarinus. With some remarks Thereon: To Which Are Added, a Few Quaeries in Answer to the Scruples of Many about the Lawfulness of this Method.* Published by Dr. Zabdiel Boylston (Boston: Sold by S. Gerrish at his shop in Corn-Hill, 1721), 21.
16 Minardi, "The Boston Inoculation Controversy," 50.
17 Stephen Coss. *The Fever of 1721* (New York: Simon and Schuster, 2016).
18 Katherine S. Koo, *Strangers in the House of God: Cotton Mather, Onesimus, and an Experiment in Christian Slaveholding* (Worcester, MA: American Antiquarian Society, 2007), 145.
19 Koo, *Strangers*, 145.
20 Minardi, "The Boston Inoculation Controversy," 63.
21 Benjamin Colman, *Some Observation on the New Method of Receiving the Small-Pox by Ingrafting or Inoculating* (Boston: Printed by B. Green for Samuel Gerrish, 1721), 16.

22 Koo, *Strangers*, 161; Jennifer E. Monaghan, "Reading for the Enslaved, Writing for the Free" in *Learning to Read and Write in Early America* (Amherst, MA: University of Massachusetts Press, 2005), 314–15.
23 Minardi, "The Boston Inoculation Controversy," 63.
24 Mather, *Diary of Cotton Mather* (New York: Ungar, 1957).
25 Robert Tindol, "Getting the Pox Out of All Their Houses: Cotton Mather and the Rhetoric of Puritan Science" *Early American Literature,* 46, no. 1 (March 2011), 7.
26 Winthrop G. Jordan, *White Over Black: American Attitudes Toward the Negro, 1550-1812* (New York: Norton, 1977), 68–69.
27 Koo, *Strangers*, 152.
28 Joanne Pope Melish, *Disowning Slavery: Gradual Emancipation and 'Race' in New England, 1780-1860* (Ithaca, NY: Cornell University Press, 1998), 18–20.
29 Koo, *Strangers*, 153.
30 Tindol, *Getting the Pox*, 11.
31 Mather, *Rules for the Society of Negroes, 1693* (Boston: B. Harris, 1693), n.p.
32 Koo, *Strangers*, 154; Lorenzo Johnston Greene, *The Negro in Colonial New England* (New York: Atheneum, 1968), 262.
33 Cotton Mather, *Diary for 1712*, ed. William Manierre, Jr. (Charlottesville, VA: University of Virginia Press, 1964), 69.
34 Koo, *Strangers in the House,* 160–61.
35 Cotton Mather Files: Box 5, Folder 1, American Antiquarian Society (Worchester, MA).
36 Larry Stewart, "The Edge of Utility: Slaves and Smallpox in the Early Eighteenth Century," *Medical History,* 29 (1985), 66.
37 Stewart, "The Edge," 66–67.
38 Stewart, "The Edge," 67.
39 Eugenia Herbert, "Smallpox Inoculation in Africa" *The Journal of African History,* 16, no. 4 (1975), 542.
40 Cadwallader Colden, "Extract of Letter from Cadwallader Colden, Esq. to Dr. Fothergill, Concerning the Throat Distemper, 1753," *The American Museum; or, Repository of Ancient and Modern Pieces, Prose and Poetical,* 3 (Philadelphia: Carey, 1788).
41 Elizabeth Donnan, *Documents Illustrative of the Slave Trade to America II* (Buffalo, NY: Wm. S. Hein & Co, 2002), 94–95.
42 Herbert, "Smallpox Inoculation," 543.
43 Kittredge, "Introduction," to *Several Reasons Proving That Inoculating or Transplanting the Small Pox, Is a Lawful Practice, and That It Has Been Blessed by God for the Saving of Many a Life.* By Increase Mather. *Sentiments on the Small Pox Inoculated.* By Cotton Mather in Boston, 1721. Cleveland, OH: 1921, 23; Herbert, "Smallpox Inoculation," 542.
44 Sir Hans Sloane, *Philosophical Transactions of the Royal Society of London,* 49 (1756), 516.
45 Mather, *Angel*, 107.
46 Reginald Heber Fitz, *Zabdiel Boylston, Inoculator, and the Epidemic of Smallpox in Boston in 1721* (Boston: Harvard, 1911), 27.
47 Genevieve Miller, "Smallpox Inoculation in England and in America: A Reappraisal" *The William and Mary Quarterly*, Series 3, 13, no. 4 (October 1956), 476–92.
48 Daniel Neal, "An Historical Introduction," to Benjamin Colman's *A Narrative of the Method and Success of Inoculating the Small-Pox in New England* (London: George Grierson, 1722), 5.
49 Neal, "An Historical," 5.

50 Douglass, *Inoculation Considered,* 20.
51 Stewart, "The Edge," 67.
52 Kittredge, "Introduction," 2–3.
53 Stewart, "The Edge," 65.
54 Stewart, "The Edge," 65.
55 James Phipps and Phipps' Court Assistants, Public Records Office T/*70/53/169* (March 1721), quoted in Stewart, "The Edge of Utility," 65.
56 Phipps et al., June 1722, quoted in Stewart, 65.
57 Bruno Latour and Steve Woolgar, *Laboratory Life: The Construction of Scientific Facts* (Princeton, NJ: Princeton University Press, 1986), 76–80.
58 Latour and Woolgar, *Laboratory Life, 77.*
59 Latour and Woolgar, *Laboratory Life*, 80.
60 Neal, "An Historical Introduction," 6.
61 Laird Okie, "Daniel Neal and the 'Puritan Revolution'" *Church History: Studies in Christianity and Culture, 55* (1986), 6.
62 Okie, "Daniel Neal," 6.
63 Okie, "Daniel Neal," 6.
64 Okie, "Daniel Neal," 6.
65 Okie, "Daniel Neal," 6.
66 Benjamin Colman, *A Narrative of the Method and Success of Inoculating the Small-Pox in New England* (Dublin, George Grierson, 1722), 31.
67 Colman, *A Narrative,* 31–32.
68 Benjamin Colman, *Some Observations*, 15–16; Colman, *A Narrative*, 31–32.
69 Colman, *A Narrative*, 32.
70 Colman, *A Narrative*, 32.
71 Cotton Mather, *Sentiments on the Small Pox Inoculated* (Boston: 1721), 74.
72 Kittredge, "Introduction," 23–24.
73 Mather, *Sentiments,* 76.
74 Anonymous Contributor, "Letter" in *New-England Courant,* ed. James and Benjamin Franklin, no. 32 (Boston: March 5–12, 1722), 2.
75 Mather, *Sentiments*, 75.
76 Mather, *Sentiments*, 75.
77 Mather, *Angel*, 107; Kittredge, "Introduction," 24.
78 Anonymous Contributor, "Letter," 1.
79 Douglass, *Inoculation Considered*, 6–7.
80 Stewart, "The Edge," 65.
81 Boylston, *An Historical Account*, 34.
82 Clifford Geertz, *Local Knowledge* (New York: Basic, 2000), 16.
83 Fitz, *Zabdiel Boylston*, 6.
84 Fitz, *Zabdiel Boylston*, 6.
85 Fitz, *Zabdiel Boylston*, 6.
86 Fitz, *Zabdiel Boylston*, 6.
87 Fitz, *Zabdiel Boylston*, 6–7.
88 John L. Blake *A General Biographical Dictionary, Comprising a Summary Account of the Most Distinguished Persons of All Ages, Nations, and Professions. Including More Than One Thousand Articles of American Biography,* 2nd ed. (New York: E. French & A.V. Blake, 1839).
89 Blake, *A General Biographical.*
90 Kittredge, "Introduction," 64.
91 Geertz, *Local Knowledge*, 4.
92 Geertz, *Local Knowledge*, 11.
93 Geertz, *Local Knowledge*, 35.
94 Geertz, *Local Knowledge*, 6.

95 Foucault, *Power/Knowledge,* 82.
96 Barbara Heifferon, *Look Who's Not Talking: Recovering the Voice of the Patient in the Clinique* (PhD Dissertation, University of Arizona, 1998).
97 Colman, *A Narrative,* 32.
98 Kelly Wisecup, "African Medicine, the Plain Style, and Satire in the 1721 Boston Inoculation Controversy" *Early American Literature,* 46, no. 1 (2011), 25–26; Michael Warner, *The Letters of the Republic: Publication and the Public Sphere in Eighteenth Century America* (Cambridge, MA: Harvard University Press, 1990), 279.
99 Warner, *The Letters of the Republic,* 279; Wisecup, "African Medicine," 26.
100 David D. Hall, *Cultures of Print* (Boston: University of Massachusetts Press, 1996); David S. Shields, *Civil Tongues and Polite Letters* (Chapel Hill, University of North Carolina Press, 2012).
101 Wisecup, "African Medicine," 26–27; Hall, *Cultures of Print,* 157.
102 Samuel Grainger, *The Imposition of Inoculation as a Duty Religiously Considered in a Leter (sic) to a Gentleman in the Country Inclined to Admit It* (Boston: Nicholas Boone and John Edwards, 1721), 3.
103 Grainger, *The Imposition of Inoculation,* 3.
104 Stewart, "The Edge," 55.
105 Berlin, *Many Thousands Gone,* 47.
106 Berlin, *Many Thousands Gone,* 47.
107 William D. Pierson, *Black Yankees: The Development of an Afro-American Sub-Culture in Eighteenth Century New England* (Amherst, MA: University of Massachusetts Press, 1988), 3–4.
108 Berlin, *Many Thousands Gone,* 48.
109 Berlin, *Many Thousands Gone,* 48.
110 Berlin, *Many Thousands Gone,* 48; Pierson, *Black Yankees,* 4–5.
111 Berlin, *Many Thousands Gone,* 59
112 Berlin, *Many Thousands Gone,* 60.
113 Douglass, *Inoculation Considered,* 3.
114 Douglass, *Inoculation Considered,* 3.
115 Douglass, *Inoculation Considered,* 3.
116 Douglass, *Inoculation Considered,* 3.
117 Pliny, *Natural History* (Medford, MA: Tufts Perseus Digital Library, 2018), Book 6, Ch. 35; Samuel Grainger, *The Imposition of Inoculation*, title page.
118 Grainger, *The Imposition of Inoculation,* 25.
119 Grainger, *The Imposition of Inoculation*, 25.
120 Cristobal Silva, *Miraculous Plagues* (Oxford, England: Oxford University Press, 2011), 1.
121 Kittredge, "Introduction," 25
122 Quoted in Kittredge, "Introduction," 25.
123 John (Mundungus) Williams. *Several Arguments, Proving, That Inoculating the Small Pox Is Not Contained in the Laws of Physick* (Boston, J. Franklin, 1721), 7.
124 Douglass, *Inoculation Considered,* 3.
125 Douglass, *Inoculation Considered,* 3.
126 Douglass, *Inoculation Considered,* 3.
127 Douglass, *Inoculation Considered,* 3.
128 Anonymous Contributor, "Letter," 2.
129 Anonymous Contributor, "Letter," 2.
130 One source suggested Francis Archibald is the author, but the letter was addressed to him and addressed him again in the closing as "Dear Francis," 8.
131 Anonymous Contributor, "Letter," 4.

132 Anonymous Contributor, "Letter," 8.
133 Isobel Grundy, *Lady Mary Wortley Montagu*, 1st ed. (Oxford, UK: Oxford University Press, 2001), 209.
134 Grundy, *Lady Mary*, 209.
135 Joseph Levine, *Doctor Woodward's Shield: History, Science, and Satire in Augustan England* (Berkeley and Los Angeles: University of California Press, 1977), 11; Genevieve Miller, *Adoption of Inoculation for England and France* (Oxford, PA: University of Pennsylvania Press, 1957), 36; Sir Hans Sloane, "An Account of Inoculation" *Royal Society's Philosophical Transactions* (1756), 516.
136 Grundy, *Lady Mary*, 210.
137 Grundy, *Lady Mary*, 210.
138 Charles Maitland, *Mr. Maitland's Account* (London, John Arbuthnot, 1722), 9–11.
139 Grundy, *Lady Mary*, 211.
140 Grundy, *Lady Mary*, 211.
141 Grundy, *Lady Mary*, 211.
142 Art Boylston, "The Newgate Guinea Pigs," in *London Historians* (London: London Historians, Ltd., 2012).
143 *London Mercury* (London: September 16, 1721).
144 Grundy, *Lady Mary*, 212.
145 *Post Man* (London: December 2, 1721) and *St. James's Evening Post* (London: December 7, 1721).
146 *Daily Post* (London: August 23, 1721).
147 Grundy, *Lady Mary*, 214.
148 Grundy, *Lady Mary*, 216.
149 William Wagstaffe, *Letter to Dr. Freind; Shewing the Danger and Uncertainty of Inoculating the Small Pox* (1722), accessed May 16, 2022, https://wellcomecollection.org/works/zjv2gx4k
150 Edward Huth, "Quantitative Evidence for Judgments on the Efficacy of Inoculation for the Prevention of Smallpox: England and New England in the 1700's" *The Journal of the Royal Society of Medicine,* 99, no. 5 (2006), 262–66.
151 Huth, "Quantitative Evidence," 262–66.
152 Grundy, *Lady Mary*, 217.
153 Grundy, *Lady Mary*, 217.
154 *Flying-Post* (London: September 13, 1722).
155 Grundy, *Lady Mary*, 217–18.
156 Claire Gherini, "Rationalizing Disease: James Kilpatrick Atlantic Struggles with Smallpox Inoculation," *Atlantic Studies,* 7, no. 4 (2010), 42.

Bibliography

Anonymous Contributor. "Letter." In *New-England Courant*, ed. James and Benjamin Franklin, no. 32 (Boston: March 5–12, 1722).

Berlin, Ira. *Many Thousands Gone: The First Two Centuries of Slavery in North America.* Cambridge, MA: The Belknap Press of Harvard University Press, 1998.

Blake, John L. *A General Biographical Dictionary, Comprising a Summary Account of the Most Distinguished Persons of All Ages, Nations, and Professions. Including More Than One Thousand Articles of American Biography*, 2nd ed. New York: E. French & A.V. Blake, 1839.

Boylston, Art. "The Newgate Guinea Pigs." In *London Historians*. London: London Historians, Ltd., 2012.

Boylston, Zabdiel. *An Historical Account of the Small-Pox Inoculated in New England*. S. Chandler at the Crosskeys in the *Poultry*. London: 1726.

Colden, Cadwallader. "Extract of Letter from Cadwallader Colden, Esq. to Dr. Fothergill, Concerning the Throat Distemper, 1753." In *The American Museum; or, Repository of Ancient and Modern Pieces, Prose and Poetical*, no. 3 (Philadelphia: Carey, 1788).

Colman, Benjamin. *A Narrative of the Method and Success of Inoculating the Small-pox in New England*. Dublin: George Grierson, 1722.

Colman, Benjamin. *Some Observation on the New Method of Receiving the Small-pox by Ingrafting or Inoculating*. Boston: Printed by B. Green for Samuel Gerrish, 1721.

Coss, Stephen. *The Fever of 1721*. New York: Simon and Schuster, 2016.

Daily Post. London: August 23, 1721.

Donnan, Elizabeth. *Documents Illustrative of the Slave Trade to America II*. Buffalo, NY: Wm. S. Hein & Co, 2002.

Douglass, William. *Inoculation of the Small Pox as Practised in Boston, Considered in a Letter to A[lexander] S[tuart], M. D. F. R. S., in Boston:* J. Franklin, 1722.

Fitz, Reginald Heber. *Zabdiel Boylston, Inoculator, and the Epidemic of Smallpox in Boston in 1721*. Boston: Harvard, 1911.

Flying-Post, London: September 13, 1722.

Foucault, Michel. *The History of Sexuality*, translated by Robert Hurley. New York: Random House, 1978.

Foucault, Michel. *Power/Knowledge*. New York: Pantheon, 1980.

Freire, Paolo. *Pedagogy of the Oppressed*. New York: Herder, 1971.

Geertz, Clifford. *Local Knowledge*. New York: Basic, 2000.

Gherini, Claire. "Rationalizing Disease: James Kilpatrick Atlantic Struggles with Smallpox Inoculation." *Atlantic Studies*, 7, no. 4 (2010) 42.

Grainger, Samuel. *The Imposition of Inoculation as a Duty Religiously Considered in a Leter (sic) to a Gentleman in the Country Inclined to Admit It*. Boston: Nicholas Boone and John Edwards, 1721.

Greene, Lorenzo Johnston. *The Negro in Colonial New England*. New York: Atheneum, 1968.

Grundy, Isobel. *Lady Mary Wortley Montagu*, 1st ed. Oxford: Oxford University Press, 2001.

Hall, David D. *Cultures of Print*. Boston: University of Massachusetts Press, 1996.

Heifferon, Barbara. *Look Who's Not Talking: Recovering the Voice of the Patient in the Clinique*. PhD. Dissertation, University of Arizona, 1998.

Herbert, Eugenia. "Smallpox Inoculation in Africa." *The Journal of African History*, 16, no. 4 (1975).

Huth, Edward. "Quantitative Evidence for Judgments on the Efficacy of Inoculation for the Prevention of Smallpox: England and New England in the 1700's." *The Journal of the Royal Society of Medicine*, 99, no. 5 (2006).

Jordan, Winthrop G. *White Over Black: American Attitudes Toward the Negro, 1550–1812*. New York: Norton, 1977.

Kittredge, George Lyman. "Introduction" to *Several Reasons Proving That Inoculating or Transplanting the Small Pox, Is a Lawful Practice, and That It Has Been Blessed by God for the Saving of Many a Life.* By Increase Mather. *Sentiments on the Small Pox Inoculated.* By Cotton Mather in Boston, 1721. Cleveland, OH: 1921.

Koo, Kathryn. S. *Strangers in the House of God: Cotton Mather, Onesimus, and an Experiment in Christian Slaveholding.* Worcester, MA: American Antiquarian Society, 2007.

Latour, Bruno, and Steve Woolgar, *Laboratory Life: The Construction of Scientific Facts.* Princeton, NJ: Princeton University Press, 1986.

Levine, Joseph. *Doctor Woodward's Shield: History, Science, and Satire in Augustan England.* Berkeley and Los Angeles: University of California Press, 1977.

London Mercury. London: September 16, 1721.

Maitland, Charles. *Mr. Maitland's Account.* London: John Arbuthnot, 1722.

Mather, Cotton. *Angel of Bethesda.* Barre, MA: American Antiquarian Society, 1972.

Mather, Cotton. Cotton Mather Files: Box 5, Folder 1, "Contract for Onesimus." American Antiquarian Society. Worchester, MA.

Mather, Cotton. *Diary of Cotton Mather.* New York: Ungar, 1957.

Mather, Cotton. *Diary for 1712*, edited by William Manierre, Jr. Charlottesville, VA: University of Virginia Press, 1964.

Mather, Cotton. *Rules for the Society of Negroes, 1693.* Boston: B. Harris, 1693.

Mather, Cotton. *Sentiments on the Smallpox Inoculated.* Boston, 1721. Reprinted for private distribution, Cleveland, 1921.

Mather, Cotton. *Some Account of What Is Said in Inoculating or Transplanting the Smallpox, By the Learned Dr. Emanuel Timonius, and Jacobus Pylarinus. With some remarks Thereon: To Which Are Added, a Few Quaeries in Answer to the Scruples of Many about the Lawfulness of this Method.* Published by Dr. Zabdiel Boylston. Boston: Sold by S. Gerrish at his shop in Corn-Hill, 1721.

Melish, Joanne Pope. *Disowning Slavery: Gradual Emancipation and 'Race' in New England, 1780–1860.* Ithaca, NY: Cornell University Press, 1998.

Miller, Genevieve. *Adoption of Inoculation for England and France.* Oxford, PA: University of Pennsylvania Press, 1957.

Miller, Genevieve. "Smallpox Inoculation in England and in America: A Reappraisal." *The William and Mary Quarterly*, Series 3, 13, no. 4 (October 1956).

Minardi, Margot. "The Boston Inoculation Controversy of 1721–1722." *William and Mary Quarterly*, 61, no. 1 (2004).

Monaghan, Jennifer E. "Reading for the Enslaved, Writing for the Free." In *Learning to Read and Write in Early America.* Amherst, MA: University of Massachusetts Press, 2005.

Neal, Daniel. "An Historical Introduction," to Benjamin Colman's *A Narrative of the Method and Success of Inoculating the Small-Pox in New England.* London: George Grierson, 1722.

Okie, Laird. "Daniel Neal and the 'Puritan Revolution'." *Church History: Studies in Christianity and Culture*, 55 (1986).

Phipps, James and Phipps' Court Assistants, Public Records Office T/70/53/169 (March 1721), quoted in Stewart, "The Edge of Utility:" Slaves and Smallpox in the Early Eighteenth Century." *Medical History*, 29 (1985).

Phipps, James and Phipps' Court Assistants. Public Records Office (June 1722), quoted in Stewart, "The Edge of Utility:" Slaves and Smallpox in the Early Eighteenth Century." *Medical History*, 29 (1985).

Pierson, William D. *Black Yankees: The Development of an Afro-American Sub-Culture in Eighteenth Century New England*. Amherst, MA: University of Massachusetts Press, 1988.

Pliny, *Natural History*. Medford, MA: Tufts Perseus Digital Library, 2018, Book 6, Ch. 35.

Post Man. London: December 2, 1721.

Schiebinger, Londa. *Nature's Body: Gender in the Making of the Modern Body*. Boston: Beacon Press, 1993.

Shields, David S. *Civil Tongues and Polite Letters*. Chapel Hill: University of North Carolina Press, 2012.

Silva, Cristobal. *Miraculous Plagues*. Oxford: Oxford University Press, 2011.

Sloane, Sir Hans. *Philosophical Transactions of the Royal Society of London*, no. 49, Royal Society Publisher,London, 1755.

St. James's Evening Post. London: December 7, 1721.

Stewart, Larry. "The Edge of Utility: Slaves and Smallpox in the Early Eighteenth Century." *Medical History*, 29 (1985).

Stoler, Ann Laura. "A Colonial Reader of Foucault: Bourgeois Bodies and Racial Selves." In *Foucault and Beyond*, edited by Vernon W. Cisney and Nicolae Morar. Chicago: University of Chicago Press, 2016.

Tindol, Robert. "Getting the Pox Out of All Their Houses: Cotton Mather and the Rhetoric of Puritan Science." *Early American Literature*, 46, no. 1 (March 2011).

Wagstaffe, William. *Letter to Dr. Freind; Shewing the Danger and Uncertainty of Inoculating the Small Pox*, 1722. Accessed May 16, 2022. https://wellcomecollection.org/works/zjv2gx4k.

Warner, Michael. *The Letters of the Republic: Publication and the Public Sphere in Eighteenth Century America*. Cambridge, MA: Harvard University Press, 1990.

Williams, John (Mundungus). *Several Arguments, Proving, That Inoculating the Small Pox Is Not Contained in the Laws of Physick*. Boston: J. Franklin, 1721.

Wisecup, Kelly. "African Medicine, the Plain Style, and Satire in the 1721 Boston Inoculation Controversy." *Early American Literature*, 46, no. 1 (2011).

Wisecup, Kelly. *Medical Encounters*. Amherst, MA: University of Massachusetts Press, 2013.

6 Then and Now

Although the inoculation project carried out by Mather and Boylston was not accepted by the populace (other than by many ministers, the successfully inoculated who had remained free from smallpox, and their group of adherents), it had an impact on medicine not only in America but also in England. The Royal Society and others in England followed the Boston implementation of the smallpox procedure eagerly. "With the involvement of Sir Hans Sloane, president of the Royal College of Physicians and vice president of the Royal Society, a 'certain exalted figure,' [most likely Princess Caroline of Wales], and James Jurin had persuaded Zabdiel Boylston ... to come to London, where he published a book giving the details of his experience of inoculation."[1] In England, Jurin had published numerous books on successful inoculations in Great Britain in 1723, 1724, 1725 and 1726. In July 1726, the Massachusetts surgeon, Boylston, published *An Historical Account of the Small-Pox Inoculated in New-England* and presented it to the Royal Society and its President, Sir Isaac Newton. Jurin's correspondence had letters and other testimonials reporting that British surgeons, apothecaries, and lay women were practicing inoculations in that time period.[2] These correspondents together with Boylston's carefully documented variolations created a fairly thorough picture of smallpox inoculatory practices during those times, for England and the Boston area in 1721–1722.

This variolation project carried out by Mather heralded the birth of what Foucault called "the medicine of social spaces," an earlier precursor to his formulation of what he called biopower.[3] European and Colonial American practices, as James B. Blake had argued convincingly, created a social space for public health as a result of the smallpox inoculation controversy and also created an exigence for an intriguing rhetorical situation.[4] This was the medicine that came into being "wherever a government body or the *polis* begins to take charge of the health and welfare of its constituents."[5] Although the smallpox vaccination had been resisted by most in the American colony at the time, it was these technologies and discipline that came together for both individuals and the body politic that heralded this advance of biopower. This was one of a number of early forays that laid the

DOI: 10.4324/9781003312369-7

foundation for our present paradigms, including what we refer to as public health today.[6] Both the political/governmental body of the Selectmen and the physicians of Boston gained power over the former parsons who had functioned as those in control of patients' bodies and the body politic. The variolation project marked the beginning of a future framework that would result in today's Western biomedicine. Biopower for Foucault, however, reached far beyond and into many other areas in the early formation.

This early inoculation project, although also tried in England, was in Boston "distinctly American: a marriage of a narrative by [enslaved people] and a nascent understanding of disease pathogens that had the potential to revolutionize American medicine when the political revolution was still over fifty years away."[7] But in early America, out of a desire to protect, as well as to garner power, the first laws were issued to regulate medical practice. In Europe, before the 18th century, bodies were controlled by monarchs for military and economic purposes. In the 18th century, a further function had been added: "the disposition of society as a milieu of physical well-being, health, and optimum longevity."[8] However, before emigration, the Puritans had already been involved in a type of social welfare as a close-knit religious group under long periods of attack in Europe. Much care of the body had been under the province of the ministers and the church. Now control over and jurisdiction regarding the body by the church had been dramatically challenged and shifted in 1720s Boston.

> According to Foucault, biopower traces its roots back to pastoral power – the power of a minister over his flock – under medieval Christianity. As he puts it, pastoral power 'gave rise to an art of conducting, directing, leading, guiding, taking in hand, and manipulating men, an art of monitoring them and urging them on step by step, an art with the function of taking charge of men collectively and individually throughout their life and every moment of their existence.'[9] 'The pastorate does not disappear with the rise of modern power forms, as he emphasizes more than once.'[10] Indeed, he makes a much stronger claim: 'I think this is where we should look for the origin, the point of formation, of crystallization, the embryonic point of the governmentality whose entry into politics … . marks the threshold of the modern state.'[11]

The discontinuation of the inoculation project was also the beginning of an attempt to regulate the practice of medicine. The attempt might appear strange to us today, given that actual medical practice of those who identified as physicians or doctors did not exist until 1760 in New York. As John B. Beck suggested about the times: "[M]any ignorant and unskillful Persons in Physick and Surgery, in order to gain a subsistence, do take upon themselves to administer Physick, and practice Surgery … endangering of the Lives and Limbs of their Patients … ."[12] The doctors and the Selectmen of Boston took on the social role of regulating smallpox inoculation, asking the ministers and the main doctor participating in the practice to make an account of themselves and then passing legislation putting a stop to the process of inoculation, although it was continued by Boylston for a time. "Among the many unusual features of the heated controversy caused by the introduction of the smallpox inoculation in 1721 was the fact that the Selectmen called on the doctors for their professional opinion," an important development.[13] At this time, the *ethos* of the Selectmen and other physicians seemed to outweigh the gravitas of Boylston and the ministers, especially the Mathers, as seen in the many texts. In addition, there was the surprising trade of discursive styles and genres of arguments, as the doctors and other Anti-Inoculators had often offered religious claims and evidence for their views, and the ministers and other supporters of inoculation had offered more precedents of the procedure and/or scientific ones.

Early Beginnings of New Paradigms

The view through the microscope that for Cotton Mather opened the inside of a pustule of smallpox in the early 1700s was not yet accepted as a valid recognition of a disease organism by most of his community. Germ theory had been discussed by a number of writers, but was still an amorphous collection of impressions and confusions. History shows that advances in medical science can lead roller-coaster existences for decades before they take hold. And in contemporary debates, such as the one addressing vaccinations in this country today, we can see this pattern of resistance and of ebb and flow yet again. One could maintain that such processes are typical of the fertility of ideas during a rupture such as one caused by an epidemic or pandemic. These controversies could reflect cultural fears and quandaries in spite of improved health practices in general. "[O]ne is dealing with mobile and transitory points of resistance, producing cleavages in a society that shift about, fracturing unities and effecting regroupings, furrowing across individuals themselves, cutting them up and remolding them, marking off irreducible regions in them, in their bodies and minds."[14]

Mather was using new instruments and looking in new places. The textual arguments in the debate had been constructed through discursive practices and cultural concepts within the colonial space. The framing of those arguments was key to their acceptance or rejection by the general populace and the medical practitioners. There were a number of reasons for the overall rejection of the project, but it would be simplistic to consider only the failure and not consider certain cultural changes driven forward as a result of the rhetorical exchanges. Mather's compendium and the actual inoculation project reveal the struggle between older humoral medicine and newer theories of medicine as a science, which created a rich and contradictory mixture of epistemes. However, the old paradigm was widely reflected within public discourse in the 1700s, and the colony was not yet ready for a new "science" of medicine. Yet the inoculation project allowed a brief glimpse of the cultural concepts that reigned side-by-side with visions of a future science of medicine.

Mather's, the Inoculators' and even some of the Anti-Inoculators' exposure to the latest developments from The Royal Society coupled with C. Mather's and other Puritans' interest in science began to interrupt the old medical paradigm of Colonial America, as well as the roles and power of both ministers and physicians. Because of Mather's avid interest in and zealous pursuit of so many topics, he was able at times to see beyond the lens of humoral medicine to the beginnings of modern disease theory, although that old lens and miasma theory, too, would continue to weave in and out for numerous decades to follow.[15] Although Mather's compendium, *The Angel of Bethesda,* was not "modern" in any sense of the word, it embodied tangible evidence of the epistemic development of the new science, especially in the chapters on smallpox vaccination and his conjectures about a new theory of the cause of disease. In the theory chapter, he quoted from some of the many earlier authors of a fledging germ theory he followed as he peered into his microscope. Cotton described what he saw and reflected on all his reading, having searched for a way to end the suffering of and perhaps in hopes of reclaiming some more respect from the Bostonians. In addition, it meant that rather than just judging the health or illness of a patient by what came out of the patient's body as in humoral medicine, the Inoculators were putting something *into* the body to immunize it against a worse case of a disease, beginning to institute a new paradigm in the practice of medicine.

1720s Debate: Religion, Legality, and the Firebombing

A brief review of the contributing factors and frames of the debate showed that even though ostensibly a failure in terms of the number of inoculations, the texts revealed not only an important medical development, but perhaps more importantly also provided a window into a rhetorical and epistemic process in American culture. There were many issues in the debate: religious, legal, common sense, racial, class-based, anti-intellectual, political, disciplinary, historical (a hysterical witchcraft debacle), technical, epistemic, paradigmatic, and shifts in power relations; these point to a complicated process of change in the field of medicine. The debate, including cultural factors, had also ignited the violent acts of firebombing Cotton Mather's home and also had threatened Boylston's life.

Chapter 1 examined how a life-saving technique in the midst of a smallpox epidemic could be rejected and had created a context for this important debate by providing a brief history of the disease of smallpox and the inoculation itself; describing the already developed quarantine system; focusing on the religious beliefs germane to the controversy; explaining the common sense trope; outlining colonial medicine and science in the 1720s; showing Mather's sources; and characterizing the two main antagonists:

a minister and a physician. This work analyzed the exigence of the epidemic and the multiplicity of factors fueling certain responses of the doctors and the public against inoculation. While the final birth of a new institution had certainly not yet happened, the slow-and-stop-and-start process of labor involved in changing and building a discipline and shifting the power away from one cultural group, a Puritan theocracy, to a fledgling profession and civic/governmental body had indeed begun. While these discursive practices reflect a multiplicity of minor processes, did they eventually lead to a "new micro-physics of power"?[16] Yes, eventually; these signs in the early 1720s signaled the start of labor and the first contractions in the birth of modern medicine in America.

Who "owns" the body now? How much agency does a patient have? Have both the social and the physical body been subjugated in the process of "medical" treatment in hospitals? To some extent the body has almost always been subjugated, although in very different ways, whether in earliest human times in small social groups or in later times under a religious institution, such as that found among the Puritans. Under current Western health and medicine, the body remains subjugated not only to the hospitals, but also to doctors' practices, government programs, large pharmaceutical corporations, public health agencies, and insurance companies. In some U.S. communities, the body continues to be also subjugated by violence and poverty. Such conditions are also still found among the impoverished in many poorer and other "first-world" countries.

Under Boston's theocracy, the long, tedious sermons of the Mathers and their colleagues, as well as the religious claims in various tracts by the Anti-Inoculators showed the attention that had been paid to minute details that carefully trained and molded the minds of colonists, particularly the leading literati, whose training through religious teachings in daily Biblical readings in churches and in homes had become the norm. In each tract of the Anti-Inoculators and in some of the rebuttals of the Inoculators, the overall impression was one of rigorous subjugation of the whole person — mind and body.

Thus, in Chapter 2 those religious and legal or religio/legal discursive practices that framed the debate were analyzed. One could speculate that part of the emphasis on the legal, in addition to the "laws" of the church and the "law of physick," which were examined and which both Inoculators and Anti-inoculators used as frames for much of the debate, could have continued to have been contextualized within the European experience of the ancestors of the colonists and the founders of the various American colonies. The Puritans valued their freedom and also valued a certain structure or set of rules. The various texts examined throughout attest to both contradictory emphases.

Colonists continued to struggle with the paradox of colonial rule under an English monarch, while asserting their own local control via the Selectmen and the General Assembly. In addition, the power of the monarch was itself not some impenetrable monolith. While there are many reasons not to liken the Puritan theocracy to a monarchy, Foucault's understanding that to function successfully as a society, various social classes tolerated a certain non-observance of rules and had acknowledged that this pattern may not have been limited to only the powerful *Ancien Regime* that he had studied.[17] The original Puritan theocracy constituted an *Ancien Regime* in colonial New England that first subjugated individual bodies and the body politic through fear of a terrible and wrath-filled deity.

In any complicated social situation, certain practices that contradict teachings and doctrines can find their way to become regularized, at least for a time, in direct opposition to societal tenets. For example, in the Puritan community, strict adherence to the "Ten Commandments" was contravened in the witchcraft persecutions and executions. The religio/legal debate of the 1720s could be said to carry a resistance having grown out of the experience of the earlier settlers in the Boston colony, who continued to want to erect a different sense of the "law" from that experienced by their forefathers in England.

The debate of the smallpox inoculation, then, happened within this wider historical frame of legality, illegality, and spaces for freedom, both real and imagined, within colonial Boston.

Even if in the past "illegality" had meant being persecuted for their religion in other countries prior to the American experience, their religious doctrine included a strict adherence to the *law* of *their* deity. Such paradoxes within lived experience could have also created spaces in which a people could take advantage of a lack of consistency to accommodate both the ideas of freedom and a desire at the same time for clear, enforceable laws that adherents could use as a measure for their lives.

This paradox can also help to explain, perhaps, why a debate that frequently centered on *law,* could then break down to produce at least one documentable, "lawless" act, that of the firebombing. That question about why Cotton Mather's house was firebombed was what had begun this investigation. Why did the citizens of Boston firebomb the home of the initiator of inoculation? That same opening of spaces created an interesting merger of legality and illegality and, finally, criminality. The same space that opened in response to the "illegality" of an English monarch ruling their lands, along with what appeared as often cruel punishment of sending diseases by their Deity, had made "room" for the convergence of illegality and criminality, whether major or petty crime. Certainly since the intent was to burn down the house of a sleeping family, even though the firebombing had been unsuccessful, numerous people could have been injured or murdered. One doesn't have to work too hard today to imagine colonial America, regardless of its insistence on legality, as a place where violent protest and lawlessness were inevitable, even as recently as January 6, 2021 at the U.S. Capitol. Who could have ever imagined that one of the key ministers, Cotton Mather, who had carried on the ancestral line of the key Puritan founders of Boston, one of the main members of the theocracy, would have suffered such an attack on him and his family? Who could have ever imagined that a U.S. President and several U.S. House of Representatives members would have organized and supported an attack on the U.S. Capitol and attempted to interfere in the peaceful transfer of power?

Perhaps the angry pamphlets, letters, and the newspaper that championed the Anti-Inoculators' cause during the inoculations, their social media and misinformation, had incited a fire bombing. Perhaps the anger and frustration in the 1720s were also part of a struggle to loosen the theocracy's hold, which had already sustained a number of attacks, as seen in Chapter 2. In addition, were they also part and parcel of a new struggle: one resulting from the dynamic changes of new paradigms, power relations, and epistemes? What was the popular response to the violent acts? Would Mather, the Inoculators and the project itself have received sympathy and some sense of reprieve in the face of such "criminality" or would the perpetrator(s) have been seen as a hero or heroes? Would the "criminal" have benefited from a spontaneous wave of sympathy? Although the historic records do not account for the responses in any great detail, other than briefly in Mather's own text, history does show that the inoculations remained "discontinued" by order of the Selectmen on July 21, 1721, even if in actuality they continued through May of 1722. Three years later in 1724 in Mather's compendium, there's no record of the perpetrator of the firebombings having been apprehended or punished. Within four years of finishing *Angel of Bethesda,* Cotton Mather died of natural causes.

Witches and Who Controls the Body?

The historical influence of the witchcraft debacle, both because of Mather's role and the later revulsion of the perpetrators and supporters, was an important factor to consider in Chapter 3. His personal history alone presented a problem with his *ethos* and credibility for many in his audience. In addition, certain rhetorical features, particularly the "invisibility trope," his having used the word *invisible* to describe what his microscope revealed in a pox, mapped onto his descriptions years earlier of witchcraft. This term had been used as further evidence of Mather's wrongheadedness in the popular view. Particularly noteworthy was that the policing of the society during the witchcraft debacle had also created issues of power over the body, both individual and social. Large portions of the testimonies and texts from those times, some of which were highlighted in that chapter, showed that the belief was that it was the power of the Devil that caused individual colonists to harm others and act in anti-social and egregious ways. The belief had been that the bodies of the victims were under the control of the witches, guided by the Devil himself, so the leaders of the colony used their judicial system to imprison the bodies of the witches, to test their bodies through torture, drownings, etc., and to force confessions. These violent actions were committed to gain back adherence to religious dogma so that the religious community could gain back power over both the social and individual colonial bodies. God through the ministers had controlled the bodies; if possessed, then the Devil through the witches had controlled the bodies.

In Salem at the time, it was as if the witches had also carried some contagious disease, one that affected children at first and later many others. The fear of one's body being taken over by some invisible force is much like the fear of one's body being taken over by an unseen disease organism. Both were unseen at first, unexpected, mysterious, not easy to forecast until a victim of the disease presented visible symptoms. Those "infected" or cursed by witches and pox infected others. As the witches were confined, so, too, would the patients be confined or quarantined. With the spread of contagion, people must be watched, must be supervised, and, with the microscope, as with the outline of future hospital space, these fears of contagion and the discoveries of technology would make it possible to observe and control in order to protect. In addition, both the individual and social body were subjugated. Interestingly, both the witchcraft debacle and the inoculation project, to a smaller degree, resulted in violent acts being taken against individuals. Although threats and a failed attempt at a bombing had been less lethal than the hangings, drownings, etc., the impulse had been to resist with physical violence and not just rhetoric.

Disciplining Bodies and Spaces

Imprisoning "witches" was not the only way disciplinary spaces were part of this inoculation debate. Both the debate and the analysis of it moved from the prison and the confinement of witches to the college, Harvard, presided over for some years by Puritan ministers. The seminary of Harvard disciplined the minds of those who were destined to be ministers in and around Boston and other colonial sites. The analysis of the debate in the 1720s illustrated both anti intellectualism on the part of Bostonians toward the college itself as well as great skepticism toward the medical roles of its early graduates: Puritan ministers. Numerous texts pointed to the desire on the part of the Anti-Inoculators for the religious leaders to stay in their pulpits and leave medical treatment in the hands of physicians, especially as stated directly in the *Academicus Dialogues*.

Changes in medical language, taxonomies, and technologies to explore the human body and nature in general had already begun to move into higher education.[18] A new way of seeing the body and a more organized and exclusive group of practitioners/observers would begin to reorganize medical language, medical practice, and science. That would change the mission and students and engender the need to reorganize the schools. Especially, as power over the human body moved from ministerial hands to those of educated doctors, new disciplinary norms would be born. Douglass was espousing the value of his own education in European universities and how that validated him, not the Mathers, to determine medical practice in the midst of a smallpox epidemic. Soon others would begin to insist on the value of doctors' knowledge of medicine over that of ministers. In addition, and importantly, the doctors were consulted by the Selectmen, who made the decision to outlaw the use of inoculation, thus government was now involved in healthcare, medicinal practices, and prevention. Care of the body and patient would no longer rest with various practitioners who were not necessarily professionals, nor would it rest with the ministers. Instead it had begun to have new actors and institutions involved in the field of healthcare and medicine even in those times.

Such incursions as the smallpox inoculation project, even though ostensibly rejected, made room for eventual changes in education, the medical profession, the roles of government and religion, science itself, and attendant technologies. "The eighteenth century ... has joined other powers – the Law, the Word (Parole) and the Text, Tradition – imposing new delimitations upon them."[19] Foucault saw surveillance, nominalization, and normalization side-by-side, as part of the same process: biopower enabled organization or reorganization of knowledge while the new norms reinforced it.

In Chapter 4, schools competed through their alumni: Mathers (Harvard) and Douglass (Utrecht, Leyden, etc.). Both medicine and education have norms. Under the older medical system, when the doctor or minister visited the patient's home, the ill person was observed as to outward symptoms, and the body products were also carefully inspected. Old urine charts from the time, one of which is shown in Chapter 1, Figure 1.2, for example, can have numerous different examples, varying in their color, consistency, and clarity, each indicating some problem with the balance of the humors. These inspections, however, because the doctor was not "in house" all the time, were not performed very regularly. Even in early hospitals, which were more like quarantine sites, poorhouses, or almshouses, doctors were rarely present. These poorhouses were also often under religious control in the various parts of Europe. In the Boston area, the hospital on Spectacle Island housed those quarantined from ships seeking entrance to the harbor. When it came to private patients, doctors treated the wealthy in their homes. Those who could pay for attention received much more observation.

When more hospitals were developed to treat diseases, the change "had two consequences: in the internal hierarchy, the physician ... begins to gain power over the religious staff and to relegate them to a clearly specified, but subordinate role in the technique of the examination; ... while the hospital itself, ... was to become a place of training ... ."[20] While Foucault did not write about medicine in the American colonies, we see a similar process. Douglass, who had been trained abroad, did not recognize the role of the religious as important as it was in the colonies at the time. In England and some other European countries, the reigning religious paradigm was literally determined by the religion of whichever monarch was on the throne, often a result of religious and other wars. And yet, the Scottish physician had recognized the religious domination of healthcare in Boston, and, as a college-educated practitioner of medicine, he had resented it.

Certain disciplinary practices of writing itself had been making a new paradigm possible. The detailed writing, the exegeses used in religious study and in higher education at the time, and the habits of mind and of practice provided certain foundational possibilities. In both Mather's compendium and Boylston's text, in which all his patients who received the inoculation were carefully observed, tracked, and recorded, the beginnings of new medicine could be found. Especially under the pressure of the debate, the doubts, the threats, and even under the auspices of rejection, these detailed reports of the inoculated so widely rejected in America would find acceptance among the British shortly thereafter. Such record keeping would eventually be of "*decisive importance* in the epistemological 'thaw' of the sciences of the individual" (emphasis added).[21]

In order to move toward scientific medicine, subjects of earlier medicine would need to become objects. Bodies would become not only docile but also "legible" in new ways unable to be read by their owners. A patient can have an x-ray, a blood test, or some other procedure that can only be read by a health professional. Just going through the process does not reveal to the patient herself what is discovered. The results must first be interpreted and then either spoken or written about for the patient to gain the knowledge. Many innovations in medical writing were organized around the accumulation of documents, and their seriation in tandem with other fields of classifications, categorizations, and standardization helped relocate power. In this 1720s inoculation effort, in which the public health was at stake during an epidemic, the old parish registers of births, marriages, and deaths and the old plague bills would eventually give way to individual records of diseases, treatments, and results. The rejected smallpox project, the lone physician in tandem with the minister had helped initiate change rejected by the majority of physicians in the 1720s colonial setting, rather than the physicians initiating such an important change in medicine.

The eventual sea change did not happen quickly. In 1800, the hospital was still not central to American healthcare. Especially those in the upper classes would not have darkened the door of a hospital, unless an accident or epidemic had landed them there.[22] Such individuals would still have been treated in their private homes. Charles E. Rosenberg insisted that the development of the hospital had been a result of technological inventions, social perceptions, economic relationships, and the rise of professions.[23] Just as writing was central in the social or political texts to understand the reasons for the "failure" of the inoculation project, medical writing would move into an even more central role in both institutions of learning and healing. These changes would further organize power, because the medical documents were no longer legible for a layperson.

The Subjugated Body of the Other

In Chapter 5, another reason for the failure of the inoculation project had been that certain types of knowledge were disallowed. The knowledge of enslaved Africans was discounted by most Bostonians; they were painted as the Other, because they were not regarded as citizens or even individuals. Knowledge by outsiders, such as Middle-Eastern Turks and even Greek practitioners of inoculation or "Mahometans," who had enabled an introduction of the procedure from Turkey to England, had also been discounted. At the same time Boylston was studying and recording each individual case, the "individuality" of those designated as "Others" was being disregarded by the Anti-Inoculators. Thus, enslaved persons had been seen as part of a disenfranchised group that included non-colonists and non-Westerners who had also had their knowledge ignored. In the first part of the 18th century, their knowledge had no status, no *ethos*, and no credibility. In the latter part of the 18th century and early 19th century, even as new procedures saved lives that would have been lost earlier, individual patients would largely lose power over their own bodies and disenfranchised groups often continued to remain outside of adequate medical treatment and/or outside of medical schools and higher education.

However, such a totalizing taxonomy was also prone to changes. Perhaps instead it should be argued that while the objectification of such privileged, microscopic views and the other disciplinarity practices that had very early beginnings in this period were indeed part of what would eventually be achieved, other power relations would also be changed to some degree. For example, under a regime in which the members of some groups automatically had their knowledge discounted *because of their group membership,* now all individuals would be sorted in other ways as well: according to disease, organ, physiological system, blood type, etc. These new boundaries would somewhat ignore but, in some arenas, still privilege the non-enslaved, the Westerner or American colonist, the male. The privileging would become different only to some extent, though; it did not mean that eventually each person would have ultimate equality within this society. In either case, our culture and its texts, its institutions, and its frames and all discursive practices that create reality and power would be changed in some way. Power over the body now has shifted from the ministers to the doctors, even as a few decades after the smallpox inoculation project, the governmental authority would change from the British crown to American colonial settlers and founders of a new nation-state. There had been a power shift toward a new discipline and profession that had begun to take root and grow in a complicated web of influences. Rather than analyze a complicated controversy as having one impetus, instead a series of rhetorical and cultural analyzes revealed the many possible reasons for cultural ruptures and resistance. As post-modernists, we realize cultural "truths" are always, already mobile and in flux, changeable, and malleable. They are colored by discourse, culture, times, technology, history, individuals' histories, and habits. Such "truths" and disciplines, however, are not easily changed as seen in the struggles to change medicine and power in Boston in the 1720s. While they might not easily lend themselves to change, such shifts had been and would eventually be possible.

Last View of the 1720s

Smallpox inoculations failed to move forward in most American colonies after the event of 1721–1722 because of the various reasons highlighted earlier. Religious beliefs were of importance because of the Calvinistic belief in predestination. In many of the tracts of the time and in the newspaper editorials, religious reasons against inoculation played key roles. In addition, Mather's reputation had clearly suffered after the revulsion experienced by Bostonians and Salemites following the witchcraft debacle. The professionalization of medicine had begun to surface. The Scottish physician, William Douglass, was clearly a leader among the Anti-Inoculators, and he found the project backed by ministers to be a clear violation or trespass of his territory. Class and status along with a strong anti-intellectual bent, particularly against the Mathers and their education at Harvard, could be read in some of the claims advanced by the Anti-Inoculators. Fear and the othering of certain types of knowledge sources also played key roles in this dramatic situation. Of interest was the strange reversal during the debate following the introduction of the inoculation project: minsters argued from empirical, testimonial, and scientific foundations for the inoculation, while the physicians and other Anti-Inoculators argued primarily using religious proofs. Various tropes were influential, whether it was common sense or *invisibility* weaving itself through rounds of the debate. Inoculation against smallpox in America was not widely accepted and remained controversial, although some had continued the intervention. In Charleston in 1738, a physician and naval surgeon inoculated 800 people, only eight of whom had died. Yet the South Carolina Assembly banned the practice and threatened to fine the inoculators and the patients 500 pounds each. The fear had been that the inoculation would spread the disease faster. New York prohibited inoculation in 1747. In 1774, inoculation had become "a political wedge issue" in the midst of another smallpox epidemic throughout the colonies on the eve of the Revolutionary War. The War itself took 25,000 American lives, while 130,000 Americans died of smallpox, over five times the amount of the military battles.[24]

One record from the time, although data was seldom recorded, shows the losses in the "New World" as the following (Table 6.1):

Table 6.1 Documented Smallpox of New World, Public Domain

1520–1527	Mexico, Central & South America	Smallpox kills millions of native inhabitants of Mexico. Unintentionally introduced at Veracruz with the arrival of Panfilo de Narvaez on April 23, 1520 and was credited with the victory of Cortes over the Aztec empire at Tenochtitlan (present-day Mexico City) in 1521. Kills the Inca ruler, Huayna Capac, 200,000 others, and weakens the Incan Empire.
1561–1562	Chile	No precise numbers on deaths exist in contemporary records but it is estimated that natives lost 20 to 25 percent of their population. According to Alonso de Góngora Marmolejo, so many Indian laborers died that the Spanish gold mines had to shut down.
1588–1591	Central Chile	A combined smallpox, measles and typhus plague strikes Central Chile contributing to a decline of indigenous populations.
1617–1619	N. American N.E. Coast	Smallpox killed 90% of the Massachusetts Bay Indians.
1655	Chillan, Central Chile	An outbreak of smallpox occurred among refugees from Chillán as the city was evacuated amidst the Mapuche uprising of 1655. Spanish authorities put this group in effective quarantine decreeing death sentences for anyone crossing Maule River north.
1674	Cherokees	Death count unknown. Population in 1674 about 50,000. After 1729, 1738, and 1753 smallpox epidemics their population was only 25,000 when they were forced to Oklahoma on the Trail Of Tears.
1692	Boston, MA	Unknown number of deaths.
1697	Boston, MA	1000 deaths out of 6000–7000 inhabitants.[25]
1702–1703	Boston, MA	300 died of smallpox. Unknown number in New York.
1721–1722	Boston, MA	Over 800 died out of 5000–6000 cases of 10,000-11,000 population.
1736	Pennsylvania	Several hundred died of smallpox.
1738	S. Carolina	300 died of smallpox out of 2000 cases of 5000 population in Charleston. One half of Cherokees died.[26]

(*Continued*)

Table 6.1 (Continued)

1770s	N.W. Coast of N. America	At least 30% (tens of thousands) of the Northwestern Native Americans die from smallpox.
1781–1783	Great Lakes	Number of deaths unknown.
1830s	Alaska	Reduced Dena'ina Athabaskan population in Cook Inlet region of southcentral Alaska by half. Smallpox also devastated Yup'ik Eskimo populations in western Alaska.
1836–1840	Great Plains	1837 Great Plains smallpox epidemic
1860–1861	Boston and Pennsylvania	Smallpox epidemics
1862	British Columbia, Washington state, & Russian America	Known as the Great Smallpox of 1862, an outbreak of smallpox in a large encampment of all indigenous peoples from around the colony on June 10, 1862, dispersed by order of the government to return to their homes, resulted in the deaths of 50–90% of the indigenous peoples in the region.
1869	Araucania, S. Chile	A smallpox epidemic breaks out among native Mapuches, just some months after a destructive Chilean military campaign in Araucanía.
1880	Tacna, Peru	Tacna hosted the combined armies of Peru and Bolivia before being defeated by Chile in the Battle of Tacna. Before it fell to Chileans in late May 1880 infectious diseases were widespread in the city with 461 deaths of smallpox in the 1879–1880 period, making up 11.3% of all registered deaths for the city in the same period.
1902	Boston, MA	Of the 1,596 cases reported in this epidemic, 270 died.

Brief Analytical Summary

This textual/rhetorical and cultural analysis has unpacked the complicated resistance toward very early medical science in its unique expression in an American colony. Perhaps by understanding how such early mechanisms work, how paradigms shift, and how power reorganizes itself, citizens can understand how bodies in such regimes experience subjugation and decide both as individuals and groups what type of power Americans want the culture to have over their bodies. Or maybe citizens will be simply manipulated into accepting their own subjugation or perhaps fashion a shared partnership between valid science and patient agency. These patterns are not a new phenomenon but were engendered in the early days of American settlement and perhaps are even now being reorganized and reborn for better or for worse.

Exactly 300 years later, the horrors of the present pandemic offer too many possible "coincidences" and "similarities" to the 1721–22 controversy to be ignored. While smallpox has been eradicated, and measles has been pretty well controlled in this country, the Covid-19 virus continues to kill and compromise people across the world; the United States has been particularly hard hit. Problems of resistance to vaccines, masking, and social distancing continue to create social problems and give the virus more opportunities to develop more transmissible and possibly deadly variants. It's difficult to believe that a significant percentage of citizens have been and are still resisting life-saving vaccination. Some of the convergences seem to erase the three hundred years between then and now. Such resistance calls for a comparison between 1721–1722 and 2020–2022. What comes next offers as many questions and inquiries as there are answers and conclusions. The hope is this: The more understanding our analyses, language, writing, media, and education can achieve, the more power citizens may have to alter the misinformation about viruses and vaccines.

The 2020s Resistance: Religion and Its Role in Vaccination Debates

Many would say that since the beginning of the Tea Party as part of the Republican Party in 2009, the role of religion has been heightened in politics, even though our *Constitution* holds that state and religion should be separate. The Puritans in Boston of course immigrated here in order to escape the dicta of both Catholic and Anglican monarchs of England. There were also Anglicans in Boston among the Puritans in the 1720s, but they, too, believed in Calvinism and its focus on predestination. In 1791 the first amendment of the *U.S. Constitution* established the separation of church and state, but the clause only applied to the federal government. Although the actual words "separation of church and state" do not appear in the First Amendment, the establishment clause was intended to separate church from state. "By 1833, all states had disestablished religion from government, providing protections for religious liberty in state constitutions. In the 20th century, the U.S. Supreme Court applied the establishment clause to the states through the 14th Amendment. Today, the establishment clause prohibits all levels of government from either advancing or inhibiting religion."[27]

In the late summer of 2009, as the recession-ravaged economy bled half a million jobs a month, the country began to experience a sea change. Organizers convened mass gatherings across the country called "tea parties."[28] The Tea Party focused on resisting Federal regulations. Lawmakers accustomed to scheduling town hall meetings where no one would show up suddenly faced shouting crowds of hundreds, some of whom brought a holstered pistol or a rifle slung over the shoulder. One demonstrator at a rally in Maryland hanged a member of Congress in effigy. A popular bumper sticker at the time captured the contempt for the federal bailout of certain homeowners. "Honk if I'm Paying Your Mortgage." The name, *tea party,* of course refers to the Boston Tea Party that heralded the resistance to taxation and then the American Revolution. Thus the name hearkens back to 1773, when Boston was itself resistant to the taxation of tea by the British overlords, a resentment that had begun to build its strength in the controversy of 1721–1722, some fifty years earlier.

In 2010, a psychographic opinion research firm called MyType conducted a large survey of 17,000 Americans and asked them about the contemporary Tea Party. The goal was to uncover the demographics, beliefs, values, and characteristics of the Tea Party's supporters. The survey revealed that the Tea Party was undergoing large changes as religious conservatives increased in numbers and were the fastest growing segment, outpacing the libertarians, who were not as religious or as traditional as the religious right, and had started leaving the Republican party.[29] The Tea Party morphed as right-wing politics gained more ground. First a Republican candidate, and then new President, took the helm in 2016.

Religious belief and racial identity were connected with vaccine politics in the early 1700s in Boston, although the ministers, heads of churches, were for inoculation, many parishioners, although not all, were against inoculation. Many Bostonian churchgoers were so against vaccination for religious reasons that the Anti-Inoculators (surgeons, apothecaries, physicians, and others) used their understanding of Biblical passages, predestination, and grace to further persuade them that undergoing the procedure against smallpox would put their souls in jeopardy. So, many of the religious in Boston in 1721–1722 were too afraid of God's wrath to risk inoculation. Many Christians that make up the Tea Party found their place in the Covid anti-vaccination camp in 2021 and 2022.

Michael Coren, a Canadian Anglican priest and broadcaster writing in *The New Statesman,* suggested that in addition to obvious changes, the pandemic has enabled a release of "all sorts of cultural toxins into the bloodstream of society, infecting the body politic and likely causing lasting and even irreparable damage."[30] Coren elucidated his argument as follows: "One of these is the empowerment of the conspiracy movement, always extant of course but never as activated and dangerous as it is now. It's manifested itself especially severely in the anti-vaccine campaign, a phenomenon that damages public health, causes civil unrest and, in some parts of the world, leads to direct violence." He claimed that it was curious, but maybe not so surprising, that an "element in the movement is conservative Christianity, which remains an extremely powerful force in the United States in particular. Specifically, the reactionary wings of the Roman Catholic and evangelical [Protestant] churches, comprised of the very people who largely voted for Donald Trump and will – if given the morbidly likely chance – do so again."[31]

National Public Radio (NPR) reported on the numbers of conservative and churched Americans who had voted for Trump in 2016. "The religious landscape in terms of voting has been remarkably stable. Since Reagan, we have essentially seen this: white Christian voters have tended to support Republican candidates, and Christians of color and everyone else, including the religiously unaffiliated, have tended to support Democratic candidates."[32] Only a slight change was registered in 2020, when about two percent of white Catholics split off from the 2016 Trump vote and voted for Joe Biden, a practicing Catholic himself.[33] Ryan Burge, a political science professor at Eastern Illinois University who follows the faith vote closely, discovered one slight change: a small decline in support for Trump among white Catholics. Burge thought that could be significant in the future because their vote is important in the swing states of Michigan, Pennsylvania, and Wisconsin, important states in close races. At the same time, Catholic support for Republicans increased in 2020 in Florida among Hispanics. Still, it was notable that 2016 exit polls showed "about 80% of white evangelical Christians supported Trump in spite of his unfamiliarity with the Bible, his divorces, his vulgar rhetoric, and his association with porn stars. Trump's reputation in moral terms hasn't changed all that much during his time in office, but there [was still] little evidence of slippage among these faith voters." In 2020 once again exit polls among early voters showed that "between 76 and 81% of white evangelical and 'born again' voters" had supported Trump, according to the National Election Pool and AP/Votecast.[34] Robert P. Jones agreed, "We essentially have White evangelicals, somewhere around 8 in 10, supporting the president, standing by their candidate, standing by their man."[35] "Their man" downplayed, lied about, and refused to support social distancing, masking, and other attempts to limit the spread of the virus. Until early in 2022, he had been eager to support the anti-vaxxers as well, even though he credited himself legitimately with expediting the vaccines.

At the same time, many faith communities, whether Islamic, Judaic, or Christian closed their houses of worship during the pandemic and reopened them with careful attention to Covid constraints. Although some congregations of orthodox Jews were adamantly against vaccinations, Israel provided an excellent model of mass vaccination. The hope was that right-wing Christians could be ultra-conservative and still support science and vaccine technologies, but many did not choose that path either in the United States or Canada. An Adventist-Canadian conservative MP, Derek Sloan, presented a petition against Covid safety protocols signed by 40,000, that declared Covid vaccines were a human experiment and not to be allowed or followed. While in Baton Rouge, Louisiana, minister Tony Spell at Life

Tabernacle Church defied state law and did not close his church, but kept it open, saying, "We're anti-mask, anti-social distancing, and anti-vaccine."

> Rick Wiles, a particularly odious homophobic and racist broadcaster who pastors a church in Florida, condemned vaccinations as part of a 'mass death campaign,' even when he, his wife and daughter-in-law were infected. 'This was a full-frontal hit from Hell. Because Jesus Christ lives in us, we shall live too. Thanks to Jesus Christ, I survived the CCP's [Chinese Communist Party's] Covid genocide on the American people.'[36]

Although the ministers in Boston in the 1720s were staunchly together behind Cotton and Increase Mather, ministers in the 2020s were more diverse, in that while many did indeed support vaccination, other heads of evangelical churches and "born again" Christians were adhering to their right-wing beliefs and those of their congregations against Covid vaccines and protocols. Still germane to the analysis is the considerable amount of liberals who identify themselves as not religious and not churchgoers, a marked difference with the 1720s Boston colony in which most likely all or nearly all identified themselves as religious. Burge also alluded to those unchurched individuals during the NPR segment: "I think the 'God Gap' is more and more the narrative when we think about the parties. Half of white liberals today identify as religiously unaffiliated, while the Right is staying very Christian."[37] Many of those "nones" were Generation Z individuals, those born after 1996. Those most adamant who made their negative views on vaccination known were in fact evangelical Christians. Their Republican presidential votes in 2016 had insured that with the former President in charge when Covid arrived in New York in March of 2020, a poorly led effort to minimize illness and death would follow.

Witchhunts, QAnon, and Satanism

During the present vaccination controversy, characterized by extreme polarization, one would assume that Americans have nothing in common any longer with any beliefs in or worry about witchcraft. Yet the former President himself often referred to any investigation of his past and more recent practices as a witchhunt. Some of the misinformation and propaganda disseminated during our Covid pandemic also invoked witchcraft or Satanic behavior, which is a persistent American theme. However, even before the pandemic and continuing in full force during the pandemic itself were woven threads of blame that sought to entangle Democrats, who were painted as worshipers of the Devil, just as Salem "witches" had been accused of worshiping the Devil. Then and now, those who supported vaccinations, whether for smallpox or the Covid virus, were painted as practicing and/or supporting witchcraft.

Those accusations, the hysteria, and the blame, just as in the 1720s have now also been associated with or followed by violent behavior. Cotton Mather had a "granado" or Molotov cocktail thrown into his home, while Boylston had to hide out for a couple of weeks as men marauded through the streets threatening to hang him. During our pandemic in the 2020s, we have seen violent attacks and threats as well, horrible ones that threaten the wellbeing of those who are of course innocent of any "Satanic" behavior. Some of those threats and attacks included the "Pizzagate" incident, the threatened but thwarted kidnap of the Governor of Michigan who enforced Covid safety protocols, the January 6, 2021 riot and insurrection at the U.S. Capitol, and the hangmen's noose outside on the Capitol grounds as insurrectionists sought to hang Vice President Mike Pence.

Violence during an epidemic both then and now seemed to be more apparent, including the violent threats or actions against government officials and the Capitol that have increased during the pandemic. Yet during the Viet Nam War the country was polarized, and there were horrendous assassinations. The war had greatly disrupted "normal" lives, and some types of violence then had taken center stage.

Even before the pandemic, QAnon had emerged in 2016–2017. When Trump won the election in 2016, QAnon could find support in a President who believed both in misinformation and conspiracy theories. The Democrats were painted with Satanic theories that were absurd. During the smallpox epidemic or pandemic in the 1720s, the Anti-Inoculators knew that just mentioning witchcraft or the Devil when writing against Cotton Mather's inoculation project would trigger more resistance against smallpox variolation. They knew enough to know that the "fear of evil forces" who might conspire to "hurt good people [was] deeply rooted in the human psyche," just as those around Trump knew that a number of supporters would also be vulnerable to just such a belief and provide a gullible audience for the conspiracy theories of QAnon.[38]

Soon after the emergence of QAnon, images of Trump supporters wearing "Q" clothing became noticeable at various rallies. Q adherents believe that a secret, civil war is happening in this country, based on "reports" by an anonymous person, "Q." "Q" claims access to classified, top-secret information about a cabal of corrupt intellectuals, the elite class, and left-wing politicians who conspire against the right-wing. The supposed "cabal" is also referred to as the "Deep State." These tropes are meant to trigger fear, anger, and violent action among Q believers and others. Part of that belief system includes an example such as what happened at "Pizzagate," which Q supporters had targeted as one of many Democrat-sponsored centers for pedophiles.

"Pizzagate" occurred in 2016, before the Covid virus pandemic started, and was based on a conspiracy theory. Part of the problem with building up resistance to masking, social distancing, and vaccinations has been directly related to other bizarre conspiracy theories. Thus, trigger words, "dog whistles," or right-wing tropes have fed directly into the resistance to vaccination ongoing today in 2022. How did this "pedophile" false rumor get started in the first place? The *New York Times* contributed an analysis of the conspiracy theory in a story at the end of 2016 and had dissected its strange origin. It centered on Hillary Clinton, who had competed in the 2016 election against Donald Trump for U.S. President. Here is their step-by-step analysis:

1 WikiLeaks began releasing emails hacked from the account of John Podesta, Hillary Clinton's campaign chairman, a month before the election.
2 Social media users on a popular Reddit forum dedicated to Donald J. Trump and 4chan's far-right fringe message board searched the releases for evidence of wrongdoing.
3 Within the emails were discussions that include the word pizza, including dinner plans between Mr. Podesta and his lobbyist brother, Tony Podesta.
4 A participant on 4chan connected the phrase "cheese pizza" to pedophiles, because on Q-type chat boards users identify the initials "c. p.," the beginning letters of "cheese" and "pizza," as denoting child pornography.
5 Following the use of "pizza," theorists focused on the Washington pizza restaurant Comet Ping Pong [also c. and p. letters]. The WikiLeaks emails revealed that John Podesta corresponded with Comet's owner, James Alefantis, who had connections to Democratic operatives.
6 The theory started snowballing, taking on the meme #PizzaGate. Fake news articles emerged and were spread on Twitter and Facebook.
7 The false stories swept up neighboring businesses and bands that had played at Comet. Theories about kill rooms, underground tunnels, Satanism, and even cannibalism emerged in fabricated stories on social media.
8 On Dec. 4, Edgar M. Welch, a 28-year-old from North Carolina, arrived at Comet with a military-style rifle and a handgun. The police said he fired the rifle inside the pizzeria, hurting no one, and surrendered after finding no evidence to support claims of child slaves being held there.
9 The shooting did not put the theory to rest. Purveyors of the theory and fake news pointed to the mainstream media as conspirators of a cover up to protect what they said was a crime ring.
10 The conspiracy theory took the internet by storm. YouTube clips pushed the false story, racking up hundreds of thousands of views. Tens of thousands of individuals subscribed to message boards, feeding into theories with fake news reports and crowd-driven detective work. The police refuted the claims of an online pedophile ring running out of Comet Ping Pong, but the theories continued.[39]

When the pandemic started here in 2020, these social media conspiracies continued among the "base" of the Republican party, even after the election of the Republican candidate, Donald J. Trump. One could argue that the new President and the party operators continued and supported the extreme conspiracies, as a way of controlling popular opinions of their base. After all, if the "base" has those who believe such bizarre ideas as Democratic pedophilia, a politician and a party can convince those voters of anything.

There have been real conspiracies in the past, "Watergate" being just one example, but that conspiracy had been real and actual, not a made-up narrative: a number of Republican operatives conspired to break into the Washington, D.C. National Democratic Headquarters to replace and repair two "bugs" that had been placed on phones earlier and were caught in the act. A conspiracy theory is different; it's a type of mass hysteria. Mass hysteria now is reminiscent of this country's history of so-called conspiracies with the "Devil." During the smallpox epidemic, the reminders of Cotton Mather's role in the witchcraft trials and his firm beliefs in the existence of witches and Satan worshippers triggered the newspaper readers and others to suspect the vaccinations for smallpox could also be connected to a new conspiracy theory of others wanting to harm Bostonians. Here, three hundred years later, believers in the wild conspiracy of Democrats as pedophiles and Satan worshippers are still resisting vaccinations. They have painted Hillary Clinton, John Podesta, and others with the same brush with which Cotton Mather and Zabdiel Boylston had been painted, even though neither had any association with witchcraft at the time of the smallpox inoculation project. Theoretically, those Bostonians who had eschewed their earlier beliefs from the 1680s and 1690s would also have no longer believed in such accusations; however, they were still made by the Anti-Inoculators and proved persuasive.

Why are vaccine conspiracies so potent in the United States, although some vaccine resistance occurs in other countries? One can imagine that support for conspiracy beliefs finds root in those people who have mental illness, or that these theories are a direct result of social media. Certainly social media accelerates the spread of misinformation, and there are those who have mental issues, but neither can be held as totally responsible. Conspiracy theories have existed before the Digital Age, and some people who are otherwise leading normal lives believe in such clearly false ideas. Scholars, such as Jan-Willem van Prooijen, Clara de Inocencio, and Karen Douglas who have studied this phenomenon suggest some people are more vulnerable after they had already believed in an earlier conspiracy.[40] Those three scholars, and also Nils Jossmann and Michele Acker "found that feelings of uncertainty, coupled with the feeling that one's life is not fully in his or her control anymore, increases conspiracy thinking. Studies by other researchers confirm that emotions reflecting uncertainty — such as fear or worry — can increase conspiracy beliefs."[41] Part of this thinking could revert back to a common saying or meme in the American society that believes, even back to Puritan times, that everything happens for a reason. There are no such things as coincidences. Instead, a deity has a plan, or one's predetermined fate has somehow already been set. It's easier, perhaps, to accept one's fear or a tragic event if everything had actually taken place according to a larger plan. Frightened persons could then have more of a sense of security if they believed certain things were happening according to some plan, even if it was a conspiracy theory. Unfortunately, it would be a false security. Frequently blame is sought, and if a person could find someone to blame, to point to as an enemy, then one could justify one's own hatred or violence against that person or group of persons (Figure 6.1).

In the early 1720s fear reigned for a very real reason as smallpox was such a horrendous disease. In the early 2020s, citizens around the world also had very rational reasons for fear, as a very new, in fact "novel," virus had suddenly appeared that would cause illness, impairment, and/or deaths. Modern medicine, in which many Americans have such trust and confidence, simply did not seem to see a pandemic coming. So this period in U.S. history *is* a time of fear, even though some of the current dependence on conspiracy theories and heightened fear and anger existed before the onset of Covid.

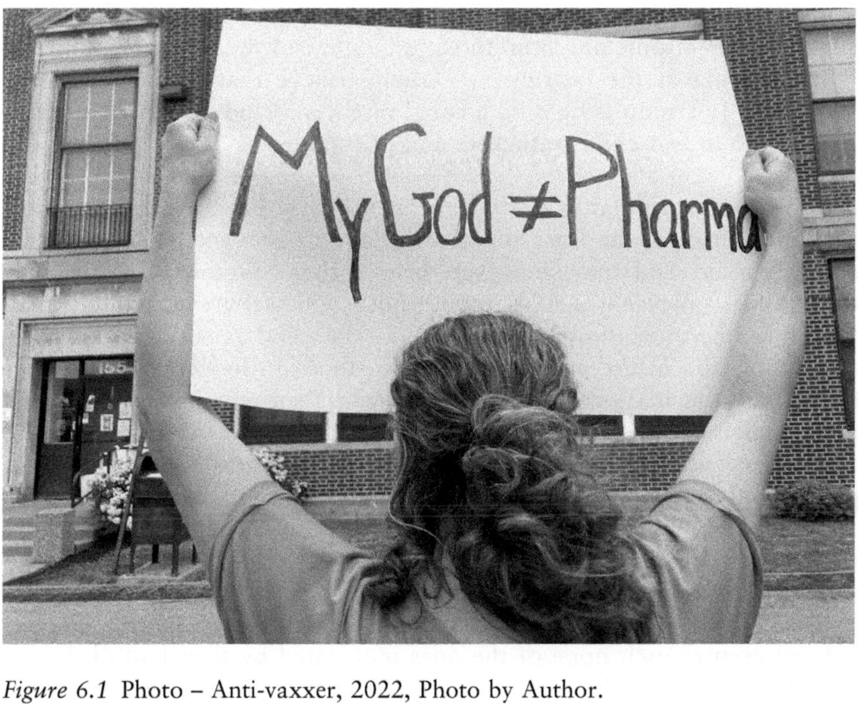

Figure 6.1 Photo – Anti-vaxxer, 2022, Photo by Author.

Conspiracy theories, however, do not relieve the anxiety people feel, and such feelings end up feeding a vicious circle of even more conspiracy theories, since the belief in an earlier one impels another. Political groups function in similar ways. For example, Joseph E. Uscinski and Joseph M. Parent showed that Democrats are more willing to believe governmental conspiracies when a Republican is president, and Republicans are more likely to believe them when a Democrat is president. QAnon, however, shows an extreme and fairly consistent pattern for the far right portraying liberals as especially dangerous and also acting in immoral ways.[42] Besides the PizzaGate debacle in 2016, television viewers got to experience QAnon more immediately as the January 6, 2021 insurrection was telecast in real time. The violence of that day resulted in deaths and numerous injuries. To at least some viewers of the 2022 Senate hearing for a nominee for the Supreme Court, Ketanji Brown Jackson, the emphasis on child pornography by several Republican senators seem to again hearken back to the QAnon claims about Democratic pedophilia.

Writers at the *New York Times* noted in their news analysis piece that indeed such questioning was yet another dog whistle to the Republican base and especially those members of QAnon:

> Republicans contended that the nominee had been especially lenient on purveyors of child sexual abuse imagery, a claim that spoke to a fixation of those wedded to the QAnon conspiracy theory. Many of its followers — some of whom took note online of the Republican line of questioning at the hearings — falsely believe that former President Donald J. Trump is fighting a cabal of elites including top Democrats who are in fact child traffickers and pedophiles.[43]

Ironically, it seemed that in 1720s, Bostonians moved away from the earlier conspiracy theories, at least those attendant to the witch trials several decades earlier. Did they, however, believe that Mather, Boylston, and others were conspiring against their health and welfare? Certainly they blamed Mather for the earlier obsession that had taken hold of their community, and in the newspaper reports, the Anti-Inoculators had triggered fear of vaccination against smallpox with their references to Mather's earlier beliefs by mentioning bargaining with the Devil. In Chapter 2 Mundungus had made a religious argument against variolation by accusing Mather and Boylston of such "bargaining." He had also charged the Inoculators with killing patients, by saying that the vaccinations were fatal. He had written that "Now to save Life, by giving Death for it, it is but a *swapping,* and very dear, though the purchaser may think he hath a good *bargain.*"[44] Williams invoked fears of death in those Boylston had inoculated even though none of the ones inoculated by then had died, and very few would later die (six out of 246) and possibly by some other disease. Also, they might have already been infected with smallpox naturally and not by the procedure. In the Colonies after the 1690s witchcraft debacle the terms "bargaining" or "swapping" were dog whistles for Satanic practices, terms that invoked deals made with the Devil.

Does the concept of a Devil or Satan have relevance with those in some branches of current religious practice? A recent study was conducted with various Christian Evangelicals to obtain a sample of their belief system. The researchers interviewed and asked for reflective writing from those who had been "churched" for an average of over 30 years and reported being diagnosed as depressed or anxious or having a personality disorder. Most of our world, in a pandemic, could indeed express depression and especially anxiety given the omnipresence and continuation of the Covid virus in our lives and its impact on our normal activities. The researcher found that "the belief that mental distress is caused by demons, sin, or generational curses is commonplace among many evangelical Christian communities."[45] Evangelical Christian communities can be found in many different denominations and types of Christian churches. The researcher used snowball sampling and cited around twenty-five other studies. Many of the participants reported feeling a sense of shame over their "mental distress" and were further stigmatized and felt shame when they requested help from their church and/or religious leaders. Some of the interviewees were also discouraged from consulting mental health facilities and counselors. "The dismissal of help-seeking outside communities of faith was another difficulty ... and led to negative experiences concerning mental health." As one participant remarked, "sometimes the attitude will be you don't trust secular psychology ... They'd probably say it's because it's based on materialism [rather than faith-based]."[46]

Here are several comments by other participants in this study: "The person who came to speak to me was the head of the pastoral team and used to be a church minister. I said that I was really very low and very depressed or feeling suicidal, and he just literally stood over me and kind of [denounced] the devil, and sort of praying the devil leaves me ... it made me feel awful, absolutely awful." Another participant reported, "Of them saying that I'm not mentally ill, I'm possessed, that it's an evil spirit ... I was even once described as demonic ... they decided that I was demonic and I was demon possessed, which is why they then went ahead with this deliverance. That just distressed me more." One interviewee analyzed his experience in this way:

> The go-to explanation for anything that's unpleasant or unwanted or difficult is to regard it as a demonic attack. Those churches, if not wisely guided, do tend to have a rather positional [attitude]; 'this is God and all the good, and there's the devil and all the bad, and mental health is bad, so that must come from the devil.' It's easy, but it can lead to a lot of very damaging behaviour.[47]

The syllogism in the quote could have been one of Mundungus's. This study and many others suggest that the route from the Tea Party in the earlier 2000s and conspiracy theories that paint "the enemies" of Trump and others as Satanic and part of demonic cults is perhaps not so surprising. Among some of the "base," such belief systems are continuous: an earlier Tea Party ideology has evolved into the current one. There are other polls and analyses that also show connections between QAnon, PizzaGate, some Christians, and the January 6, 2021 insurrection with the belief in Satanism.

This text has already described "Q" as head of a social media group who claims insider knowledge as a government and security operative. 4chan is an anonymous and rather primitive image-board website and is a hub of Internet subculture, whose anonymous community is influential in forming Internet memes, comics, hacktivist, and political movements. *The Guardian* in 2008 said it was "lunatic, juvenile ... brilliant, ridiculous and alarming."[48] All postings (called drops) are usually not traceable back to an actual person, as there is no registration, and posters are allowed to upload images and leave their names blank. One week after his first posts, Q quoted the 23rd Psalm: "The LORD is my shepherd, I lack nothing." It's unclear how many of those who attacked the Capitol on January 6th believe the conspiracy of democratic pedophilia or in "Q." They were certainly part of the group, and at times stood out, such as the man with the furs, war paint, and animal horns on his head.

The 2021 American Enterprise Institute's American Perspectives Survey queried 2000 Americans with a series of statements to discover how accurate they were for each of them. In answering the following: "Donald Trump has been secretly fighting a group of child sex traffickers that include prominent Democrats and Hollywood elites," 27 percent of those who rated that as "mostly" or "completely" accurate were white evangelical Christians; 31 percent of those who identified as white evangelical Republicans rated that statement as "mostly" or "completely" accurate. The U.S. population is made up of 25% Christian evangelicals, so they were at least somewhat over represented, thus there is an overlap between that type of Christian and Q followers.[49] A survey conducted in October, 2020 by Paul Djupe and colleagues from Denison University sampled 1700 Americans and discovered that 50 percent of white evangelical Christians "agreed" or "strongly agreed" with QAnon beliefs; other surveys also exhibited a correlation between conspiratorial thinking and Christian nationalism.[50] According to an earlier (2014) poll by Pew Research Center, 56 percent of evangelical Christians identified as Republicans, and in January 2021, 24 percent of Republicans believed in QAnon. Beliefs, though, dropped somewhat in months after the January 6th insurrection.

The news media is not held in high esteem by evangelicals. A 2019 Pew survey showed that while 44 percent of the general public thought journalists were known for high ethical standards, only 27 percent of white evangelicals thought that. However, in October 2020, 80 percent of evangelicals supported Trump. Compared to the general public, that religious group also believed him to be honest, trustworthy, and even ethical.[51] QAnon has cast the former president in the role of hero in their strange myth, in which he is the one who will save everyone else from the evil "Deep State." Such myths are archetypal, and especially if his supporters think they are misunderstood and victims of the elite class, then they see him as a warrior who can win that fight against the intellectuals and the elites.

Certainly in the 1720s there was also a type of class warfare, and although it was somewhat ironic, the physicians led by the European university-educated doctor had joined the group of people in Boston who had a similar reaction to their elite ministerial citizens. The preachers had enjoyed enormous power for numerous decades and had had the education and ability to go to Harvard, even though it was still a fledgling school then. By joining with Mundungus, who could well represent the people who felt themselves also not appreciated and not having the same privileges, the Anti-Inoculators, mostly physicians, other than Boylston, had been successful in gathering a majority of Bostonians into their anti-vaccination camp. Even though the American colonies had not been quite as class conscious as their home country of England, classes still existed and continue to exist in this country today. Although today's legitimate media can explain and "fact-check" conspiracy theories from the right, that has clearly not been effective enough to curb the disruptive ruses. It will be increasingly important to understand people's motivations and concerns, because conspiracy theories will continue to attract those who feel as if someone or something else, like a governmental body, a satanic group, or the Deep State is attempting to take charge of their lives.

The comparison of the two eras side-by-side, especially the witchcraft debacle and the unusual symbols and theories that are found on 4chan, which is used by QAnon, points to a suspension of practical thinking and reality. A likeness between things "witches" supposedly did and the descriptions of the QAnon conspiracy theories exists. Both are centered on Satanism: the devil is responsible for the evil and uses people to commit heinous acts. "The QAnon movement has suffered multiple failed prophecies, predictions for events that never came to pass. To continue holding onto beliefs in spite of those disappointments, followers need something many evangelicals have in spades: faith."[52] When the former president did not win the election and the inauguration for his second term, the Q followers blamed the "Deep State," and most of the followers did not leave QAnon. The executive director of the Wheaton College Billy Graham Center, evangelical minister Ed Stetzer, remarked: "QAnon is a train that runs on the tracks that religion has already put in place."[53]

To be clear, though, not all QAnon members are evangelical Christians, and not all evangelical Christians are QAnon members. In the early 2020s, the majority of those in the United States did elect to receive the vaccination (or some of the series), but the evangelicals and those following conspiracy theories were less apt to get the shots and relied on such misinformation as Ivermectin being the best medicine for treating Covid, which is a worming medication for livestock. Also, an active and vocal subset of the far-right conservatives have pushed for religious exemptions from masking and vaccine mandates, believing that life-saving measures and breakthroughs in medical science interfere with their religious freedom.[54]

Freedom, Politics, and Education Then and Now

Having compared religious and the Satanist similarities and differences between the early 2020s and three hundred years ago, it's important to also compare political tenets. The author Stephen Coss believes that the controversy of 1721–1722 was in essence the first salvo of the Revolutionary War that was to follow over 50 years later. In the beginning year of the smallpox infestation, the elected members of the Massachusetts assembly were pushing back against the Governor appointed by the Crown. This had not been the first time Bostonians had revolted against a Governor. As noted in an earlier chapter, the *New-England Courant* had become the first independent newspaper in Boston; the others had adhered closely to views held by the British Crown. James and Ben Franklin's newspaper had set out not just to oppose vaccination but also to insist that the *Courant* would not pledge allegiance to the Crown. The paper had begun to include controversial political views and discussions and had insisted on freedom of the press, the first newspaper to have done so in Massachusetts.[55] It would have been easy to presume that epidemics and politics would not have been bedfellows. The evidence was and is clear, then and now, how in fact these two can go hand-in-hand.

In the early days of the pandemic in the United States, in late 2019 and throughout the election year, 2020, a former president was very keen on playing down the virulence of the Covid-19 virus. In Bob Woodward's book, Trump is telling Woodward one thing about the pandemic, while telling the American people the opposite. He had acknowledged in early February 2020 how deadly the novel virus could become in an interview with the author; in Woodward's book *Rage,* Trump had said that "You just breathe the air and that's how it's passed. And so that's a very tricky one. That's a very delicate one. It's also more deadly than even your strenuous flu."[56] But a few days later, Trump was publicly saying that the virus was less of a concern, telling New Hampshire supporters, "Looks like by April, you know, in theory, when it gets a little warmer, it miraculously goes away." He also had tweeted in late February 2020 that the virus was "very much under control in the USA."[57] By May, 2022, over one million people in the United States had died of Covid. In March of 2020, Trump in a Fox interview had said that "We've never closed down the country for the flu," unwilling to do what was necessary to save hundreds of thousands of lives. "I wanted to always play it down," Trump also said then, telling Woodward that he "still [likes] playing it down, because I don't want to create a panic."[58] Because of the vaccination issue, Trump's relationships with Jim Mattis, his defense secretary, as well as with other former cabinet members, were fraught. According to Woodward, Mattis had prayed for the country and had called the former president "unfit" and even "dangerous" because of his attitude, rhetoric, and actions regarding Covid-19.[59] Trump's adherents followed his lead in down-playing the virus, and cemented an anti-vaxxers' position, willing to sacrifice their own health and possibly incur death, along with the wellbeing and lives of others.

As in the 1720s, those against vaccinations were fighting against science, although William Douglass and some of the other physicians must have thought Mather and Boylston had some evidence in their favor. However, the two Inoculators, a minister and a surgeon, had seemed to have been imposing on the physicians' territory by bringing new medical knowledge and techniques forward. Boylston had been known for the first recorded surgery to remove a cancerous breast in 1718. The husband of the patient, Sarah Winslow, had written a testimonial in a letter to Zabdiel Boylston published in the *Boston News-Letter* in 1720.[60] The *New-England Courant*, because of its advocacy for independence and freedom from England along with being adamantly against the Mathers and other Puritan ministers of long-standing, had combined both the epidemic contagion and politics in its first issue and in those that followed.

In the 2020s science was more broadly accepted, but Trump's White House Corona Virus Task Force became deeply frustrated by his refusal to value their input, and he had seemed more interested in raising the ire against modern medicine in his huge outdoor rallies during the epidemic. Large crowds of supporters gathered maskless and even though sometimes at outdoor rallies infected each other with the virus. A former task force member has recently spoken out. "Dr. Deborah Birx, who had been one of the White House's chief coronavirus response coordinators, admitted she considered quitting under former President Donald Trump, whose cavalier attitude toward combatting the disease created consternation among public health officials."[61]

> Her comments came a day after Dr. Anthony Fauci, one of the government's other top public health experts, said he feels free to speak honestly about Covid-19 now that Trump is out of office. Fauci said that the new [Biden] administration was committed to being "completely transparent, open and honest," a sharp break from the Trump White House in which Fauci said he often felt there would be repercussions for speaking honestly about the pandemic.[62]

Because the Mathers and other ministers were on the side of vaccination, the Franklins felt compelled to be against. Media has and had played a large role in both the 1720s and 2020s. The *Courant* had helped gather, legitimize, and forward what would ultimately erupt into the drive for American independence from England. Sadly, most likely those in QAnon and other right-wing groups and individuals who stormed the U.S. Capitol on January 6, 2021 thought they, too, were patriots fighting for freedom against the Democrats and the "Deep State." 4chan, Fox News and Tucker Carlson, and other social media sites mirror the ability to influence that *The New-England Courant* and James and Ben Franklin wielded in the 1700s. Fauci and Birx could represent Mather and Boylston. The social media possible in a digital world play similar roles to the *Courant,* broadsheets, town criers, and gossip in the pubs. The country is perhaps even more polarized now than it was in the Boston's colonial era, but with the enormous reach of social media, such a spread of a diseased message is easier, even as the spread of a real disease is now global and more far-reaching.

U.S. citizens by law do not have the right to injure and kill other Americans, install gallows for politicians, and deface a public and governmental building, even as Bostonians had no right to attempt to kill Cotton Mather or threaten Zabdiel Boylston's life and both of their families. Given the state of the United States now, is there danger of another revolution, one that would seem to advocate for freedom, but that could entail freedom much more exclusively for white Christian males? Matthew Dowd, now a political analyst for MSNBC and former campaign strategist for Bush-Cheney (2004), recently called the current insurrectionists "Christian Nationalists" during an interview with Nicole Wallace, saying "Trump opened the door" to them rather than "causing" their movement; he "released" a virus or toxin that already existed in the United States but had been dormant or under wraps. Dowd believes now "75-80% of the Republicans believe that democracy doesn't matter as long as they get what they want" and "what they want is white Christian Nationalism."[63] The future is, of course, not yet clear. The clock has not been turned back to the early 1700s before real freedom of the press, of speech, and religion were achievable goals. The greatest irony would be if what in 1721–1722 had been a move toward an American revolution with democracy in mind in Boston would reverse itself nationally to return to or to reinstate a narrower theocratic and autocratic state that denied the right to vote to people of color; the right to healthcare for women, LBGTQ, and transgendered youth; and the right to read and hear about America's actual past. The global balance of power seems to be leaning in the direction of authoritarian or autocratic governments; autocracies tend to spread to or support others. Large population groups in other countries are now under such control. A more thorough understanding of the politics in the early 1720s and its seeding of a later revolution is relevant for America now.

In addition to the role played by the Franklin's *Courant* newspaper, there had also been a division in the early colonial assembly that had some control vis-à-vis the crown-appointed Governor. The Massachusetts assembly, like other colonies' assemblies, had the duty to make local laws and ordinances, although the ones they created could not have been inconsistent with British laws. A number of these assemblies, including the Massachusetts assembly, sought to limit some of the powers of the crown and the Governor. Early in the colony when first under sole control of the ministers, Puritans had created their own government or theocracy. At that time in the early 1630s, every aspect of life was dictated by religious beliefs in that particular colony. Soon there had been a tri-cameral government: The Governor was the executive, and the Massachusetts General Assembly was the legislative branch, and there was a local Court. The Selectmen that had ruled against Boylston's vaccinations were the equivalent of a city council, ruling in Boston. The Governor could veto any law or ordinance passed by the legislature that he disagreed with. In addition, he could also suspend the Assembly at will as well as shut down the Court. Although in day-to-day life, religion still exercised very strong control over the body, in the early 1700s the theocracy had been faced with more instances of losing its power. New religions were coming in, especially the Congregationalists and Anglicans. More and more comments against the Papists (a slur denoting Catholics) and the Quakers had appeared over time in Mather's diaries, but the Congregationalists had been more accepted even though they faced competition with some of the Puritan ministers.

The relations between England and the American colonies had never remained smooth for very long. England had revoked an early charter in 1684; a new one had been enacted in 1691 with a loophole regarding the Governor's salary. One Puritan-hating Governor had faced much opposition when he tried to nullify Puritan practices or force the churches to hold services for the Church of England, especially during Christmas, a holiday which the Puritans did not recognize in the same way as the Anglicans. That Governor had been packed off back to England by the colonists when King James was overthrown. Both Elisha Cooke, Sr. and Jr. had been much involved in the struggles against various Governors, and both had gained followers in the assembly.[64]

During the smallpox epidemic of the 1720s, one of the main assembly leaders had been Elisha Cooke, Jr. who had very quickly gathered followers against the current Governor. The election that put Cooke and his followers so decisively in control of the assembly in 1719 reflected a "seismic" change in the voting structure of the colony: namely that voters had come out in droves, exhibiting "America's first urban political machine" with connections to other caucuses that eventually resulted in the American Revolution.[65] Cooke had worked the pubs, as had Mundungus, to get patrons/voters angry both about Governor Shute, the crown-appointed executive at the time, as well as against the Mathers, who had often seemed to have played up to the British representative, as well as urging them to take a stand against inoculation. The president elected in 2016 had, like Cooke and Mundungus, pitched his campaign toward the working class, even though he himself had never been part of that demographic. However, as has been shown, much of the underlying animosity toward England and its Governors had been stewing for a long time, practically since the beginning of American colonization; it, of course, did not result in revolution until the later 1700s. In the 2020s in the United States, animosity toward the elite and intelligentsia, as well as against blacks, immigrants, the working poor had also been brewing for a long time, even though those who were angry, racist, and xenophobic were often part of the working class themselves.

Those who were privileged enough to be educated at Harvard in the 1700s came under fire from those who were against vaccination then. Both then and now, it would be difficult to separate education and politics. Along with being against vaccinations and science in general, today to be part of the conservative party means to be against "Critical Race Theory." The irony is that most of those against it have no idea about its history or its limited use in education. Those demanding that it be removed from all curriculum have lumped it together with teaching about white privilege and any mention of race or the history of slavery. Such parents also criticize the use of pictures of brown and black children in elementary readers. There appears to be no understanding of small children who might like to see pictures of other children who look like them.

Although parents are often represented as those most outraged at curriculum about diversity in schools, they tend to be the same ones espousing the tenets of a right-wing agenda. The focus tends to be more toward energizing the base.

> But the specific focus on banning the teaching of racial history smacks of political motivation by a party that is trying to ignore this nation's rising diversity and appeal to its largely white, culturally conservative voter base. In fact, the term 'critical race theory' — a much narrower academic framework than what is commonly taught in K-12 courses on American racial history — is intentionally used as a scare tactic to appeal to that base.[66]

The main instigators of new laws banning books about race had been initiated by Governors of the more conservative states and those with more Republican legislatures: Ron DeSantis of Florida, Greg Abbott of Texas, and the more recently elected Youngkin of Virginia.[67] A CBS poll done at the end of February in 2022 found that a large majority of Americans, in the 80 percentile, do not believe books should be banned because they teach about racism or the history of slavery. Even books that criticize U.S. history in general should not be banned according to 83% of Americans.[68] Clearly, here is an example in the 2020s that shows among a small minority not just the convergence of the creation of hostility toward education with politics, but also includes racism in the mix. It's as if conservative and/or right-wing leaders want to revise the education to produce more white supremacists who agree with their own biases. One could add even another issue to the mix, the threats of violence that many school board members and teachers face from right-wing community members. School board meetings have sometimes had to move online because of the threats. Reuters found examples of 220 threats of violence and hostile messages from anonymous harassers over culture-war issues such as race, gender, and mask mandates to protect from students from the virus. Reuters contacted 31 school boards in 15 states to uncover the 220 threats and hate-filled messages. Many school districts have had to add security for board members and school children, as children of the board members were also threatened. A number of those who serve on school boards have resigned or decided not to run for reelection.[69]

Xenophobia, Racism, and Misogyny Then and Now

White supremacism has very deep historical roots in the United States. America's Civil War history speaks to the animosity between North and South in the 1800s. That resentment existed after the revolution in which the states struggled to work together to unify this country between the plantation-dependent states and those with other types of enslaved, economic, and trade structures; following the revolution, all states had some form of enslavement. From the early 1720s, xenophobia and racism or fear and "othering" of those unlike themselves were woven deeply into the fabric of the American colonies and then the United States. This racism and resistance to other ethnicities had come through clearly in the resistance to inoculation 300 years ago because the practice had come to America with Africans and from reports of the Turkish, Arabic, and Greek practices.

Just before and then during the Covid-19 pandemic, how strange it had been to see a virulent racism and hostility toward Arabs, immigrants, and African Americans in the Black Lives Matter movement in the 2020s mirroring the hostility toward the "Mahometans," Africans, Arabs, Turks, and Greeks in the 1720s. What is it about the fear attendant to a viral pandemic that creates such a re-entrenchment and multiple espousals of hatred toward the "other," whether that other has a black or brown skin or a non-Christian religion? One theory suggests that the racism was refueled, as if it had ever lacked fuel, with the election of our first black president. The person who was elected president after Obama's second term, although only a television persona with experience as a businessman, began in 2011 during Obama's first term with his questioning of the black president's birthplace as well as inciting fears of his being a Muslim. White nationalism raised its head during the presidential terms of Barack Obama with the encouragement of the former President Trump. Those espousing such an ideology seemed to have felt threatened by an African-American President, and birtherism, the belief that Obama was not born in the United States, was also a conspiracy theory espoused by the man who would then run for the 2016 election and win. Birtherism was one of the recognizable conspiracy theories that received a lot of traction during that time before the pandemic.

> Birtherism is the baseless conjecture that the 44th president of the United States not only was born abroad and was therefore ineligible for the presidency, but also was a secret Muslim planning to undermine America from within. It is the combination of these two elements that transformed birtherism from mere false speculation about Obama's birth to a statement of values about who belongs in America, and who does not. Conspiracy theories are meant to explain the unexplainable. Birtherism's explanatory power was negligible, but as a worldview, its appeal to conservatives was enduring. By 2011, about half of Republican voters believed Obama was born abroad.[70]

Trump then had begun his own presidency by banning Arabs from entering the country under Executive Order # 13769, titled "Protecting the Nation from Foreign Terrorist Entry into the United States" in 2017. This ban included seven different predominantly Muslim countries including those refugees seeking asylum from Syria. The ban initiated and necessitated multiple legal battles going back and forth for three years, and Trump had to re-ban for a second and then third time until in 2020 the Supreme Court upheld the third ban.[71] This anti-religious and xenophobic response fit well with the religious right that supported a Christian nationalistic agenda. The former Republican President fanned racist flames as well against other minorities and religions, such as Judaism, by supporting the white supremacist movements that gained more and more public notice.

During this pandemic, there were counter movements that have shown a light on racism and xenophobia; at the same time, there have been those who began to advocate for a different and peaceful path with the Black Lives Matter movement. Compared to the 1960s, the protests by Afro Americans had much participation and support by white protesters, especially younger people, who marched side-by-side with them. At the same time some young white men choose to inflict mass casualties with weapons of war on black and brown bodies. Is it just a coincidence that these other fissures in our society come to the surface when a country is threatened by a viral pandemic that showered other fears along with its infections? What is there about a fear that lets loose all the other odious germs of disintegration of a society, and at the same time helps the country makes gains in some civil rights if those gains can be maintained in the polarization now? It would seem, though, in the past in the advance of other horrific diseases, such as polio, the country had pulled together. Some have suggested that because the children were not so affected with Covid, more support for vaccination was not easily achieved. However, in the 1720s, children were very much affected by smallpox, yet what could have saved their lives had not been trusted for the most part.

From Chapter 5 we learned of one of William Douglass's anti-inoculation texts that expressed his own negative view of African sources of wisdom regarding variolation. In addition to the atrocious description of story-telling, Douglass had indeed referred to enslaved people as a "Race" and included yet another slur against their verity. Samuel Grainger, too, also an Anti-Inoculator, clearly had chosen to attack the vaccination project because of its African and Eastern sources. Empirically, the Inoculators' references made up a snowball sampling research method in which one trusted enslaved person would recruit another who had also had a similar experience with variolation. It's clear not all Africans had experienced the procedure; many had arrived to the shores of America with smallpox scars still obvious from a natural and more terrible case of the disease. The enslaved-to-be were often captured along different shorelines from diverse tribes and multiple African languages in order to insure no early chance of group cohesion both aboard ships and then on plantations. Some captives had arrived from areas that had not had inoculation as a choice or possibility. Some had. The writings of the Anti-Inoculators had moved from xenophobic and anti-Black attitudes to religious prejudice against Islam, a religion long held as an enemy to European and English Christians. White supremacists in the 2020s expressed racist, anti-Muslim, and anti-immigrant sentiments along with anti-Semitism. It should be noted that African-American Christians today, just as in earlier times in the United States, vastly outnumber the number of African-American Muslims.

Earlier in the text, Minardi was quoted as having suggested that "race" was not really a concept until much later than the 1720s, so perhaps it was not technically correct to write that the Bostonians were racist when they had written against vaccination on the basis of testimonials by Africans. A recent lecture by Henry Louis Gates, Jr. and Andrew S. Curran shed more light on the construction of race as a "category" within a larger taxonomy. The co-authors spoke about their research of the topic, which is also the theme of their new book: *Who Is Black and Why?* The text features a 1739 essay contest sponsored by Bordeaux's Royal Academy of Sciences in which contributors or contestants were to "explain the sources of 'blackness.'" Gates and Curran contextualized the contest and its results within the history of the period, and how the essays spoke to the origins of anti-Black racism and colorism in the West. Some of the questions the essays were to address were: "What is the physical cause of blackness and African hair" and "what is the cause of Black degeneration?" In a "search for a 'scientific' understanding of race," physicians, amateurs, theologians, and naturalists had written their answers to the questions. "By the time answers were received two years later, more than four million Africans had been kidnapped and shipped across the Atlantic into a life of brutal enslavement in cities, farms, and plantations on the other side of the world."[72] These essays were never published before Gates and Curran discovered them. They truly "provide an indispensable record of the Enlightenment-era thinking that normalized the sale and enslavement of Black human beings."[73]

The Enlightenment that featured such writers/thinkers as Rousseau, Voltaire, Kant, and Locke has also been referred to the as The Age of Reason, in which science was to replace blind faith, and reason was to replace superstition. Our Western world has been dominated by that philosophy and our education dependent on it ever since the very late 1700s, which is why the "scientific" categorization of "race" first was organized and became a taxonomy of human types. That process then is why scholars such as Minardi, Gates, and Curran understand "racism" as not being "racism" until that time. The issue, in addition to the labeling of humans and regarding that exercise as important, while at the same time setting up an extensive system of cruelty and oppression, points to the most important take-away: The Enlightenment thinking that the West holds in such high regard not only contains the seeds of, but also enables the systems of racism. An attendant philosophy that goes with Enlightenment thinking is positivism, which often applies to scientific progress and the law. The tenet that any rational assertion that can be verified by science, mathematical, or logical proof can therefore be justified, leaves out morals, beliefs, and ethics. Also, if a law comes from an appropriate authority or again from logic, then morality can't limit its operation. In addition, the West that has been over-determined by this philosophy has long felt itself superior and that anything made by the West is a sign of progress. In essence, the main argument of positivism is that progress is constantly being made; science has improved everything. This idea is of course both false and true. When one observes the horror of racism, and the other problems and attitudes covered in this text, one's doubt of Western progress is greatly increased. That is the best gem delivered by Gates and Curran and their studies of that time period: one that challenges the blind trust in the Enlightenment itself.

Now the clock has even started to turn back against women's rights, although misogyny had never been removed from the culture. The Supreme Court's decision on Roe vs. Wade will subject women to needless suffering and in some cases death. The decisions made by men have shown who controls women's bodies, although the Supreme Court now has more women on it than ever before. About 75% of the women, however, voted against the recent decision, and the lone woman supporter of the decision on the Supreme Court had religious reasons fueling her choice. As has been pointed out earlier, the response in England in the 1720s, although misogynistic in its public embrace of inoculation, had been less apt to tear the country apart. English women worked behind the scenes to advocate for, educate about, and schedule vaccinations there. In the 2020s, other countries were horrified by the U.S. Supreme Court's decision to overturn *Roe v. Wade*.

At the same time, the conundrum becomes even thornier. When it comes to vaccination and refusing vaccination, the balance between science and QAnon must be reset. The inoculation against Covid-19 has contributed its life-saving gift again and again to the United States and other countries; it's a result of our brilliant scientists, who broke all-time records to get this protection to U.S. citizens. Superstition in the form of conspiracy theories is at an all-time high. The opposites could not be further apart. The question continues unanswered: How do such extremes exist and do pandemics and epidemics of disease draw forth and infect politics, economics, and create social unrest? Foucault had a partial answer, perhaps when he described the "productivity" of a "rupture." Wars, epidemics, pandemics, economic collapses, and soon climate changes can be and have all been ruptures. In these Covid years, people talk about a "return to normal life." That is what has been ruptured and disrupted. When Foucault wrote about the productivity of rupture, he did not mean all "productivity" was good. In fact, if it's suggested that Covid-19 is "productive" of great fear that aided a release of racist, misogynistic, biased venom, it was indeed productive of social attitudes that are extremely negative. The best insight that Foucault gave, however, can be found in his *Archaeology of Knowledge*:

> For many years now historians have preferred to turn their attention to long periods, as if, beneath the shifts and changes of political events, they were trying to reveal the stable, almost indestructible system of checks and balances, the irreversible processes, the constant readjustments, the underlying tendencies that gather force, and are then suddenly reversed after centuries of continuity, the movements of accumulation and slow saturation, the great silent, motionless bases that traditional history has covered with a thick layer of events.[74]

In fact, it's best to think that instead of trying to visualize, insist on, or else reconstitute large "periods" or even "centuries, Americans should see their history and current time as: "phenomena of rupture, of discontinuity" rather than continuity.[75] The problem, Foucault writes "is no longer one of tradition, of tracing a line, but one of division, of limits."[76] Rather than presenting a monolithic vision of a period in time, he advocates for discovering how a period in time reveals:

> Several pasts, several forms of connexion (sic), several hierarchies of importance, several networks of determination, several teleologies, for one and the same science, as its present undergoes change: those historical descriptions are necessarily ordered by the present state of knowledge, they increase with every transformation and never cease, in turn, to break with themselves.[77]

To add to this description, those disruptions as they occur do not travel in the same direction, but can move back over themselves, reversing what once was, returning it to an earlier state, or some altered set of events that a culture may not have or even could not have anticipated. There are no smooth, uninterrupted, unruptured periods of time or space, at least not for the length of time that would be endlessly sustainable. Instead, it's possible to move forward in ways that save and greatly improve human life, as well as for what once was to fold back on itself and be unrecognizable or eerily familiar in a negative way.

Most likely, this "conclusion" did not provide many answers to certain quandaries but instead has produced more questions. Those questions will hopefully inspire others to take up more research, analysis, and study in search of answers to complex problems in our culture, especially those that involve life and death issues and especially in times of pandemics or other major crises. The analytical tools used throughout this text can be applied to other controversies. Understanding and careful analyses help groups make changes not only discursively but also in cultural and individual practices. A pattern of resistance has been revealed here in the very earliest days of our country's history that continues to play out today: against vaccinations, abortions, stem cell use, civil rights, immigration and other areas where religion, class, history, and prejudice prevent logical arguments, ethical behavior, and clear thinking. Rhetorical analyses or close textual readings can contribute much to the wider society, and public messages need careful crafting to be successful to multiple audiences. It is important to continue to conduct additional thorough research into historical as well as current epistemological processes within the fields of rhetoric, cultural studies, science, and scientific medicine.

Notes

1 Arthur W. Boylston and A. E. Williams, "Zabdiel Boylston's Evaluation of Inoculation Against Smallpox" in *JLL Bulletin: Commentaries on the History of Treatment Evaluation* (2008), n.p.
2 *Royal Society Classified Papers* (London: Royal Society Archives, 1660–1741).
3 Michel Foucault, *Birth of the Clinic: An Archaeology of Medical Perception.* Trans. A. M. Sheridan Smith (New York: Vintage, 1973), 19.
4 James B. Blake, *Public Health in the Town of Boston, 1630-1822.* Boston: Harvard University Press, 1959; Lloyd Bitzer, "The Rhetorical Situation," *Philosophy and Rhetoric*, 1 (1968).
5 Barbara Heifferon, "The New Smallpox: An Epidemic of Words?" in *Rhetoric Review* 25: no. 1 (January 2006), 84.
6 Heifferon, "The New Smallpox?" 84.
7 Heifferon, 88.
8 Michel Foucault, "The Politics of Health in the Eighteenth Century," in *Foucault Studies*, no. 18 (October 2014), 272.
9 G. Hull, "The Subject and Power of Bioethics," in *Ethics, Medicine, and Public Health,* 2017, no. 4. Michel Foucault, *Security, Territory, Population: Lectures at the College de France, 1977-1978*, trans. G. Burchell (Basingstoke and New York: Palgrave Macmillan, 2007), 165.
10 Foucault, *Security,* 148–150. Quoted in G. Hull.
11 Hull, "The Subject," 165.
12 John B. Beck, *Medicine in the American Colonies* (Albuquerque: Horn and Wallace, 1966), 90.
13 Blake, *Public Health*, 46.

14 Foucault, *The History of Sexuality,* trans. Robert Hurley (New York: Random House, 1978), 96.
15 Blake, *Public Health.*
16 Michel Foucault, *Discipline and Punish: The Birth of the Prison* (New York: Vintage, 1979), 138–139.
17 Foucault, *Discipline,* 82.
18 Blake, *Public* Health, 7–8.
19 Foucault, *Discipline,* 184.
20 Foucault, *Discipline,* 185–186.
21 Foucault, *Discipline*, 190–191.
22 Charles E. Rosenberg, *The Care of Strangers: The Rise of America's Hospital System* (Baltimore, MD: Johns Hopkins University Press, 1995), 4.
23 Rosenberg, *The Care of Strangers,* 7.
24 Elizabeth A. Fenn, *Pox Americana: The Great Smallpox Epidemic of 1775–1782* (New York: Farrar, Straus, and Giroux, 2002), 275.
25 Samuel Bayard Woodward, M.D., "Annual Oration of 1932." Massachusetts Medical Society. Accessed June 23, 2022. https://www.massmed.org/About/MMS-Leadership/History/The-Story-of-Smallpox-in-Massachusetts/
26 Donald R. Hopkins, *The Greatest Killer: Smallpox in History,* (Chicago: University of Chicago Press, 2002), 244.
27 Freedom Foreign Institute. Laurel, MD. (2022) Accessed March 26, 2022. https://www.freedomforuminstitute.org/about/faq/the-first-amendment-says-nothing-about-separation-of-church-and-state-or-a-wall-of-separation-between-church-and-state-where-did-this-idea-come-from-is-it-really/
28 Jeremy W. Peters, "The Tea Party Didn't Get What It Wanted, but It Did Unleash the Politics of Anger" in *The New York Times.* (August 30, 2019).
29 Tim Koelkebeck, "Is the Religious Right Overtaking the Tea Party?" in the *Huffington Post.* (October 27, 2010).
30 Michael Coren, "How the Christian Right is Driving the Anti-Vax Movement." In *The New Statesman.* Accessed March 26, 2022. https://www.newstatesman.com/international-politics/society-international-politics/2021/12/how-the-christian-right-is-driving-the-anti-vaxx-movement
31 Coren, "How the Christian."
32 Robert P. Jones, CEO of the Public Religion Research Institute. On NPR, December 8, 2020. Robert P. Jones, *White Too Long: The Legacy of White Supremacy in American Christianity* (New York: Simon & Schuster, 2021).
33 Jennifer Rubin, "What the Election Tells Us About Religion in America" in *The Washington Post* (November 12, 2020). Accessed May 20, 2022. https://www.washingtonpost.com/opinions/2020/11/12/what-election-tells-us-about-religion-america/
34 NPR and Associated Press Votecast. AP-NORC Center for Public Affairs Research. (May, 2021). "AP VoteCast 2020." Accessed March 26, 2022. https://apnorc.org/projects/ap-votecast-2020-general-elections/
35 Robert P. Jones, on NPR, December 8, 2020.
36 R. P. Jones, on NPR, December 8, 2020.
37 NPR and Associated Press Votecast.
38 Jan-Willem van Prooijen, "The Psychology of QAnon," on NBC News *Think,* August 13, 2018. Accessed Mar. 26, 2022. https://www.nbcnews.com/think/opinion/psychology-qanon-why-do-seemingly-sane-people-believe-bizarre-conspiracy-ncna900171
39 Gregor Aisch, Jon Huang and Cecilia Kang, "Dissecting the #PizzaGate Conspiracy Theories" in the *New York Times,* December 10, 2016.
40 van Prooijen, "The Psychology QAnon."

41 van Prooijen, "The Psychology QAnon."
42 Joseph E. Uscinski and Joseph M. Parent, *American Conspiracy Theories* (London, Oxford UP, 2014).
43 Jonathan Weisman and Jazmine Ulloa, "Judging a Judge on Race and Crime, GOP Plays to Base and Fringe," *The New York Times,* March 22, 2022. Accessed March 29, 2022. https://www.nytimes.com/2022/03/22/us/politics/ketanji-brown-jackson-race.html?name=styln-scotus-nominations&region=TOP_BANNER&block=storyline_menu_recirc&action=click&pgtype=Article&variant=0_Control&is_new=false
44 John Williams [Mundungus], *Several Arguments, Proving, that Inoculating the Small Pox Is Not Contained in the Laws of Physick*. Boston, MA: J. Franklin, 1721, 6.
45 Christopher E. M. Lloyd, "Contending with Spiritual Reductionism: Demons, Shame, and Dividualising Experiences Among Evangelical Christians with Mental Distress in the *Journal of Religious Health* 60.4 (May 2021): 2702–2727, Accessed on Pub Med Central: March 31, 2022, https://www.ncbi.nlm.nih.gov/pmc/articles/PMC8270825/
46 Lloyd, "Contending."
47 Lloyd, "Contending."
48 Sean Michaels, "Taking the Rick," in *The Guardian*, London: July 24, 2008.
49 Kaleigh Rogers, "Why QAnon Has Attracted So Many White Evangelicals," in *538, ABC News*, March 4, 2021. https://fivethirtyeight.com/features/why-qanon-has-attracted-so-many-white-evangelicals/
50 Rogers, "Why QAnon."
51 Rogers, "Why QAnon."
52 Rogers, "Why QAnon."
53 Rogers, "Why QAnon."
54 Maggie Siddiqi, "Covid Vaccine and Mask Mandates Expose Alt-Right Christian Hypocrisy" in *Think Newsletter,* NBC News, December 26, 2021.
55 Stephen Coss, *The Fever of 1721: The Epidemic That Revolutionized Medicine and American Politics* (New York: Simon and Schuster, 2016), ix, x.
56 Bob Woodward, *Rage* (New York: Simon and Schuster, 2021). And in *NPR* Broadcast, "Trump Admits Playing Down Covid's Severity, According to New Woodward Book," Sept. 9, 2020. Accessed April 2, 2022, https://www.npr.org/2020/09/09/911109247/trump-admitted-to-playing-down-the-cornaviruss-severity-per-new-book
57 Woodward, *Rage.*
58 Woodward, *Rage.*
59 Woodward, *Rage.*
60 Edward Winslow, "Letter to Z. Boylston" in *The Boston News-Letter* (Boston: December 5, 1720), no. 873.
61 *NBC News*. January 22, 2021. Accessed April 2, 2011. https://www.nbcnews.com/politics/donald-trump/dr-deborah-birx-trump-s-covid-19-coordinator-said-she-n1255413
62 *NBC News*. Jan. 22, 2021.
63 MSNBC, Nicole Wallace, "Deadline: White House," Podcast. Apr. 6, 2022. https://podcasts.apple.com/us/podcast/just-doesnt-fly-on-any-kind-of-logical-basis/id1367201919?i=1000556470642
64 Coss, *The Fever*, 12–14.
65 G. B. Warden, *Boston, 1689–1776* (Boston: Little, Brown, and Co., 1970), 91–93.
66 William H. Frey, "Anti-CRT Bills Are Aimed to Incite the GOP Base—Not Parents" in *Brookings* (March 30, 2022). Accessed May 18, 2022. https://www.brookings.edu/research/anti-crt-bills-are-aimed-to-incite-the-gop-base-not-parents/

67 Frey, "Anti-CRT Bills."
68 Fred Backus, Anthony Salvanto, "Big Majorities Reject Book Bans—CBS News Poll. (February 22, 2022). Accessed May 18, 2022. https://www.cbsnews.com/news/book-bans-opinion-poll-2022-02-22/
69 Gabriella Borter, Joseph Ax, and Joseph Tanfani, "School Boards Get Death Threats Amid Rage Over Race, Gender, Mask Policies in *A Reuters Special Report*. (February 15, 2022). Accessed May 18, 2022. https://www.reuters.com/investigates/special-report/usa-education-threats/
70 Adam Serwer, "Birtherism of a Nation," in *The Atlantic*, May 13, 2020. Accessed Mar. 29, 2022. https://www.theatlantic.com/ideas/archive/2020/05/birtherism-and-trump/610978/
71 American Civil Liberties Union, "Timeline of the Muslim Ban" (Washington, D. C.: February, 2020) Accessed April 7, 2020. https://www.aclu-wa.org/pages/timeline-muslim-ban
72 Henry Louis Gates, Jr. and Andrew S. Curran: The Robert B. Silvers Lecture. New York: New York Public Library, March 10, 2022. Accessed March 20, 2022 & April 9, 2022. https://www.nypl.org/events/programs/2022/03/14/henry-louis-gates-jr-andrew-s-curran?nref=56896
73 Gates, Jr. and Curran: Silvers Lecture, March 10, 2022.
74 Michel Foucault, *The Archaeology of Knowledge* (New York: Routledge, 1972), 3.
75 Foucault, *Archaeology*, 4.
76 Foucault, *Archaeology*, 5
77 Foucault, *Archaeology*, 5.

Bibliography

Aisch, Gregor, Jon Huang and Cecilia Kang. "Dissecting the #PizzaGate Conspiracy Theories" in the *New York Times*, December 10, 2016.

American Civil Liberties Union. "Timeline of the Muslim Ban" Washington, D. C.: February, 2020. Accessed April 7, 2020. https://www.aclu-wa.org/pages/timeline-muslim-ban

Backus, Fred and Anthony Salvanto. "Big Majorities Reject Book Bans—CBS News Poll." (February 22, 2022). Accessed May 18, 2022. https://www.cbsnews.com/news/book-bans-opinion-poll-2022-02-22/

Beck, John B. *Medicine in the American Colonies*. Albuquerque: Horn and Wallace, 1966.

Bitzer, Lloyd. "The Rhetorical Situation" in *Philosophy and Rhetoric*, 1 (1968).

Blake, James B. *Public Health in the Town of Boston, 1630–1822*. Boston: Harvard University Press, 1959.

Borter, Gabriella, Joseph Ax, and Joseph Tanfani. "School Boards Get Death Threats Amid Rage Over Race, Gender, Mask Policies" in *A Reuters Special Report*. (February 15, 2022). Accessed May 18, 2022. https://www.reuters.com/investigates/special-report/usa-education-threats/

Boylston, Arthur W. and A. E. Williams. "Zabdiel Boylston's Evaluation of Inoculation Against Smallpox" in *JLL Bulletin: Commentaries on the History of Treatment Evaluation* (2008).

Coren, Michael. "How the Christian Right is Driving the Anti-Vax Movement" in *The New Statesman*. Accessed March 26, 2022. https://www.newstatesman.com/international-politics/society-international-politics/2021/12/ how-the-christian-right-is-driving-the-anti-vaxx-movement

Coss, Stephen. *The Fever of 1721: The Epidemic That Revolutionized Medicine and American Politics*. New York: Simon and Schuster, 2016.

Curriculum Concepts International, "Slave Revolt of 1712" in *Mapping the African American Past*. New York: Columbia University. Accessed April 7, 2022. https://maap.columbia.edu/place/34.html

Douglass, William. *Inoculation of the Small Pox as Practised in Boston, Considered in a Letter to A[lexander] S[tuart], M. D. F. R. S.*, Boston: J. Franklin,, 1722.

Fenn, Elizabeth A. *Pox Americana: The Great Smallpox Epidemic of 1775–1782*. New York: Farrar, Straus, and Giroux, 2002.

Foucault, Michel. *The Archaeology of Knowledge*. New York: Routledge, 1972.

Foucault, Michel. *Birth of the Clinic: An Archaeology of Medical Perception*, trans. A. M. Sheridan Smith. New York: Vintage, 1973.

Foucault, Michel. *Discipline and Punish: The Birth of the Prison*. New York: Vintage, 1979.

Foucault, Michel. *The History of Sexuality*, trans. Robert Hurley. New York: Random House, 1978.

Foucault, Michel. "The Politics of Health in the Eighteenth Century" in *Foucault Studies* vol. 3, no. 18 (October 2014).

Foucault, Michel. *Security, Territory, Population: Lectures at the College de France, 1977–1978*, trans. G. Burchell. Basingstoke and New York: Palgrave Macmillan, 2007.

Freedom Foreign Institute. Laurel, MD. (2022) Accessed Mar. 26, 2022. https://www.freedomforuminstitute.org//about/faq/the-first-amendment-says-nothing-about-separation-of-church-and-state-or-a-wall-of-separation-between-church-and-state-where-did-this=idea-come-from-is-it-really/

Frey, William H. "Anti-CRT Bills Are Aimed to Incite the GOP Base—Not Parents" in *Brookings* (March 30, 2022). Accessed May 18, 2022. https://www.brookings.edu/research/anti-crt-bills-are-aimed-to-incite-the-gop-base-not-parents/

Gates, Jr. Henry Louis and Andrew S. Curran, *The Robert B. Silvers Lecture*. New York: New York Public Library, March 10, 2022. Accessed March 20, 2022 & April 9, 2022. https://www.nypl.org/events/programs/2022/03/14/henry-louis-gates-jr-andrew-s-curran?nref=56896

Heifferon, Barbara. "The New Smallpox: An Epidemic of Words?" in *Rhetoric Review* 25, no. 1 (January 2006).

Hull, G. "The Subject and Power of Bioethics" in *Ethics, Medicine, and Public Health* vol. 3, no. 4. (2017).

Jones, Robert P. CEO of the Public Religion Research Institute on NPR, December 8, 2020.

Jones, Robert P. *White Too Long: The Legacy of White Supremacy in American Christianity*. New York: Simon & Schuster, 2021.

Koelkebeck, Tim. "Is the Religious Right Overtaking the Tea Party?" in the *Huffington Post*. (October 27, 2010).

Lloyd, Christopher E. M. "Contending with Spiritual Reductionism: Demons, Shame, and Dividualising Experiences Among Evangelical Christians with Mental Distress in the *Journal of Religious Health* 60.4 (May 2021): 2702–2727, Accessed on Pub Med Central: March 31, 2022, https://www.ncbi.nlm.nih.gov/pmc/articles/PMC8270825/

Michaels, Sean. "Taking the Rick," in *The Guardian*, London: July 24, 2008.

MSNBC, Nicole Wallace. "Deadline: White House," Podcast. April 6, 2022. https://podcasts.apple.com/us/podcast/just-doesnt-fly-on-any-kind-of-logical-basis/id1367201919?i=1000556470642

NBC News. January 22, 2021. Accessed April 2, 2011. https://www.nbcnews.com/politics/donald-trump/dr-deborah-birx-trump-s-covid-19-coordinator-said-she-n1255413

NPR and Associated Press Votecast. AP-NORC Center for Public Affairs Research. (May, 2021). "AP VoteCast 2020." Accessed March 26, 2022. https://apnorc.org/projects/ap-votecast-2020-general-elections/

Peters, Jeremy W. "The Tea Party Didn't Get What It Wanted, but It Did Unleash the Politics of Anger" in *The New York Times* (August 30, 2019).

van Prooijen, Jan-Willem. "The Psychology of QAnon," on NBC News *Think*, Aug. 13, 2018. Accessed March 26, 2022. https://www.nbcnews.com/think/opinion/psychology-qanon-why-do-seemingly-sane-people-believe-bizarre-conspiracy-ncna900171

Rogers, Kayleigh. "Why QAnon Has Attracted So Many White Evangelicals" in *538, ABC News*, March 4, 2021. https://fivethirtyeight.com/features/why-qanon-has-attracted-so-many-white-evangelicals/

Rosenberg, Charles E. *The Care of Strangers: The Rise of America's Hospital System*. Baltimore, MD: Johns Hopkins University Press, 1995.

Royal Society Classified Papers. London: Royal Society Archives, 1660–1741.

Rubin, Jennifer. "What the Election Tells Us About Religion in America" in *The Washington Post* (November 12, 2020). Accessed May 20, 2022. https://www.washingtonpost.com/opinions/2020/11/12/what-election-tells-us-about-religion-America

Serwer, Adam. "Birtherism of a Nation," in *The Atlantic*, May 13, 2020. Accessed March 29, 2022. https://www.theatlantic.com/ideas/archive/2020/05/birtherism-and-Trump/610979/

Siddiqi, Maggie. "Covid Vaccine and Mask Mandates Expose Alt-Right Christian Hypocrisy" in *Think Newsletter*, NBC News, December 26, 2021.

Uscinski, Joseph E. and Joseph M. Parent. *American Conspiracy Theories*. London: Oxford University Press, 2014.

Warden, G. B. *Boston, 1689–1776*. Boston: Little, Brown, and Co., 1970.

Weisman, Jonathan and Jazmine Ulloa. "Judging a Judge on Race and Crime, GOP Plays to Base and Fringe" in *The New York Times*, March 22, 2022. Accessed March 29, 2022. https://www.nytimes.com/2022/03/22/us/politics/ketanji-brown-jackson-race.html?name=styln-scotus-nominations&region=TOP_BANNER&block=storyline_menu_recirc&action=click&pgtype=Article&variant=0_Control&is_new=false

Williams, John [Mundungus]. *Several Arguments, Proving, that Inoculating the Small Pox Is Not Contained in the Laws of Physick*. Boston, MA: J. Franklin, 1721.

Winslow, Edward. "Letter to Z. Boylston" in *The Boston News-Letter* no. 873. Boston: December 5, 1720.

Woodward, Bob. *NPR* Broadcast, "Trump Admits Playing Down Covid's Severity, According to New Woodward Book," September 9, 2020. Accessed April 2, 2022. https://www.npr.org/2020/09/09/911109247/trump-admitted-to-playing-down-the-cornavirussseverity-per-new-book

Woodward, Bob. *Rage*. New York: Simon and Schuster, 2021.

Index

Note: Citations of tables are indicated in **bold** and citations of figures are in *italics*.

For Product Safety Concerns and Information please contact our EU representative GPSR@taylorandfrancis.com
Taylor & Francis Verlag GmbH, Kaufingerstraße 24, 80331 München, Germany

www.ingramcontent.com/pod-product-compliance
Ingram Content Group UK Ltd.
Pitfield, Milton Keynes, MK11 3LW, UK
UKHW020143200926
475702UK00005B/895
9781032320120